OXFORD MEDICAL PUBLICATIONS

Smoking and Hormone-Related Disorders

This publication represents the proceedings of a symposium 'Smoking and hormone-related disorders' held on 31 October–2 November 1988 at the Ciba Foundation, 41 Portland Place, London, W1N 4BN, and sponsored by the UK Department of Health, Hannibal House, Elephant and Castle, London SE1 6TE.

Smoking and Hormone-Related Disorders

Edited by

NICHOLAS WALD
St Bartholomew's Medical College

and

JOHN BARON
Dartmouth Medical School

Oxford New York Tokyo
OXFORD UNIVERSITY PRESS

This book has been printed digitally and produced in a standard specification in order to ensure its continuing availability

OXFORD
UNIVERSITY PRESS

Great Clarendon Street, Oxford OX2 6DP
Oxford University Press is a department of the University of Oxford.
It furthers the University's objective of excellence in research, scholarship,
and education by publishing worldwide in

Oxford New York

Auckland Cape Town Dar es Salaam Hong Kong Karachi
Kuala Lumpur Madrid Melbourne Mexico City Nairobi
New Delhi Shanghai Taipei Toronto
With offices in
Argentina Austria Brazil Chile Czech Republic France Greece
Guatemala Hungary Italy Japan South Korea Poland Portugal
Singapore Switzerland Thailand Turkey Ukraine Vietnam

Oxford is a registered trade mark of Oxford University Press
in the UK and in certain other countries

Published in the United States
by Oxford University Press Inc., New York

Reprinted 2011

ISBN 978-0-19-261935-8

Printed and bound in Great Britain by CPI Antony Rowe,
Chippenham and Eastbourne

Foreword

The Independent Scientific Committee on Smoking and Health was established in 1973 to provide unbiased advice to Health Ministers (who appoint the members) and, where appropriate, the tobacco companies, on the scientific aspects of matters concerning smoking and health. This advice is used in negotiating the 'voluntary agreements' between government and the tobacco industry which is the method of tobacco product regulation favoured in the United Kingdom.

The quality of the Committee's advice depends *inter alia* on its comprehensiveness. For the past seven years the Committee has been enabled to sponsor research projects from substantial funds made available by the industry through the Tobacco Advisory Council and the Committee's fund-administration instrument, the Tobacco Products Research Trust. These have greatly increased our knowledge of, particularly, the relationship between smoking-related diseases and the constitution of tobacco products (Independent Scientific Committee on Smoking and Health 1988). We have also organized international symposia focused on particular and crucial areas of concern. The first was held in November 1986 and was funded by the monies from the Tobacco Advisory Council (Wald and Froggatt 1989). The present book is the Proceedings of the second symposium and was funded by the Department of Health, the other party to the 'voluntary agreements'.

The latest in the series of 'voluntary agreements' on product modification formally expired at end-December 1987. No new one has yet been negotiated because of an impending European Community Council Directive on limiting tar yields of cigarettes. No new money is therefore at present available to the Committee but I am confident that the future symposia already planned will take place. Without these, government and the industry cannot receive from the Committee scientific advice of the calibre they would require, our terms of reference dictate, society would expect, and the public health require.

The Committee is grateful to Nicholas Wald, one of its members, and John Baron for their skilful editing of these Proceedings, and to the Department of Health for funding the Symposium and publication.

Peter Froggatt
Chairman, Independent Scientific Committee on Smoking and Health

References

Independent Scientific Committee on Smoking and Health. (1988). *Fourth Report*. London, HMSO.

A Draft Council Directive on the Approximation of the Laws, Regulations, and Administrative Provisions of the Members States Concerning the Maximum Tar Yields of Cigarettes. 9695 FAN 129 PRO CO-OP 168.

Wald, N. and Froggatt, P. (ed.) (1989). *Nicotine, Smoking and the Low Tar Programme*. Oxford University Press, Oxford.

Preface

In recent years cigarette smoking has been linked with a number of disorders that have in common the suggestion that they are caused by an excess or deficiency of hormones. The range of these disorders is wide, and their association with smoking has often been unexpected. Some of the disorders are more common in smokers and may therefore be caused by the habit, while with others the disorder is less common in smokers suggesting that smoking may be protective. Oestrogen-related problems, in particular, have been a focus of interest, since women who smoke cigarettes behave, physiologically and pathologically, as though they were relatively oestrogen deficient. The hypothesis that smoking exerts such an anti-oestrogenic effect allows certain predictions to be made. For example, one might expect that problems associated with oestrogen deficiency, such as osteoporosis or frequency of menopausal symptoms, would be more common in smokers while disorders that are due to oestrogen excess, such as endometrial cancer, may be less common.

The purpose of the Symposium organized by the Independent Scientific Committee on Smoking and Health, held in October 1988, was to consider in detail the epidemiological, biological, and laboratory evidence relating cigarette smoking and various hormone-related conditions, with a particular emphasis on the effect of smoking on sex hormone-related disorders.

The effects of smoking on cancer of the breast and endometrium were of particular interest. Many studies had reported on endometrial cancer and, while the evidence for a decreased risk of endometrial cancer in smokers was compelling (indicating that women who smoke have about half the risk of women who have never smoked), there was uncertainty on whether the effect was more or less pronounced after the menopause and whether the reduced risk persisted after people gave up smoking.

The evidence on smoking and breast cancer was quite uncertain and it was hoped that the Symposium would help clarify the position. The relative risk estimates ranged from about 0.6 to 1.7 and seemed to cluster around 1.0. Since breast cancer is the commonest cancer in women (if not exceeded by lung cancer) in most economically developed countries in which smoking among women is common, even a small effect on the risk of breast cancer could have important public health implications.

It was recognized that women who smoke cigarettes have, on average, a natural menopause about one year earlier than women who have never smoked but the effect among ex-smokers needed clarification. A number of miscellaneous oestrogen-dependent conditions appeared to be prevented by cigarette smoking, including uterine fibroids, endometriosis, and hyperemesis gravidarum. Women who smoke have also been reported as having a higher frequency of conditions possibly associated with oestrogen deficiency, such as irregular menstrual periods, an increased frequency of menopausal symptoms, hirsutism, and increased wrinkling of the skin, perhaps due to a deficiency of subcutaneous collagen. These associations justified further examination.

Osteoporotic fractures are an important public health problem, particularly in elderly women. Several epidemiological studies had examined the relationship between cigarette smoking and osteoporosis (bone mineral density), or with osteoporotic fractures. Some showed that cigarette smokers have about double the risk of having a fracture than non-smokers, both in men and women. It was uncertain whether the relationship was causal or whether it was an indirect association arising because smokers, on average, drink more alcohol and have lower body weight than non-smokers. Moreover, studies comparing bone density in smokers and non-smokers have tended to show lower bone density in male smokers and post-menopausal female smokers compared to non-smokers, but no differences in pre-menopausal women. These observations also needed clarification, in particular whether the possibly lower bone density of smokers could be accounted for by their lower average body weight.

The associations between inflammatory bowel disease and smoking are confusing. There is a negative association with ulcerative colitis and a positive one with Crohn's disease. It was important to determine whether these suggestions were soundly based, and if so, whether they represented cause and effect relationships that could be explained by plausible biological mechanisms.

The association between a reduced risk of Parkinson's disease and cigarette smoking was well known, with indications that this represented a protective effect of smoking. The Symposium provided an opportunity to review this evidence and see if there was any reason to alter the conclusion that the link was causal.

A number of other possible associations with smoking were included in the list of topics to be considered in the Symposium, for example, the possible links between smoking and gallstones, and smoking and prostatic hypertrophy. The opportunity was also taken to review results from some large prospective studies, those performed by the American Cancer Society, the Nurses' Health Study, and the Southern California Leisure World Retirement Community Study. Special attention was also devoted to elucidating the mechanisms that might explain the epidemiological associations.

Coronary heart disease presented a special problem. Its relationship with smoking is well recognized and well described. It was acknowledged that there was evidence that coronary heart disease appeared to be related to sex hormones, although the details of the relationship were not clear. For example, in post-menopausal women exogenous oestrogens are almost certainly protective while in men they are probably causative. While there is undoubted scientific interest in the hormonal aspects of smoking and coronary heart disease, smoking and coronary heart disease was excluded from our list of topics because so much had been written on the subject and we wished to concentrate on some of the other, less well documented, associations.

As with the publication of the Proceedings of the first ISCSH Symposium on Nicotine, Smoking and the Low Tar Programme, we hope that this book will present an intelligible summary of the present position on smoking and hormone related disorders, so that it will form a base on which informed discussion can proceed and useful further research can be planned.

We would like to thank those who took part in the Symposium, the members and scientific secretariat of the Independent Scientific Committee on Smoking and Health (Chairman: Sir Peter Froggatt), the Department of Health for their financial support, and Robert Waller, who was so helpful in assisting with the preparation of the Symposium. In particular, we wish to pay tribute to Mrs Cheryl Swann for the editorial work she has put into this volume and the care with which she has assembled these Proceedings.

London and Dartmouth N.W.
November 1989 J.B.

Contents

V SMOKING AND HORMONE-RELATED CANCERS

VI MECHANISMS: HORMONAL DIFFERENCES IN SMOKERS AND NON-SMOKERS

Contributors

David Back
Department of Pharmacology and Therapeutics, University of Liverpool, New Medical Building, Ashton Street, PO Box 147, Liverpool L69 3BX, UK.

Simon Ball
Department of Pharmacology and Therapeutics, University of Liverpool, New Medical Building, Ashton Street, PO Box 147, Liverpool L69 3BX, UK.

Robert Barbieri
Department of Obstetrics and Gynecology, Laboratory of Human Reproduction and Reproductive Biology, Harvard Medical School, Boston, MA 02115, USA.

John Baron
Departments of Medicine and Community and Family Medicine, Dartmouth Medical School, Hanover, NH 03756, USA.

Elizabeth Barrett-Connor
Department of Community and Family Medicine, University of California, San Diego, La Jolla, CA 92037, USA.

Leslie Bernstein
Department of Preventive Medicine, University of Southern California School of Medicine, Los Angeles, CA 90033, USA.

Paolo Boffetta
Department of Epidemiology and Statistics, American Cancer Society, 1180 Avenue of the Americas, New York, NY 10036, USA.

Leon Bradlow
Laboratory of Biochemical Endocrinology, Rockefeller University Hospital, 1230 York Avenue, New York, NY 10021, USA.

Mark Brincat
Department of Obstetrics and Gynaecology, St George's Hospital, Blackshaw Road, London SW17, UK.

Jacob Canick
Department of Pathology and Laboratory Medicine, Brown University, Women and Infants Hospital, Providence, RI 02905, USA.

Christopher Chute

Department of Epidemiology, Harvard School of Public Health, Boston, MA 02115, USA.

Graham Colditz

Channing Laboratory, Department of Medicine, Harvard Medical School, Boston, MA 02115, USA.

Cyrus Cooper

Rheumatology Unit, Bristol Royal Infirmary, Bristol BS2 8HW, UK.

Sir Richard Doll

Imperial Cancer Research Fund, Cancer Epidemiology and Clinical Trials Unit, University of Oxford, Gibson Building, Radcliffe Infirmary, Oxford OX2 6HE, UK.

Peter Elmes

Dawros House, Dinas Powis, St Andrews Road, South Glamorgan CF6 4HB, UK.

Jack Fishman

IVAX Corporation, 8800 NW 36th Street, Miami, FL 33178, USA.

Lesley Forrester

Imperial Cancer Research Fund, Laboratory of Molecular Pharmacology and Drug Metabolism, Department of Biochemistry, Edinburgh EH8 9XD, UK.

Sir Peter Froggatt

3 Strangford Avenue, Belfast BT9 6PG, UK.

Lawrence Garfinkel

Department of Epidemiology and Statistics, American Cancer Society, 1180 Avenue of the Americas, New York, NY 10036, USA.

Brian Henderson

Department of Preventive Medicine, University of Southern California School of Medicine, Los Angeles, CA 90033, USA.

Charles Hennekens

Channing Laboratory, Department of Medicine, Harvard Medical School, Boston, MA 02115, USA.

Malcolm Law

Department of Environmental and Preventive Medicine, St Bartholomew's Medical College, Charterhouse Square, London EC1M 6BQ, UK.

Richard Logan

Department of Community Medicine and Epidemiology, University of Nottingham Medical School, Queens Medical Centre, Nottingham NG7 2UH, UK.

Stephanie London
Department of Epidemiology, Harvard School of Public Health, Boston, MA 02115, USA.

Brian MacMahon
Department of Epidemiology, Harvard School of Public Health, Boston, MA 02115, USA.

Michael Marmot
Department of Community Medicine, University College of London and Middlesex Hospital Medical School, 66-72 Gower Street, London WC1E 6EA, UK.

Jon Michnovicz
Institute for Hormone Research, 55 East 34th Street, New York, NY 10016, USA.

Alan Morrison
Department of Community Health, Brown University, Division of Biology and Medicine, Providence, RI 02912, USA.

Annlia Paganini-Hill
Department of Preventive Medicine, University of Southern California School of Medicine, Los Angeles, CA 90033, USA.

Malcolm Pike
Department of Preventive Medicine, University of Southern California School of Medicine, Los Angeles, CA 90033, USA.

David Poswillo
Department of Oral Surgery, Guy's Hospital, St Thomas Street, London SE1 9RT, UK.

Thomas Rohan
NCIC Epidemiology Unit, Faculty of Medicine, McMurrich Building, University of Toronto, Toronto, Ontario M5S 1A8, Canada.

Bernard Rosner
Channing Laboratory, Department of Medicine, Harvard Medical School, Boston, MA 02115, USA.

Ronald Ross
Department of Preventive Medicine, University of Southern California School of Medicine, Los Angeles, CA 90033, USA.

Robert Sandler
Division of Digestive Diseases and the Core Medical Center in Diarrheal Diseases, University of North Carolina School of Medicine, Chapel Hill, NC, USA.

Susan Skene

Department of Health, Hannibal House, Elephant and Castle, London SE1 6TE, UK.

Frank Speizer

Channing Laboratory, Department of Medicine, Harvard Medical School, Boston, MA 02115, USA.

Meir Stampfer

Channing Laboratory, Department of Medicine, Harvard Medical School, Boston, MA 02115, USA.

Martin Vessey

Department of Community Medicine and General Practice, Radcliffe Infirmary, Oxford, UK.

Nicholas Wald

Department of Environmental and Preventive Medicine, St Bartholomew's Medical College, Charterhouse Square, London EC1M 6BQ, UK.

Robert Waller

Department of Health, Hannibal House, Elephant and Castle, London SE1 6TE, UK.

Noel Weiss

School of Public Health and Community Medicine, Department of Epidemiology, University of Washington, Seattle, Washington 98195, USA.

Carol Wickham

MRC Environmental Epidemiology Unit, University of Southampton, Southampton General Hospital, Southampton SO9 4XY, UK.

Walter Willett

Channing Laboratory, Department of Medicine, Harvard Medical School, Boston, MA 02115, USA.

Roland Wolf

Imperial Cancer Research Fund, Laboratory of Molecular Pharmacology and Drug Metabolism, Department of Biochemistry, Edinburgh EH8 9XD, UK.

I

Results from Three Prospective Studies

1. Smoking and oestrogen-related sites. Data from American Cancer Society Studies

Lawrence Garfinkel and Paolo Boffetta

Abstract

Data from two American Cancer Society prospective studies—Cancer Prevention Study I, 1959–72 (CPS I), and Cancer Prevention Study II, 1982–6 (CPS II)—were used for an analysis of cigarette smoking and oestrogen-related sites of cancer. Smoking and cancer of the colon-rectum and of the gall bladder and biliary passage were also evaluated. Smoking was negatively related to endometrial cancer in both CPS I and CPS II, and increased the risk of cervical cancer in CPS I (RR 1.41, 95 per cent CI 1.20–1.65) and in CPS II (RR 2.27, 95 per cent CI 1.27–3.74). Breast cancer and ovarian cancer were not related to smoking. Colon-rectum cancer was negatively related in CPS I (RR 0.89, 95 per cent CI 0.82–0.98) but positively related in CPS II (RR 1.16, 95 per cent CI 0.99–1.37). Cancer of the biliary passages was related to smoking in CPS I (RR 1.81, 95 per cent CI 1.19–2.63) but too few deaths in smokers occurred in CPS II to see if there was any relationship. Adjusting for known risk factors did not substantively change the relative risk ratios.

1.1. Introduction

Evidence from the literature strongly supports an association between cigarette smoking and early natural menopause (see Adena and Gallagher 1982 for review), and lower levels of urinary oestrogens have been found among smokers (MacMahon *et al.* 1982). The hypothesis of an anti-oestrogenic effect of smoking led to a number of epidemiological studies on the association between smoking and breast and endometrial cancers (see Baron 1984 for review). Winkelstein (1977), on the other hand, proposed the hypothesis of a causal effect of smoking on cervical cancer on the basis of biological considerations and sparse epidemiological data. Since then, a large number of studies have tested this hypothesis.

The evidence of a causal effect of smoking on cervical cancer derives from at least 11 studies that showed in different populations that the association was not confounded by other known aetiological factors. (Wright *et al.* 1978; Garfinkel 1980; Harris *et al.* 1980; Clarke *et al.* 1982; Berggren and Sjostedt 1983; Lyon *et al.* 1983; Trevathan *et al.* 1983; Greenberg *et al.* 1985; Baron *et al.* 1986; Brinton *et al.* 1986a; Hellberg *et al.* 1986; La Vecchia *et al.* 1986). Two studies, however, did not confirm this result (Stellman *et al.* 1980; Marshall *et al.* 1983). Smoking seems to have an effect on pre-malignant cervical lesions as well (Harris *et al.* 1980; Trevathan *et al.* 1983; Clarke *et al.* 1985; Greenberg *et al.* 1985).

A history of smoking was protective with respect to endometrial cancer risk in seven studies (Weiss *et al.* 1980; Lesko *et al.* 1985; Baron *et al.* 1986; Franks *et al.* 1987a; Lawrence *et al.* 1987; Levi *et al.* 1987; Stockwell and Lyman 1987), while no association was found in at least three other studies (Williams and Horm 1977; Garfinkel 1980; Tyler *et al.* 1985), and one more study provided limited evidence of a protective effect (Smith *et al.* 1984). In two positive studies, however, the decrease in risk was present among post-menopausal women only (Lesko *et al.* 1985; Stockwell and Lyman 1987).

The effect of smoking on the most important oestrogen-related cancer is more controversial: breast cancer has been traditionally considered a non-smoking-related disease, and because of that, breast cancer patients have contributed to the control series in many case-control studies on the effect of smoking on other cancers. No association between smoking and breast cancer was detected in several large case-control or cohort studies (MacMahon and Feinleib 1960; Williams and Horm 1977; Garfinkel 1980; Kelsey *et al.* 1981; Hiatt *et al.* 1982). During the last 10 years, however, a number of studies have suggested a protective effect of smoking (Doll *et al.* 1980; Vessey *et al.* 1983; O'Connell *et al.* 1987), although this was not confirmed by other results (Garfinkel 1980; Kelsey *et al.* 1981; Hiatt *et al.* 1982; Rosenberg *et al.* 1984; Smith *et al.* 1984; Baron *et al.* 1986; Brinton *et al.* 1986b; Stockwell and Lyman 1987). A few studies even provided a suggestion of an increase in breast cancer risk among smokers, especially among pre-menopausal women (Schechter *et al.* 1985; Hiatt and Fireman 1986; Brownson *et al.* 1988).

The association between ovarian carcinoma and smoking has been rarely addressed: a positive association was found in one cohort study (Doll *et al.* 1980), which was not confirmed by at least six other investigations (Byers *et al.* 1983; Cramer *et al.* 1984; Smith *et al.* 1984; Baron *et al.* 1986; Stockwell and Lyman 1987; Franks *et al.* 1987b).

Carcinomas of colon–rectum, gall bladder, and biliary tract are also considered not to be smoking-dependent. However, two reasons justify the inclusion of these diseases in this analysis:

(1) they share risk factors, such as obesity, with oestrogen-related cancers;

(2) some suggestions of a link between these cancers and smoking habit have been published recently: colon cancer patients who were smokers had more advanced stages than non-smokers (Daniell 1986); a correlation between smoking and colorectal polyps has been suggested (Hoff *et al.* 1987); and a negative association between smoking and cancer of the biliary tract has been found in a case-control study (Yen *et al.* 1987).

The present analysis is aimed to test the hypotheses of a negative association between endometrial cancer and smoking and a positive association between cervical cancer and smoking, as well as to investigate the relationships of smoking and breast, ovary, colon–rectum, gall bladder, and biliary tract cancer in two large prospective mortality studies conducted since 1959 by the American Cancer Society.

1.2. Materials and methods

Data for this analysis come from two prospective studies organized by the American Cancer Society: Cancer Prevention Study I (CPS I) and Cancer Prevention Study II (CPS II). The design of both studies is similar. American Cancer Society volunteers were asked to enroll friends, neighbours, and relatives to fill out a detailed questionnaire on their life styles and exposures. The volunteers avoided recruiting people who tended to move often (military personnel, construction workers, etc.). Only households with at least one member aged 45 and over were eligible, although all family members in such households age 30 were asked to complete the questionnaire. The volunteer 'researchers' reported periodically if the persons they enrolled (an average of 15 persons) were alive or dead, and noted any changes in address. If dead, they recorded date and place of death, and death certificates were obtained from state health departments. For those who died of cancer, an attempt was made to obtain further information from cancer registries or certifying physicians or hospitals.

CPS I was started in the autumn of 1959 when 68 000 volunteers in 25 states enrolled more than 1 000 000 persons. Death rates for study participants were generally lower than for the whole country for several reasons:

(1) the subjects were better educated;
(2) low socioeconomic groups, illiterates, itinerant workers, and institutionalized populations were under-represented;
(3) seriously ill persons were not fully represented, although in some instances a family member did complete the questionnaire for the sick person.

Follow-up in CPS I was conducted annually for 6 years, to 1965. Every other year, in 1961, 1963, and 1965, a short supplemental questionnaire was completed including information on hospitalizations, cancer diagnosis, current smoking habits, changes in residence, and a few additional questions. Follow-up was successfully completed on more than 98 per cent of the subjects, and 95 per cent of the survivors returned supplemental questionnaires. In 1971, 6 years after the completion of the 1965 follow-up, another follow-up was started, and in 1972 a final follow-up was launched, including another supplemental questionnaire. Up to 1971, 98.5 per cent of the subjects were traced, and 92.5 per cent were traced up to 1972. More details on the CPS I follow-up have been reported (Garfinkel 1985).

In 1982 a new prospective study, CPS II, was started to answer a number of questions on life styles and exposures not adequately covered in CPS I. These included specific questions on diet, vitamins, involuntary smoking, occupational exposures, drugs and medications, reproductive history, and a number of other factors.

CPS II enlisted the help of 77 000 volunteer researchers in all 50 states, District of Columbia and Puerto Rico. More than 1.2 million subjects were enrolled and completed the detailed four-page confidential questionnaire. Follow-up in CPS II was conducted on a biennial basis. The second follow-up started in September 1986 and was completed 18 months later. A total of 98.5 per cent of the subjects were successfully traced and 4.2 per cent (over 50 000) of persons had been reported dead. Death certificates had been received for nearly 92 per cent of the reported deaths at the time of this analysis.

This analysis examines the relative risks (RRs), expressed as the ratio of observed vs. expected deaths, of smoking in oestrogen-related sites in women in both CPS I and CPS II. CPS I covered 12 years of follow-up (1960–72) and CPS II included 4 years of follow-up (1982–6). Expected number of deaths was computed by multiplying the 5-year age-specific attained age rates of non-smokers by the person years in each 5-year category of smokers, and

Table 1.1. Relative risks of current smoking for cancer of oestrogen-related sites and other selected sites in women—Cancer Prevention Study I, years 1–12

Site	Number of deaths*	Relative risk	95% confidence interval
Breast	1048	0.95	0.89–1.01
Cervix	160	1.41	1.20–1.65
Endometrium	54	0.88	0.66–1.14
Uterus, NOS	67	1.02	0.79–1.29
Ovary	339	1.01	0.90–1.12
Colon–rectum	511	0.89	0.82–0.98
Gall bladder	24	0.83	0.53–1.24
Biliary passages	27	1.81	1.19–2.63

* Among smokers.

dividing the observed by the expected number of deaths to obtain the RR. The sites include: breast; cervix; endometrium; uterus, not otherwise specified (NOS); and ovary. Gall bladder and biliary passages cancers were also included, and colon-rectum cancer as well.

Ninety-five per cent confidence intervals (95 per cent CI) for RRs were computed according to the approximation by Byar (Rothman and Boice 1979), and chi-square tests for trend in RRs were also computed (Mantel 1963). Multivariate analysis based on logistic regression was performed in order to control for known or suspected risk factors (Breslow and Day 1980).

1.3. Results

Table 1.1 shows the RRs for women who were current smokers at the start of CPS I. Excess risks were found for cervical cancer (RR = 1.41) and cancer of the biliary passages (RR = 1.81). Both of these were statistically significant at the 5 per cent level, with the lower limit of the 95 per cent CI higher than 1.00. Cancer of the endometrium had a RR of 0.88, and gall bladder cancer, 0.83, but neither of these were statistically significant. The RR for colon-rectum cancer was 0.89, based on 511 deaths in current smokers, and this was statistically lower than 1.00 ($P<0.05$). Breast cancer, ovarian cancer, and cancer of the uterus, NOS, all had relative risks close to unity.

Table 1.2 shows the RRs of current smokers and ex-smokers under and over 50 years of age at the start of the study. In current smokers there were few differences in RRs between women under and over age 50 for breast and endometrial cancer. Relative risks were higher in women over 50 who died of ovarian cancer (1.04) than in women under age 50 (0.83). For colon-rectum cancer, RRs were 0.77 for under age 50, and 0.91 for over age 50. The RRs for cervical cancer in current smokers, on the other hand, were higher in the younger women (1.54) than in women 50 years and older (1.38). Both these RRs were statistically different from 1.00.

In ex-smokers, RRs were higher than in current smokers for cancers of the breast ($P<0.05$), endometrium, ovary, colon-rectum, gall bladder, and biliary tract (under age 50). They were lower in ex-smokers under age 50 than in current cigarette smokers for cervical cancer. For breast, ovarian, and colon-rectum cancer, the RRs were higher in women 50 years and older than in those under age 50.

In Table 1.1 women were classified according to their smoking habits at the start of CPS I. During the course of the 12 years study, many women quit smoking, and in these women the classification of smoking status may not have been correct for the entire 12 years. Therefore a separate analysis was made for the deaths of current smokers in years 1-6 (based on smoking status at entry), and in years 7-12 (based on a smoking questionnaire received at the time of the 6th-year follow-up in 1965). Results are shown in

Table 1.2. Relative risks of smoking in cancer of oestrogen-related sites and other selected sites in women, under and over 50 years of age at start of study—Cancer Prevention Study I

Site	Age group	Current smokers		Ex-smokers	
		Number of deaths*	Relative risk	Number of deaths	Relative risk
Breast	<50	177	0.93	38	1.06
	50+	871	0.95	244	1.21†
Cervix	<50	37	1.54†	6	1.34
	50+	123	1.38†	28	1.39
Endometrium	<50	4	0.90	—	—
	50+	50	0.87	14	1.05
Uterus, NOS	<50	3	0.57	1	1.04
	50+	64	1.06	12	0.85
Ovary	<50	42	0.83	9	0.95
	50+	297	1.04	75	1.18
Colon-rectum	<50	43	0.77	10	0.90
	50+	468	0.91	136	1.11
Gall bladder	<50	1	—	—	—
	50+	23	0.80	7	0.96
Biliary passages	<50	2	0.86	1	2.27
	50+	25	1.98**	5	1.56

* Among smokers.
† Lower limit of 95% confidence interval higher than 1.00.

Table 1.3. For breast cancer the RR of 0.89 for the period 7–12 years is statistically significant. Cervical cancer had an elevated risk for current smokers in both periods. The RRs for cancer of the endometrium, ovary, and colon–rectum increased modestly over the observation period. Cancer of biliary passages had a high RR of 2.03 in the period 7–12 years.

A test of the consistency of the RRs is shown in Table 1.4 where the RR for ex-smokers and current smokers who smoked less than 20 and more than 20 cigarettes a day is presented. Cervical cancer showed a consistent upward trend in RRs (1.00 for never smoked; 1.38 for ex-smokers; 1.34 for less than 20 a day cigarette smokers; and 1.50 for women who smoked 20 or more cigarettes a day). Cancer of the biliary passages similarly showed an upward trend in RR (1.00, 1.65, 1.63, and 2.10, respectively). Both these trends are statistically significant ($P<0.01$). Colon–rectum cancer, endometrial cancer, and gall bladder cancer all showed a downward trend, but only the

Table 1.3. Relative risks of current smoking for cancers of oestrogen-related sites and other selected sites in women, by time period—Cancer Prevention Study I

Site	Years 1–6			Years 7–12		
	Number of deaths*	Relative risk	95% confidence interval	Number of deaths*	Relative risk	95% confidence interval
Breast	570	0.93	0.83–1.02	398	0.89	0.80–0.98
Cervix	92	1.26	1.01–1.54	57	2.12	1.60–2.74
Endometrium	28	0.89	0.59–1.29	20	0.99	0.60–1.53
Uterus, NOS	22	0.76	0.48–1.15	34	1.23	0.88–1.72
Ovary	159	0.96	0.82–1.12	156	1.15	0.98–1.34
Colon–rectum	211	0.84	0.73–0.96	231	0.93	0.81–1.06
Gall bladder	10	0.88	0.42–1.61	10	0.83	0.40–1.52
Biliary passages	6	1.16	0.42–2.53	17	2.03	1.18–3.25

* Among smokers.

Table 1.4. Trends in relative risks of smoking in oestrogen-related sites of cancer and other selected sites in women—Cancer Prevention Study I

Site	Never smoked	Ex-smokers	Current smokers <20 cigarettes a day	Current smokers ≥20 cigarettes a day
Breast	1.00	1.19	0.93	0.98
Cervix*	1.00	1.38	1.34	1.50
Endometrium	1.00	0.99	0.91	0.81
Uterus, NOS	1.00	0.86	0.99	1.07
Ovary	1.00	1.15	0.99	1.03
Colon-rectum †	1.00	1.09	0.94	0.82
Gall bladder	1.00	0.96	0.83	0.84
Biliary passages*	1.00	1.65	1.63	2.10

* Increase in trend statistically significant at $P<0.01$.
† Decrease in trend statistically significant at $P<0.01$.

Table 1.5. Relative risks of current smoking for breast, ovary, or colon-rectum cancer in women, by tar/nicotine (T/N) levels of cigarettes smoked at start of follow-up interval—Cancer Prevention Study I

	Low T/N	Medium T/N	High T/N
Smoked <20 cigarettes a day			
Breast	1.03	0.87*	1.03
Ovary	0.96	1.05	0.88
Colon-rectum	1.00	0.95	0.73*
Smoked ≥20 cigarettes a day			
Breast	0.97	0.98	0.96
Ovary	1.07	0.87	1.16
Colon-rectum	0.73*	0.71*	1.06

* Upper limit of 95% confidence interval less than 1.00.

trend for colon-rectum cancer is statistically significant ($P<0.01$). No trends were observed for breast cancer, ovarian cancer, or uterus, NOS.

Current smokers were classified into three groups (low, medium, high) according to the tar/nicotine (T/N) content of the cigarettes they smoked at the start of the study. In CPS I, low T/N was defined as cigarettes with 17.5 mg or tar of less; high T/N meant cigarettes with greater than 25.8 mg tar; and medium, all other cigarettes. It was hypothesized that the RR would show a decreasing trend from low T/N to high T/N. Results are shown in

Table 1.5 for breast, ovarian, and colon–rectum cancer, the only sites with large enough numbers to test the hypothesis. Although some of the RRs below 1.00 are statistically lower than 1.00 no trend by T/N could be observed.

Several investigators of smoking in relation to oestrogen-related sites have adjusted for known risk factors in evaluating the results of case-control studies. In Table 1.6, RRs are shown for breast, endometrium, ovary, and colon–rectum cancer cases who had none of the specified risk factors shown at the bottom of the table. The RRs changed little from those shown in Table 1.1. The RR of smokers for breast cancer changed from 0.95 for all subjects to 0.90 for those without risk factors; from 0.88 to 0.87 for endometrial cancer; from 1.01 to 1.08 for ovarian cancer; and from 0.89 to 0.90 for colon–rectum cancer. The upper limit for the 95 per cent CI was still below 1.00 for smokers with colon–rectum cancer shown in Table 1.6.

As stated above, the number of deaths reported in CPS II is based upon 4 years of follow-up rather than 12 years as in CPS I, so the number of deaths are much fewer. Table 1.7 shows the RRs for current smokers in CPS II. The RR for breast cancer was 0.92, similar to the RR of 0.95 shown for CPS I in Table 1.1. The RR for cervical cancer was 2.27 based on only 15 smokers' deaths, which was statistically significant at the $P<0.05$ level. Endometrial cancer had a RR of 0.58, lower than the RR of 0.88 in CPS I, and the upper limit of the 95 per cent CI was less than 1.00. The RRs for uterus, NOS were similar in CPS I (1.01) and CPS II (0.93). However, the RR for colon–rectum cancer in CPS II was 1.16 (95 per cent CI 0.99–1.37), quite different from the statistically significant RR in CPS I of 0.89. Cancer of the gall bladder and biliary passages had few deaths with wide 95 per cent CIs.

Table 1.6. Relative risks of current smoking for cancers of selected sites with exclusions for risk factors—Cancer Prevention Study I

Site	Number of deaths*	Relative risk	95% confidence intervals
Breast †	268	0.90	0.80–1.32
Endometrium ‡	21	0.87	0.54–1.32
Ovary ‡	148	1.08	0.91–1.26
Colon–rectum§	449	0.90	0.81–0.98

* Among smokers.

† Excludes subjects with menopause starting after age 55, weight 20% or more above average weight, college education or higher, and history of breast cancer in mother or sister.

‡ Excludes women with hysterectomy, late menopause, college education or higher, and weight 20% or more above average weight.

§ Excludes history of colon–rectum cancer in parents and siblings.

Table 1.7. Relative risks of current smoking for cancer of oestrogen-related sites and other selected sites in women—Cancer Prevention Study II

Site	Number of deaths*	Relative risk	95% confidence interval
Breast	294	0.92	0.82–1.03
Cervix	15	2.27	1.27–3.74
Endometrium	18	0.58	0.35–0.92
Uterus, NOS	12	0.97	0.50–1.69
Ovary	86	0.93	0.74–1.15
Colon–rectum	150	1.16	0.99–1.37
Gall bladder	8	1.05	0.45–2.02
Biliary passages	2	0.56	0.06–2.03

* Among smokers.

Table 1.8 shows RRs for current smokers and ex-smokers broken down by those under and over 50 years of age. Among women over 50 years old, the RRs of current and ex-smoking for endometrial cancer were 0.57 and 0.67, respectively, both statistically different from 1.00. The RRs in women over 50 years of age for colon–rectum cancer was 1.27 and 1.26, respectively, both significantly greater than 1.00. It is interesting that current smokers under age 50 had a RR for colon–rectum cancer of 0.48 (based on eight deaths), which is similar to what was found in CPS I. There were eight deaths of cervical cancer under age 50 with a high RR of 3.88 (95 per cent CI 1.67–7.65). In ex-smokers over age 50, the RR for cervical cancer was 2.23.

Table 1.9 shows for CPS II trends in RRs over amount smoked. The increasing trend for cervical cancer was statistically significant ($P<0.05$), as was the decreasing trend for endometrial cancer.

Low T/N in CPS II was classified as cigarettes with less than 12 mg tar; medium T/N, 12–15 mg tar; and high T/N, 16 mg and greater. An analysis of trends for low, medium, and high T/N smokers for breast, ovary, and colon–rectum cancer showed no consistent trends and none of the individual RRs were statistically different from 1.00 (Table 1.10).

Table 1.11 shows the results of a logistic regression model for smoking and breast, ovary, and colon–rectum cancer. Each case was matched with three controls on age. In the regression model, various potential confounding factors were controlled for. For breast these included age, education, history of breast cancer, age of first birth, mother or sister with breast cancer, relative weight, menopausal status, and use of oestrogens. For ovary and colon–rectum cancer, the factors included age, education, history of cancer, relative weight, and menopausal status. The relative risks were very close to those controlled for age alone shown in Table 1.7.

Table 1.8. Relative risks of smoking for cancers of oestrogen-related sites and other selected sites in women under and over 50 years of age at start of study—Cancer Prevention Study II

Site	Age group	Current smokers		Ex-smokers	
		Number of deaths*	Relative risk	Number of deaths*	Relative risk
Breast	<50	53	0.78	62	0.98
	50+	241	0.96	364	1.16†
Cervix	<50	8	3.88†	1	0.54
	50+	7	1.54	13	2.23†
Endometrium	<50	1	1.00	—	—
	50+	17	0.57‡	26	0.67‡
Uterus, NOS	<50	3	1.49	—	—
	50+	9	0.86	14	0.97
Ovary	<50	14	1.36	18	1.87*
	50+	72	0.87	105	1.03
Colon-rectum	<50	8	0.48‡	12	0.77
	50+	142	1.27†	191	1.26†
Gall bladder	<50	1	2.17	—	—
	50+	7	0.98	6	0.60
Biliary passages	<50	—	—	—	—
	50+	2	0.56	4	0.85

* Among smokers.
† Lower limit of 95% confidence interval more than 1.00.
‡ Upper limit of 95% confidence interval less than 1.00.

Table 1.9. Trends in relative risks of smoking for cancer of oestrogen-related sites and other selected sites in women—Cancer Prevention Study II

Site	Never smoked	Ex-smokers	Smoked <20 cigarettes a day	Smoked ≥20 cigarettes a day
Breast	1.00	1.13	0.90	0.93
Cervix*	1.00	1.82	2.24	2.29
Endometrium†	1.00	0.66	0.56	0.59
Uterus, NOS	1.00	0.86	0.92	1.00
Ovary	1.00	1.10	0.92	0.94
Colon-rectum	1.00	1.22	1.08	1.23

* Increasing trend statistically significant, $P<0.05$.
† Decreasing trend statistically significant, $P<0.05$.

Table 1.10. Relative risks of current smoking for breast, ovary, or colon-rectum cancer in women, by tar/nicotine (T/N) level—Cancer Prevention Study II

	Low T/N	Medium T/N	High T/N
Smoked <20 cigarettes a day			
Breast	1.02	0.86	0.84
Ovary	1.21	0.75	1.03
Colon-rectum	1.31	0.81	1.18
Smoked ≥20 cigarettes a day			
Breast	1.02	0.78	0.98
Ovary	0.98	0.80	1.33
Colon-rectum	1.29	1.11	1.37

Table 1.11. Relative risks of current smoking for cancers of selected sites based on logistic regression model—Cancer Prevention Study II

	Relative risk	95% confidence interval
Breast*	0.95	0.81-1.12
Ovary †	0.91	0.66-1.25
Colon-rectum †	1.09	0.84-1.41

* Controlled on age, education, history of breast cancer, age at first birth, mother or sister with breast cancer, relative weight, menopausal status, and use of oestrogens.

† Controlled for age, education, history of cancer, relative weight, and menopausal status.

1.4. Discussion

Table 1.12 summarizes the relationship of cigarette smoking to cancer at oestrogen-related sites and other selected sites in the two American Cancer Society Studies. The table shows the RRs of current smokers and ex-smokers (compared to non-smokers) in three studies: the first 6 years and second 6 years of experience in CPS I, and the 4-year follow-up in CPS II. This provides an opportunity to evaluate the consistency of the RRs.

The RRs of breast cancer were lower than 1.00 in current smokers in all three studies (years 7–12 was 0.89, $P<0.5$). However, all the risks for ex-smokers were more than 1.00 (1.12, 1.25, and 1.13), and the latter two RRs were statistically significant. The RR was higher in women over age 50, and about the same in light (under 20 cigarettes a day) and in heavy (more than

Table 1.12. Summary of relative risks for current smokers and ex-smokers from CPS I and CPS II

	Current smoker			Ex-smoker		
	CPS I		CPS II	CPS I		CPS II
	Years 1–6	Years 7–12		Years 1–6	Years 7–12	
Breast	0.93	0.89*	0.92	1.12	1.25*	1.13*
Cervix	1.26*	2.12*	2.27*	1.64*	1.70	1.82*
Endometrium	0.89	0.99	0.58*	(1.23)	0.92	0.66*
Uterus, NOS	0.76	1.23	0.97	(0.74)	1.44	0.86
Ovary	0.96	1.15	0.93	1.27	0.93	1.10
Colon–rectum	0.84*	0.93	1.16	1.05	1.06	1.22*
Gall bladder	0.88	0.83	(1.05)	(3.03)	(1.02)	(0.58)
Biliary passages	(1.16)	2.03*	(0.56)	(1.50)	(1.40)	(0.85)

* Statistically different from 1.00, $P<0.05$.
( ), less than 10 deaths.

20 cigarettes a day) current smokers. Adjusting for risk factors made little change in RRs for breast cancer. Thus the inconsistency of the RRs adds little to the unclear picture of previous studies.

The smoking risk for cervical cancer was higher than 1.00 for current smokers and ex-smokers in all three studies and the elevation in risk was statistically significant in all but one of the figures in Table 1.12. Current smokers under age 50 had higher RRs than those over 50, and there was an increase in risk associated with increased number of cigarettes smoked per day. Although RRs in CPS I and CPS II confirm the pattern found in other studies, the RRs are generally lower than in other published papers.

The pattern of smoking and endometrial cancer paralleled the findings in other studies. Table 1.12 shows that with one exception (because of small numbers) the RRs were all under 1.00, and in CPS II the RRs of 0.58 for current smokers and 0.66 for ex-smokers were statistically significant ($P<0.05$).

The category 'uterus, NOS' as stated on the death certificates, represents an unknown combination of cervix and endometrium cancer. We were unable in these cases to obtain additional clarifying information from certifying physicians, hospitals, or cancer registries. The RRs for this category do not show any clear pattern.

The RRs of smokers for ovarian cancer also show no consistent excess or decrease compared to non-smokers in the three studies. RRs for smokers aged 50 and over were higher than those under 50 in CPS I, but lower than those under 50 in CPS II. Adjusting for known risk factors changed the RRs only slightly.

Cancer of the colon–rectum was also studied in this analysis. Even though it is not oestrogen-related, it shares many epidemiological attributes with endometrial cancer and breast and ovarian cancer. In CPS I, RRs for smokers with colon–rectum cancer were under 1.00 ($P<0.05$); but were over 1.00 (1.16 and 1.22 for current and ex-smokers, $P>0.05$) in CPS II. In CPS I there was a downward trend for colon–rectum cancer with number of cigarettes smoked per day; in CPS II there was an upward trend, not statistically significant. Based on these analyses it is difficult to determine if smokers have a higher or lower mortality rate from cancer of the colon–rectum than non-smokers.

Gall bladder cancer RRs for current and ex-smokers in CPS I were under 1.00, but were over 1.00 (based on small numbers) in CPS II. The RR for cancer of the biliary passages in smokers was high in CPS I (RR 1.81, $P<0.05$) but there were too few deaths in CPS II to determine if this finding could be confirmed.

Some of the differences in RRs between CPS I and CPS II may have been due to temporal trends in smoking patterns between the start of CPS I (1959) and the start of CPS II (1982). In CPS II, higher proportions of female smokers inhaled or smoked heavily. Moreover, in the later cohort, the mean age of starting smoking was lower (Garfinkel and Stellman 1988). These differences may have increased the actual smoking exposure among those who smoked, resulting in lower RRs for endometrial cancer, and higher RRs for cervical cancer.

References

Adena, M. A. and Gallagher, H. G. (1982). Cigarette smoking and the age at menopause. *Annals of Human Biology*, 9, 121–30.

Baron, J. A. (1984). Smoking and estrogen-related disease. *American Journal of Epidemiology*, 119, 9–22.

Baron, J. A., Byers, T., Greenberg, E. R., Cummings, K. M., and Swanson, M. (1986). Cigarette smoking in women with cancers of the breast and reproductive organs. *Journal of the National Cancer Institute*, 77, 677–80.

Berggren, G. and Sjostedt, S. (1983). Preinvasive carcinoma of the cervix uteri and smoking. *Acta Obstetrica Gynecologica Scandinavica*, 62, 593–8.

Breslow, N. E. and Day, N. E. (1980). *Statistical methods in cancer research*, Vol. 1, The analysis of case-control studies, IARC Scientific Publications No. 32. International Agency for Research on Cancer, Lyon.

Brinton, L. A., *et al.* (1986a). Cigarette smoking and invasive cervical cancer. *Journal of the American Medical Association*, 255, 3265–9.

Brinton, L. A., Schairer, C., Stanford, J. L., and Hoover, R. N. (1986b). Cigarette smoking and breast cancer. *American Journal of Epidemiology*, 123, 614–22.

Brownson, R. C., Blackwell, C. W., Pearson, D. K., Reynolds, R. D., Richens, J. W., and Papermaster, B. W. (1988). Risk of breast cancer in relation to cigarette smoking. *Archives of Internal Medicine*, **148**, 140–4.

Byers, T., Marshall, J., Graham, S., Mettlin, C., and Swanson, M. (1983). A case-control study of dietary and nondietary factors in ovarian cancer. *Journal of the National Cancer Institute*, 71, 681–6.

Clarke, E. A., Morgan, R. W., and Newman, A. M. (1982). Smoking as a risk factor in cancer of the cervix: additional evidence from a case-control study. *American Journal of Epidemiology*, **115**, 59–66.

Clarke, E. A., Hatcher, J., McKeown-Eyssen, E., and Lickrish, G. M. (1985). Cervical dysplasia: association with sexual behavior, smoking, and oral contraceptive use? *American Journal of Obstetrics and Gynecology*, **151**, 612–16.

Cramer, D. W., Welch, W. R., Hutchison, G. B., Willett, W., and Scully, R. E. (1984). Dietary animal fat in relation to ovarian cancer risk. *Obstetrics and Gynecology*, **63**, 833–8.

Daniell, H. W. (1986). More advanced colonic cancer among smokers. *Cancer*, **58**, 784–7.

Doll, R., Gray, R., Hafner, B., and Peto, R. (1980). Mortality in relation to smoking: 22 years' observations on female British doctors. *British Medical Journal*, **280**, 967–71.

Franks, A. L., Kendrick, J. S., Tyler, C. W., and The Cancer and Steroid Hormone Study Group (1987a). Postmenopausal smoking, estrogen replacement therapy, and the risk of endometrial cancer. *American Journal of Obstetrics and Gynecology*, **156**, 20–3.

Franks, A. L., Lee, N. C., Kendrick, J. S., Rubin, G. L., Layde, P. M., and The Cancer and Steroid Hormone Study Group (1987b). Cigarette smoking and the risk of epithelial ovarian cancer. *American Journal of Epidemiology*, **126**, 112–17.

Garfinkel, L. (1980). Cancer mortality in nonsmokers: prospective study by the American Cancer Society. *Journal of the National Cancer Institute*, **65**, 1169–73.

Garfinkel, L. (1985). Selection, follow-up, and analysis in the American Cancer Society prospective studies. *National Cancer Institute Monograph*, **67**, 49–52.

Garfinkel, L. and Stellman, S. D. (1988). Smoking and lung cancer in women. Findings in a prospective study. *Cancer Research*, **48**, 6951–5.

Greenberg, E. R., Vessey, M., McPherson, K., and Yeates, D. (1985). Cigarette smoking and cancer of the uterine cervix. *British Journal of Cancer*, **51**, 139–41.

Harris, R. W. C., *et al.* (1980). Characteristics of women with dysplasia or carcinoma in situ of the cervix uteri. *British Journal of Cancer*, **42**, 359–69.

Hellberg, D., Valentin, J., and Nilsson, S. (1986). Smoking and cervical intraepithelial neoplasia. *Acta Obstetrica Gynecologica Scandinava*, **65**, 625–31.

Hiatt, R. A. and Fireman, B. H. (1986). Smoking, menopause, and breast cancer. *Journal of the National Cancer Institute*, 76, 833–8.

Hiatt, R. A., Friedman, G. D., Bawol, R. D., and Ury, H. K. (1982). Breast cancer and serum cholesterol. *Journal of the National Cancer Institute*, **68**, 885–9.

Hoff, G., Vatn, H., and Larsen, S. (1987). Relationship between tobacco smoking and colorectal polyps. *Scandinavian Journal of Gastroenterology*, **22**, 13–16.

Kelsey, J. L., *et al.* (1981). Exogenous estrogens and other factors in the epidemiology of breast cancer. *Journal of the National Cancer Institute*, **67**, 327–33.

La Vecchia, C., Franceschi, S., Decarli, A., Fasoli, M., Gentile, A., and Tognoni, G.

(1986). Cigarette smoking and the risk of cervical neoplasia. *American Journal of Epidemiology*, **123**, 22–9.

Lawrence, C., *et al.* (1987). Smoking, body weight, and early-stage endometrial cancer. *Cancer*, **59**, 1665–9.

Lesko, S. M., *et al.* (1985). Cigarette smoking and the risk of endometrial cancer. *The New England Journal of Medicine*, **313**, 593–6.

Levi, F., La Vecchia, C., and Decarli, A. (1987). Cigarette smoking and the risk of endometrial cancer. *European Journal of Cancer and Clinical Oncology*, **23**, 1025–9.

Lyon, J. L., Gardner, J. W., West, D. W., Stanish, W. M., and Hebertson, R. M. (1983). Smoking and carcinoma in situ of the uterine cervix. *American Journal Public Health*, **73**, 558–62.

MacMahon, B. and Feinleib, M. (1960). Breast cancer in relation to nursing and menopausal history. *Journal of the National Cancer Institute*, **24**, 733–53.

MacMahon, B., Trichopoulos, D., Cole, P., and Brown, J. (1982). Cigarette smoking and urinary estrogens. *The New England Journal of Medicine*, **307**, 1062–5.

Mantel, N. (1963). Chi-square tests with one degree of freedom: extensions of the Mantel-Haenszel procedure. *Journal of the American Statistical Association*, **58**, 690–700.

Marshall, J. R., Graham, S., Byers, T., Swanson, M., and Brasure, J. (1983). Diet and smoking in the epidemiology of cancer of the cervix. *Journal of the National Cancer Institute*, **70**, 847–51.

O'Connell, D. L., Hulka, B. S., Chambless, L. E., Wilkinson, W. E., and Deubner, D. C. (1987). Cigarette smoking, alcohol consumption, and breast cancer risk. *Journal of the National Cancer Institute*, **78**, 229–34.

Rosenberg, L., *et al.* (1984). Breast cancer and cigarette smoking. *The New England Journal of Medicine*, **310**, 92–4.

Rothman, K. J. and Boice, J. D. (1979). *Epidemiologic analysis with a programmable calculator*. Epidemiology Resources Inc., Chestnut Hill, MA.

Schechter, M. T., Miller, A. B., and Howe, G. R. (1985). Cigarette smoking and breast cancer: a case-control study of screening program participants. *American Journal of Epidemiology*, **121**, 479–87.

Smith, E. M., Sowers, M. F., and Burns, R. L. (1984). Effects of smoking on the development of female reproductive cancers. *Journal of the National Cancer Institute*, **73**, 371–6.

Stellman, S. D., Austin, H., and Wynder, E. L. (1980). Cervix cancer and cigarette smoking: a case-control study. *American Journal of Epidemiology*, **111**, 383–8.

Stockwell, H. G. and Lyman, G. H. (1987). Cigarette smoking and the risk of female reproductive cancer. *American Journal of Obstetrics and Gynecology*, **157**, 35–40.

Trevathan, E., Layde, P., Webster, L. A., Adams, J. B., Benigno, B. B., and Ory, H. (1983). Cigarette smoking and dysplasia and carcinoma in situ of the uterine cervix. *Journal of the American Medical Association*, **250**, 499–502.

Tyler, C. W., Webster, L. A., Ory, H. W., and Rubin, G. L. (1985). Endometrial cancer: how does cigarette smoking influence the risk of women under age 55 years having this tumor? *American Journal of Obstetrics and Gynecology*, **151**, 899–905.

Vessey, M., Baron, J., Doll, R., McPherson, K., and Yeates, D. (1983). Oral contraceptives and breast cancer: final report of an epidemiological study. *British Journal of Cancer*, 47, 455–62.

Weiss, N. S., Vernon, T. F., Szekely, D. R., English, D. R., and Kiviat, N. (1980). Oestrogens and endometrial cancer: effect of other risk factors on the association. *Maturitas*, 2, 185–90.

Williams, R. R. and Horm, J. W. (1977). Association of cancer sites with tobacco and alcohol consumption and socioeconomic status of patients: Interview study from the Third National Cancer Survey. *Journal of the National Cancer Institute*, 58, 525–47.

Winkelstein, W. (1977). Smoking and cancer of the uterine cervix: hypothesis. *American Journal of Epidemiology*, 106, 257–9.

Wright, N. H., Vessey, M. P., Kenward, B., McPherson, K., and Doll, R. (1978). Neoplasia and dysplasia of the cervix uteri and contraception: a possible protective effect of the diaphragm. *British Journal of Cancer*, 38, 273–9.

Yen, S., Hsieh, C. C., and MacMahon, B. (1987). Extrahepatic bile duct cancer and smoking, beverage consumption, past medical history, and oral-contraceptive use. *Cancer*, 59, 2112–16.

2. Smoking and Hormone-related disorders in the Nurses' Health Study

Meir J. Stampfer, Graham A. Colditz, Stephanie J. London, Christopher G. Chute, Bernard Rosner, Walter C. Willett, Charles H. Hennekens, and Frank E. Speizer

Abstract

Cigarette smoking alters levels of oestrogens and other hormones, and could therefore affect the incidence of disorders thought to be hormonally related. This issue is addressed in the Nurses' Health Study. A cohort of 121 700 nurses was established in 1976, and followed through biennial questionnaires. In 1976, 34.4 per cent of the cohort were current smokers, a proportion very similar to the general US population of women. Smokers had a dose-related earlier menopause than non-smokers, independent of leanness. Cigarette smoking was an important risk factor for both stroke and coronary heart disease, with a pronounced dose effect. Even one to four cigarettes per day led to a relative risk of coronary heart disease of 2.4 (95 per cent confidence interval 1.1–1.5). Approximately half the cases of fatal coronary disease and non-fatal myocardial infarctions were attributable to cigarette smoking. These effects were not materially altered by menopausal status or use of post-menopausal hormones. Smokers who currently used oral contraceptives had a relative risk of coronary heart disease of 5.0 (confidence intervals 2.7–9.0) compared to non-smoking women who never used them. No effect of past use of oral contraception was observed on risk of cardiovascular diseases in both pre- and post-menopausal women. There was a strong protective effect of post-menopausal oestrogen use for coronary disease that was similar in both smokers and non-smokers. No material association was found between smoking and colorectal cancer, breast cancer, endometrial cancer, or fractures. The effect of smoking on endometrial cancer and fractures cannot be considered conclusive because of the relatively young age of the cohort.

These data demonstrate that smoking has a pronounced dose-related adverse impact on several important health outcomes. Smoking does not have a major impact on the hormonally related disorders that were studied among these middle-aged women, apart from the occurrence of menopause.

2.1. Introduction

Cigarette smoking affects the production of oestrogens and some other hormones among both men and women. Any 'anti-oestrogenic' effect of smoking might therefore have consequences, either adverse or beneficial, for disorders that may be related to hormone levels. Since cigarette smoking is the leading avoidable cause of death in industrialized countries, no direct public health implications derive from such findings. None the less, these issues are of considerable interest and importance, since other, less lethal methods to alter hormone levels could be developed to achieve the benefits, if any.

The Nurses' Health Study has examined the relationship of cigarette smoking with a number of disorders potentially related to hormone levels.

2.2. Methods

The Nurses' Health Study cohort

The Nurses' Health Study began in 1976 when all married, female, registered nurses 30 to 55 years of age, living in 11 large US states, were mailed a questionnaire that included items concerning medical history, exogenous hormone use, cigarette smoking, and other factors which might influence risks of cancer (Willett *et al.* 1987a) and cardiovascular disease (Stampfer *et al.* 1985). The list was obtained from the American Nursing Association. Of the 172 413 questionnaires that were delivered, 121 964 (71 per cent) nurses responded (Belanger *et al.* 1978). In the ensuing years 264 were out of the eligible age range, were male, or were duplicate responders, leaving a total cohort of 121 700.

Follow-up questionnaires were sent every 2 years to update information on various exposures of interest, and to ascertain the incidence of newly diagnosed illnesses. In each questionnaire cycle, up to five repeated mailings to non-respondents were sent. Every other year, when questionnaires were not mailed, an informational letter was sent to all cohort members about the progress of the study. This letter included a questionnaire for persistent non-responders, and also served to maintain current information on the addresses and vital status of the participants.

The scope of the study was broadened in 1980 when a detailed dietary assessment was added to the questionnaire. Dietary information was updated in 1984 and 1986. The cohort continues to be followed in this manner; the sixth mailing cycle of biennial questionnaires began in June 1988. The follow-up rates have remained high. A total of 111 099 (91 per cent) participants responded to the 1978 questionnaire. In 1980, 98 769 completed the full questionnaire (including dietary assessment), and another 4591 completed an abbreviated questionnaire, for a total 103 360 responses (86 per cent follow-up of living subjects). In 1982, the overall response rate remained essentially unchanged (101 174 responded), and attempts to telephone the approximately 19 000 living non-respondents were made. Telephone numbers were found for 77 per cent of non-respondents and 92 per cent of these women were contacted, or 71 per cent of the non-respondents. Thus at the end of 1982 there was current information on 116 160 (95 per cent) of the original cohort. In 1984, 100 239 responses were received to the questionnaire, and in 1986 there was current information on 86 per cent of the participants. The overall follow-up is higher than these response rates suggest because of intermittent rather than continuous non-response by many participants.

Ascertainment of exposures

The baseline and subsequent follow-up questionnaires included these items: menopause—natural, or surgical and whether none, one, or both ovaries were removed; use of post-menopausal hormones; reproductive variables (including age at menarche and number of pregnancies); and a variety of other factors thought to possibly influence risks of breast cancer or cardiovascular disease. Of particular interest for this report, baseline inquiry included smoking status—current, past, or never; for current and past smokers the age of starting and typical number of cigarettes smoked per day; and for past smokers, the age of stopping. On the follow-up questionnaires, any changes in smoking status were updated, and also brand of cigarette sought.

Ascertainment of outcomes

Whenever a participant reported the new diagnosis of a disease of interest (e.g. cancer, myocardial infarction, stroke, etc.) on a follow-up questionnaire, permission was sought to obtain the relevant medical records. These records were reviewed by physicians blinded to exposure data reported by the participant; in addition to confirming the report, the records were also used to categorize endpoints. For example, for breast cancer this included the histological type, the size of the tumour at diagnosis, presence or absence of local or distant metastases, and results of hormone receptor assays. Repeated efforts were made to obtain these records for all reported endpoints, and the follow-up for endpoint confirmation has been quite high.

Deaths were reported usually by relatives or postal authorities. After each biennial questionnaire cycle, the National Death Index (Stampfer *et al.* 1984) was searched for non-respondents who may have died. Before the National Death Index was established in 1980, the vital statistics records of the 11 states were searched. Death certificates for all deceased participants were obtained; for any death possibly due to cancer or cardiovascular disease not documented before death, the family was contacted for permission to obtain the relevant medical records. Based on a comparison of ascertainment of deaths using independent sources, 98 per cent of the deaths in the cohort have been identified.

As expected, these nurses provide accurate information. A variety of studies were conducted in which detailed records were obtained to validate the accuracy of the self-reports of hypertension, hypercholesterolaemia, diabetes, and age and type of menopause, including whether one or both ovaries were removed (Colditz *et al.* 1986, 1987). In general, the self-reports were accurate. In the reports of outcomes, the accuracy was highest for cancers in which the pathology reports were usually unequivocal, such as breast cancer; as expected, the accuracy was less for endometrial cancer in which the diagnostic procedure is often curative (Colditz *et al.* 1986). All of the analyses of outcomes included only documented cases.

Data analysis

For most analyses, age-specific and age-adjusted relative risks were calculated by estimating the ratio of the incidence of disease in the exposure category of interest, to the corresponding rate in the reference group. The incidence rates were estimated as the number of new cases occurring in the population at risk in the exposure category of interest, divided by the person-years of follow-up for that group. The follow-up time was derived by counting the months from the receipt of the baseline questionnaire until return of the subsequent follow-up questionnaire, or the occurrence of an endpoint. Follow-up time was allocated according to the most recent exposure category, and updated with information on each successive questionnaire. Follow-up time ceased with death, the occurrence of an endpoint, or the end of the interval chosen for analysis.

To control for confounding and to assess the possibility of effect modification, stratified analyses within and across categories of other variables were performed (Rothman and Boice 1979). Finally, proportional hazards analyses were conducted to control for a variety of risk factors simultaneously (Cox 1972).

2.3. Results

Age cohort effects for prevalence, starting and stopping smoking in the Nurses' Health Study

A detailed analysis of this issue has been published by Myers *et al.* (1987). In 1976, after exclusion of those with cancer, coronary disease, hypertension, and diabetes, 34.4 per cent of the cohort were current smokers and 23.4 per cent were former smokers. The percentage of current smokers was very similar to the 32 per cent prevalence among women over age 20 in the

US in general at that time (Report of the Surgeon General 1979). Several studies have shown a somewhat higher prevalence of smoking among nurses (National Clearinghouse for Smoking and Health 1976; Report of the Surgeon General 1980); Myers' findings probably reflect the tendency for smokers to be less likely to volunteer for epidemiologic studies.

The prevalence of smoking was remarkably similar across all five 5-year birth cohorts. However, this finding masked strong divergences among the birth cohorts in attaining a similar ultimate prevalence of smoking. In general, the older age cohorts tended to start smoking at a later age; by age 20, 24.4 per cent of the nurses in the oldest cohort, born 1921–6 had begun to smoke, whereas the corresponding figure for those in the youngest age cohort, born 1942–6, was 38.7 per cent. In every age cohort, women who started smoking earlier had lower rates of quitting. Despite this, women in the younger cohorts stopped smoking at a faster rate. For example, among women who started to smoke between ages 17–21, the proportion stopping within 10 years was 8.7 per cent in the oldest and 29.5 per cent in the youngest cohort.

The drop in cigarette use observed in this cohort has persisted. In succeeding intervals, the proportion of current smokers (without exclusions for illnesses) has dropped from 33.2 per cent at baseline in 1976, to 29.0 per cent in 1980, and 27.7 per cent in 1984. In part this may reflect, to a small extent, selective survival and response to questionnaires, but most of the decline probably reflects continuing cessation of smoking.

Smoking and menopause

The interrelationships of cigarette smoking and relative weight with the occurrence of natural menopause were examined during the subsequent 2 years among Nurses' Health Study participants who were pre-menopausal in 1976. These data have been published in detail elsewhere (Willett *et al.* 1983). A subset of the cohort was studied, namely women who provided complete information on smoking, weight, height, and menopause in 1976; who were pre-menopausal in 1976; who completed the 1978 questionnaire; and who did not have a surgical or radiation-induced menopause in the interval. Of the 66 663 pre-menopausal women who met these criteria, 5004 became post-menopausal (defined as an affirmative response to the question, 'Have your menstrual periods ceased permanently?').

In each 5-year age category, current cigarette smokers were more likely to have had the menopause than those who never smoked. As in previous studies, current smokers were leaner than those who had stopped or never smoked. Both leanness and cigarette smoking were independently associated with an increased chance or 'risk' of having had the menopause, but the effect of leanness was most pronounced among smokers. The increased relative 'risk' associated with smoking diminished with increasing age: after adjustment for relative weight, for ages 30–39 the relative risk (RR) was 1.9

(95 per cent confidence interval 1.1–3.3); for 40–44, 2.2 (1.7–2.7); for 45–49, 1.5 (1.4–1.7); and for 50–55, 1.2 (1.1–1.3). The rate of menopause was closely linked to intensity of smoking among current smokers. There was a monotonic increase in risk with an increasing number of cigarettes smoked per day. For those in the 40–49 year age category, the age-adjusted RR ranged from 1.3 for 1–14 cigarettes per day to 2.0 for 35 or more cigarettes per day.

In each age category, the RR for former smokers was slightly elevated, reaching statistical significance only for the 40–44 category, with a RR of 1.3 (1.0–1.7). In an analysis of former smokers, the effect was limited to women who stopped smoking within the past several years.

Smoking, exogenous hormone use, and cardiovascular disease

As reported earlier, cigarette smoking increases risks of coronary heart disease (Willett *et al.* 1987b) and stroke (Colditz *et al.* 1988) in the Nurses' Health Study. The analysis of smoking and coronary disease included 65 cases of fatal coronary disease and 242 non-fatal myocardial infarcations that occurred in 6 years of follow-up of cohort participants free from diagnosed coronary disease at baseline. Approximately half of the cases were attributable to cigarette smoking. The elevated RRs were apparent only for current smokers, and those who stopped very recently. An elevated risk was significant even for current smokers of only one to four cigarettes per day, RR = 2.4 (1.1–5.0). The RR estimates increased steadily with increased number of cigarettes, reaching 10.8 (5.5–21.1) among those who smoked 45 or more cigarettes per day.

Generally, similar findings were observed for stroke (Colditz *et al.* 1988). This analysis was based on 8 years of follow-up and included 274 strokes. For all stroke, the RR for current smokers steadily increased with the number of cigarettes per day. The RR associated with 1–14 cigarettes per day was 2.2 (1.5–3.3) and with 45 or more, it was 6.2 (2.6–14.9). The elevated risks were observed both for ischaemic and haemorrhagic stroke, and were particularly pronounced for subarachnoid haemorrhage.

For both coronary heart disease and stroke, there was no apparent difference in risk due to cigarette smoking between pre-menopausal and post-menopausal women, after adjustment for age. In addition, no effect modification by use of oestrogens among post-menopausal women was found.

As others have found, an increase in risk of coronary heart disease among current users of oral contraceptive agents in both retrospective (Rosenberg *et al.* 1980) and prospective data (Stampfer *et al.* 1988) was observed. In a case-control design using the baseline data collected in 1976, for current oral contraceptive use the RR was 1.6 (1.0–2.6).

An interaction between cigarette smoking and current oral contraceptive use was observed; among women with no other risk factors, those who smoked and currently used oral contraceptives had a RR of 5.0 (2.7–9.0) compared to non-smoking women who never used oral contraceptives. Due to the age distribution of women enrolled in the cohort, few participants currently used oral contraceptives in 1976 and beyond. Hence, despite 8 years of follow-up, the prospective data for current use were limited (2.4 per cent of the total of 921 960 person-years). An elevated RR of current use of oral contraceptives for coronary heart disease was apparent but the confidence intervals were broad (RR = 2.5, 1.3–4.9). No increase in risk of coronary disease or stroke among past users of oral contraceptive agents was found. Among past oral contraceptive users, the RR for non-fatal myocardial infarction or coronary death was 0.8 (0.6–1.0), and for stroke (all forms combined) it was 1.0 (0.7–1.3). The absence of an effect of past oral contraceptive use was seen among both smokers and non-smokers.

In this cohort, post-menopausal women who used oestrogen replacement therapy had a decreased risk of non-fatal myocardial infarction and coronary death. An analysis based on 4 years of follow-up has been published by Stampfer *et al.* (1985); this included 25 cases of fatal coronary disease and 65 non-fatal myocardial infarctions. The age-adjusted RR was 0.5 (0.3–0.8) for ever users of oestrogen therapy, and 0.3 (0.2–0.6) for current users. After adjustment for a wide range of coronary risk factors, the RRs were very similar: 0.6 (0.3–1.1) among past users and 0.3 (0.1–0.6) among current users. The apparent benefit of ever use of oestrogens was similar for cigarette smokers and non-smokers. For non-fatal myocardial infarction, the RR for oestrogen use among smokers was 0.5 (0.3–0.9) and for those who never smoked it was 0.5 (0.1–1.8). For fatal coronary disease, the RR for oestrogen use among smokers was 0.7 (0.3–1.3) and among non-smokers, 0.6 (0.1–6.7). However, the number of endpoints was small, especially among those who never smoked, so the confidence intervals around those estimates are wide. It is possible that some quantitative difference in the effect of oestrogens on smokers and non-smokers might emerge with further follow-up, but it seems unlikely that the benefit is limited only to one or the other group. An analysis based on 10 years of follow-up is planned.

Smoking and colorectal cancer

Colon cancer is not commonly considered to be hormonally related, but several investigators have postulated possible mechanisms whereby hormones might influence bile acid secretion and risk of bowel cancer. Chute (1988) provides a detailed study of reproductive variables and risk of colorectal cancer in the Nurses' Health Study. In this analysis, incident cases of colorectal cancer occurring during the first 8 years of follow-up are included. Participants with a prior history of cancer except non-melanoma skin cancer were excluded. Eligible subjects were followed from the time of return of the 1976 questionnaire until the diagnosis of colorectal cancer, death, or 31 May 1984, whichever came first; there were 191 cases of colon cancer and 49 cases of rectal cancer.

Overall, there was no material association between cigarette smoking and the risk of colon cancer. For ever smokers, the RR for colon cancer was 1.0 (0.7–1.4). Separate analyses for former and current smokers yielded similar null results. Among former smokers, the RR was 1.2 (0.9–1.7). For current smokers of up to 14 cigarettes per day, the RR was 1.0 (0.6–1.7), for 15–24 per day, 1.0 (0.6–1.5), and for 25 or more, it was 0.9 (0.5–1.6). An examination of the site-specific relative risks did not identify any region in the bowel that showed a consistent association with cigarette smoking. Similar null findings were observed for rectal cancer.

Breast cancer

Considerable interest has focused on whether smoking may affect risk of breast cancer. A comprehensive analysis of this issue in the Nurses' Health Study is provided by London *et al.* (1989), and preliminary results fail to suggest any material association. In this analysis, all women free from cancer at the start of the study who provided information on smoking and potential risk factors for breast cancer are included. There were 1799 incident cases that occurred in slightly over one million person-years of follow-up, from 1976 to 1986.

Because the pattern of breast cancer incidence, as well as the impact of adiposity, varies between pre-menopausal and post-menopausal women, separate analyses were conducted within those categories. The impact of cigarette smoking was examined on risk of breast cancer after adjustment for age in 5 year categories, age at menarche, age at first birth, parity, Quetelet index, oral contraceptive use before first pregnancy, mother or sister history of breast cancer, and benign breast disease in proportional hazards models. For past smokers, the RR was 1.1 (1.0–1.2), for current smokers of up to 14 cigarettes per day, it was 1.0 (0.8–1.2), for 15–24 cigarettes per day, it was 1.0 (0.9–1.2), and for 25 or more, it was 1.0 (0.9–1.2). These findings were quite similar to the results adjusted for age alone. Nearly identical point estimates were observed for both post-menopausal and pre-menopausal women after the same multivariate adjustment.

Because alcohol is a risk factor for breast cancer, and tends to be associated with cigarette smoking, any effect of cigarette smoking present after adjustment for alcohol intake was investigated. Alcohol intake was assessed by a semi-quantitative food frequency questionnaire sent to the cohort in 1980. This questionnaire has been well studied, and its validity and reproducibility were particularly high for alcohol (Willett *et al.* 1985, 1987a). In these analyses, only cases diagnosed in the 1980–4 interval were included. After adjustment for alcohol and the other factors listed, among post-menopausal women, former smokers had a RR of 1.06 (0.77–1.46); for current smokers it was 1.02 (0.74–1.42). For pre-menopausal women, the RR was 1.05 (0.83–1.48) for past smokers, and for current smokers it was 1.04 (0.76–1.41).

Endometrial cancer

Risk factors for endometrial cancer in the Nurses' Health Study are currently under study; only preliminary results are currently available. This analysis is limited to nurses who were free from cancer at the start of the study, and who had an intact uterus. All confirmed cases that occurred between 1976 and 1982 are included. A total of 96 365 women met the criteria in 1976, and 150 cases occurred in 548 026 person-years of follow-up. Of the cases, 80 were diagnosed in post-menopausal women, and 70 occurred in pre- and peri-menopausal women.

As expected, use of post-menopausal oestrogens increased the risk, especially for current users, in whom the RR was 4.2 (2.5–7.2). In addition, there was a strong trend of increasing risk with increased duration of use, $X_{trend} = 6.4$ for current users, and 3.1 for past users. There was a non-significant decrease in risk among past users of oral contraceptives (RR = 0.7, 0.5–1.1), and significant trends for decreased risk with increased duration of oral contraceptive use, and decreased protection with increasing interval since last use of oral contraceptives.

There was no effect of cigarette smoking on risk of endometrial cancer. Compared to women who never smoked, both current and past users had identical RRs: 1.0 (0.7–1.5). In addition, there was no effect of number of cigarettes per day; among current smokers, the X_{trend} for risk according to number of cigarettes smoked per day was 0.2. In a separate analysis restricted to women over age 50, the RR associated with current smoking was 1.0 (0.7–1.6). However, there was a suggestion of a possible difference of effect by stage of the tumour: for tumours localized to the endometrium, the RR was 1.4 (0.8–2.6), but for cancers invading the myometrium, the RR was 0.5 (0.2–1.2). These results are adjusted for age alone. Nevertheless, in this cohort, there is no strong association between cigarette smoking and use of oestrogens that might mask a protective effect of smoking. Moreover, smokers tend to be leaner than non-smokers, and since obesity is a risk factor for endometrial cancer (RR = 2.0, 1.2–3.3 between extreme quintiles), adjustment for this variable could not lead to any apparent benefit of cigarette use.

Fractures

A preliminary report on life style and fractures (Hemenway *et al.* 1988) was based on fractures of the hip or forearm sustained between return of the 1980 questionnaire and May 1984. Nurses were included if they completed the 1980 questionnaire, were free from cancer in 1980, and completed a follow-up questionnaire in 1982 or 1984. There were 925 fractures reported among the 96 508 eligible participants.

There was no apparent effect of cigarette use on fracture risk. Compared with never smokers, past smokers had a RR of 1.0 (0.8–1.1); among current smokers of 1–14 cigarettes per day it was 1.0 (0.7–1.2); for 15–24 cigarettes per day, 1.0 (0.8–1.2); and for 25 or more, it was 1.0 (0.8–1.3). In an analysis limited to the 16 126 women 55–60 years of age (291 cases), there was no effect of smoking; the rates of fracture per 10 000 person-years were 45.4 among never smokers and 47.0 for smokers of 25 or more cigarettes per day.

2.4. Discussion

In the Nurses' Health Study cohort, the pattern of cigarette smoking is comparable to US women in general. In this prospective study, there was a pronounced, dose-related adverse impact of smoking on several important health outcomes. An effect of cigarette smoking on hormonally related disorders is clearly evident only for its association with earlier menopause; smokers typically experience natural menopause about 2 years earlier than non-smokers. It is possible that this relates to a direct toxic effect on the oocyte rather than being mediated through hormonal function. Other disorders potentially related to hormonal function do not appear to be materially affected. Although smoking markedly increases the risk of cardiovascular outcomes, there appears to be no apparent alteration in its effect according to menopausal status or post-menopausal oestrogen usage.

There was no apparent effect of cigarette smoking on colon cancer, a site usually considered to be unrelated to that exposure. Also no effect for breast cancer, both among pre-menopausal and post-menopausal women was observed. The large number of cases yielded fairly narrow confidence intervals about the null value; the data reported here are generally incompatible with more than about a 10 per cent decrease in risk in smokers, and the point estimates for the RRs, after adjustment for various breast cancer risk factors, are very slightly above 1.0. These findings are in general agreement with much of the literature (MacMahon, Chapter 15).

The lack of an effect of smoking on endometrial cancer cannot be considered conclusive. There were 150 cases of which 80 occurred in post-menopausal women, so further follow-up is required.

A similar limitation holds for the data on fractures. Many of the fractures occurred among pre-menopausal women, and none of the nurses in the analysis was over age 63. If cigarette smoking has an important effect on osteoporosis, its impact would be best observed in older post-menopausal women who sustain fractures after only a minor impact. Further analyses of fracture are in progress; these will consider menopausal status, oestrogen use, and degree of impact associated with the fracture occurrence among women up to age 65.

In conclusion, based on current data, cigarette smoking does not have a major impact on the hormonally related disorders reported here among middle-aged women, apart from occurrence of menopause. It is possible that such effects may become apparent with further follow-up as the cohort ages; at present, however, there is no suggestion of any such effects.

A number of other smoking-related cancers and chronic disease outcomes are currently under investigation in the Nurses' Health Study. These include lung cancer, pancreas cancer, pulmonary embolism, and most recently chronic respiratory disease. It is clear that cigarette smoking is the leading avoidable cause of death and chronic disease in the US. Recent estimates suggest that over 320 000 deaths per year are directly attributable to cigarette smoking (US Centers for Disease Control 1987). It is imperative that whenever cigarette smoking is considered, the total context of smoking as a risk factor must be borne in mind.

Acknowledgement

The authors gratefully acknowledge the Nurses' Health Study participants for their continuing outstanding level of co-operation, and the expert help of Stephanie Bechtel, Gary Chase, Sue-Wei Chiang, Karen Corsano, David Dysert, Barbara Egan, Lori Egan, Maureen Ireland, Marion McPhee, Mark Shneyder, Steven Stuart and Donna Vincent.

Supported by research grants CA 40935 and HL 34594 from the National Institutes of Health.

References

Belanger, C. F., Hennekens, C. H., Rosner, B., and Speizer, F. E. (1978). The Nurses' Health Study. *American Journal of Nursing*, **78**, 1039–40.

Chute, C. G. (1988). A prospective study of body mass, height, and smoking on the risk of colorectal cancer in women. (Not published). Doctoral Dissertation. Department of Epidemiology, Harvard School of Public Health.

Colditz, G. A., *et al.* (1986). Validation of questionnaire information on risk factors and disease outcomes in a prospective cohort study in women. *American Journal of Epidemiology*, **123**, 894–900.

Colditz, G. A., *et al.* (1987). Reproducibility and validity of self-reported menopausal status in a prospective cohort study. *American Journal of Epidemiology*, **126**, 319–25.

Colditz, G. A., *et al.* (1988). Cigarette smoking and elevated risk of stroke in a cohort of U.S. women. *New England Journal of Medicine*, **318**, 937–41.

Cox, D. R. (1972). Regression models and life-tables. *Journal of the Royal Statistical Society*, **34**, 187–220.

Hemenway, D., Colditz, G. A., Willett, W. C., Stampfer, M. J., and Speizer, F. E. (1988). Fractures and life-style: Effect of cigarettes, alcohol and relative weight on the risk of hip and forearm fractures in middle-aged women. *American Journal of Public Health*, **78**, 1554–8.

London, S. J., Colditz, G. A., Stampfer, M. J., Willett, W. C., Rosner, B. A., and Speizer, F. E. (1989). A prospective study of smoking and risk of breast cancer. *Journal of the National Cancer Institute*, **81**, 1625–31.

Myers, A. H., *et al.* (1987). Smoking behavior among participants in the Nurses' Health Study. *American Journal of Public Health*, 77, 628–30.

National Clearinghouse for Smoking and Health (1976). *Study of the smoking behavior of physicians, dentists, nurses, and pharmacists in the United States*, 1975. DHEW, Washington, DC.

Report of the Surgeon General (1979). *Smoking and health*, DHEW Pub. No. 79-50066. Government Printing Office, Washington, DC.

Report of the Surgeon General (1980). *The health consequences of smoking for women*, DHHS Pub. No. 0-326-003. Government Printing Office, Washington, DC.

Rosenberg, L., Hennekens, C. H., Rosner, B., Belanger, C., Rothman, K. J., and Speizer, F. E. (1980). Oral contraceptive use in relation to nonfatal myocardial infarction. *American Journal of Epidemiology*, **111**, 59–66.

Rothman, J. K. and Boice, J. D. (1979). *Epidemiologic analyses with a programmable calculator*, NIH Publication No. 79-1649. Public Health Service, Washington, DC.

Stampfer, M. J., *et al.* (1984). Test of the National Death Index. *American Journal of Epidemiology*, **119**, 837–9.

Stampfer, M. J., Willett, W. C., Colditz, G. A., Rosner, B., Speizer, F. E., and Hennekens, C. H. (1985). A prospective study of postmenopausal estrogen therapy and coronary heart disease. *New England Journal of Medicine*, **313**, 1044–9.

Stampfer, M. J., Willett, W. C., Colditz, G. A., Speizer, F. E., and Hennekens, C. H. (1988). A prospective study of past use of oral contraceptive agents and risks of cardiovascular diseases. *New England Journal of Medicine*, **319**, 1313–17.

US Centers for Disease Control (1987). Smoking-attributable mortality and years of potential life lost—the United States, 1984. *Morbidity and Mortality Weekly Report*, **36**, 693–7.

Willett, W. C., *et al.* (1983). Cigarette smoking, relative weight, and menopause. *American Journal of Epidemiology*, **117**, 651–8.

Willett, W. C., *et al.* (1985). Reproducibility and validity of a semiquantitative food frequency questionnaire. *American Journal of Epidemiology*, **122**, 51–65.

Willett, W. C., Stampfer, M. J., Colditz, G. A., Rosner, B., Hennekens, C. H., and Speizer, F. E. (1987a). Moderate alcohol consumption and risk of breast cancer. *New England Journal of Medicine*, **316**, 1174–80.

Willett, W. C., *et al.* (1987b). Relative and attributable risks of coronary heart disease among women who smoke cigarettes. *New England Journal of Medicine*, **317**, 1303–9.

3. Effects of cigarette smoking on 'hormone-related' diseases in a Southern California retirement community

Ronald K. Ross, Leslie Bernstein, Annlia Paganini-Hill, and Brian E. Henderson

Abstract

The associations of cigarette smoking with several sex-hormone related disorders were investigated in a cohort study conducted in a large retirement community near Los Angeles, California. Post-menopausal women who smoked cigarettes had a lowered risk of endometrial cancer, especially when smoking at the time of last menstrual period was considered. There was no relationship between smoking and breast cancer but smokers had an increased risk of hip fracture. In men the data suggested a weak link between smoking and prostatic hyperplasia requiring surgical treatment and cancer of the prostrate, although there was no consistent relationship with amount smoked or duration of smoking.

3.1. Introduction

It has been suggested that smoking produces an anti-oestrogenic effect and therefore would influence the incidence of oestrogen-related diseases, particularly breast and endometrial cancers, two diseases thought to be related to oestrogen excess, and osteoporotic fractures, a disease related to oestrogen deficiency (Baron 1984). In addition to effects on oestrogen secretion or metabolism, it appears that smoking may affect metabolism of other sex steroids, such as testosterone, and thereby may influence the incidence of diseases such as prostate cancer and benign prostatic hypertrophy.

For endometrial cancer, smokers have been shown consistently to be at lower risk relative to non-smokers, although only one study (Weiss *et al.* 1980) provides data that are statistically significant. In a recent literature review, Baron (1984) suggested that confounding by such factors as social class and obesity remain plausible explanations for the observed association, and that possible bias introduced by control selection strategies has not been addressed adequately in published studies.

The literature relating smoking to a reduced risk of breast cancer is less convincing. Of the 10 case-control studies recently reviewed by Baron (1984), five showed a small (less than 20 per cent) reduction in risk, but only two reached statistical significance (Paffenbarger *et al.* 1979; Vessey *et al.* 1983). The data derived from cohort studies provide the same inconsistent pattern and none have found a statistically significant reduction in risk among cigarette smokers.

Even for post-menopausal osteoporotic fractures, for which smoking is widely accepted as a risk factor (Lobo 1987), the available epidemiologic data are not highly convincing. Although three or four studies addressing this issue found evidence of a high risk among smokers, results were statistically significant only in one (Daniell 1976).

The exact relationship between smoking and development of any of these important diseases remains unclear. Insufficient data currently exist on dose–response relationships and on the effects of smoking cessation on risk. The interrelationships of smoking with other oestrogen-related risk factors, such as weight, age at menopause, and ovarian status, have not been adequately addressed for any of these diseases.

Several cross-sectional studies have found cigarette smoking to be associated with high circulating testosterone levels in middle-aged men (Dai *et al.* 1981; Deslypere and Vermeulen 1984) but it is unclear whether this is a causal relationship (Honda *et al.* 1988). In fact, some investigators have found no such relationship (Tsitouras *et al.* 1982), and others have found evidence for the opposite effect (Briggs 1973).

There is considerable evidence supporting a hormonal aetiology for benign prostatic hypertrophy and prostate cancer (Ross *et al.* 1983), involving particularly testosterone and its metabolite dihydrotestosterone.

Cigarette smoking has not been associated with prostate cancer in most previous epidemiologic studies. These have been primarily hospital-based case-control studies using controls who were not screened for diseases potentially associated with smoking (Wynder *et al.* 1971; Armenian *et al.* 1975). However, in a population-based case-control study in Los Angeles, cigarette smoking, in a duration-related fashion, was found to be a risk factor for prostate cancer in middle-aged men (Honda *et al.* 1988).

Since 1981, a cohort study of about 14 000 residents of a retirement community in Southern California has been underway. Although a cohort design is no more reliable in principle than a case-control design in evaluating the association between a familiar exposure, such as cigarette smoking, and disease outcomes following a long latency, such as the hormone-related diseases discussed above, the two methods clearly supplement one another and both can make valuable contributions to understanding the relationship between smoking and these hormone-related diseases. In addition to baseline data on smoking, including amount and duration smoked, and on potential confounding variables and risk modifiers, such as weight, age at menopause, and ovarian status, this elderly cohort provides substantial numbers of cases of each of these disease outcome.

3.2. Methods

The study population consisted of a large retirement community located about 50 miles south of Los Angeles, California. Leisure World, Laguna Hills, was established in 1964 and has grown to a comparatively stable population of about 20 000. The residents of Leisure World are almost entirely Caucasian and tend to be of the upper-middle socio-economic class. Women comprise about two-thirds of the population.

Using a complete roster of community residents provided by the community business office, a detailed health questionnaire was sent to all residents of the community in June 1981. New residents who moved into the community after this date were sent this survey in June 1982, June 1983, and October 1985. To encourage responses, newspaper advertisements describing the study were placed in the community newspaper at the time of each of the three mailings. Non-respondents were then telephoned (if a phone number was listed in the local directory) to elicit participation. A total of 13 987 (61 per cent) of the residents returned questionnaires; of these, 8881 respondents were women.

The health questionnaire requested basic demographic information as well as information on medical history, including previous cancer diagnoses and fractures; use of selected medications; personal habits, including use of cigarettes and alcohol; exercise habits; dietary intake of certain foods; height and weight; and, for women, a detailed menstrual and reproductive history. The cigarette smoking history included usual amount smoked, age began regular smoking, age stopped smoking if an ex-smoker, and, for women, whether regular smoking occurred during the peri-menopausal years.

Morbidity follow-up has been conducted by routine review of discharge summaries of the major hospitals serving the community. Over 85 per cent of inpatient care occurred at a single hospital adjacent to the community.

Deceased cohort members were identified by review of the files of the local county health department and the obituary column of the community newspaper. Death certificates were sought for all decedents to determine cause of death. Follow-up questionnaires were sent to the surviving cohort members in 1983 and 1985. In only 13 cohort members, for whom there was no evidence of death, was no postal address obtained. Record linkage with the files of the National Death Index did not identify any of these individuals.

Age-adjusted incidence rates were computed by direct standardization using an internal standard (i.e. the person-years distribution of the total cohort under study). Relative risks and 95 per cent confidence intervals (CI) were obtained with the use of a regression method that assumed that the occurrence of disease could be regarded as a Poisson process (implicit in the calculation of person-years at risk) with a constant hazard rate for a given person (Breslow *et al.* 1983). The Generalized Linear Interactive Modeling (GLIM) statistical software program was used to make these calculations (Royal Statistical Society 1978).

For the endometrial cancer analysis, women reporting a prior hysterectomy were excluded; for all the conditions considered below, persons reporting a previous history of that condition were excluded from that specific analysis (i.e. hip fractures for hip fracture analysis, breast cancer for breast cancer analysis, etc.). Among all female cohort members approximately 46 000 person-years of follow-up have been accumulated to date; about 28 000 of these have occurred among women with intact uteri. Follow-up among males totals about 24 000 person-years.

3.3. Results

As of mid-1988, 179 breast cancers and 304 hip fractures had occurred among female cohort members and 55 endometrial cancers among that subgroup with intact uteri. One hundred and thirty-eight incident prostate cancers and 381 hospitalizations for treatment of benign prostatic hypertrophy (BPH) were identified.

Endometrial cancer

As expected, the most important risk factor identified for endometrial cancer was use of oestrogen replacement therapy (ORT) (Paganini-Hill *et al.* 1989). Roughly half of all women in the cohort gave a history of use of oestrogen at some time post-menopausally; all but five of the 55 cases of endometrial cancer occurred among these women. The age-adjusted relative risk was 12 for oestrogen users compared to never users. The risk of endometrial cancer was strongly related to duration of use of oestrogen; the relative risk approached 20 for more than 8 years of ORT. Risk also increased with increasing age at last menstrual period; women whose menopause was at age 53 or later had a 50 per cent higher risk of endometrial cancer than women whose menopause was at age 45 or earlier. Weight was not a risk factor for endometrial cancer in this cohort, but very few women were in the upper extreme of weight in this community.

Women who had smoked cigarettes regularly at some time in their lives were at lower risk of endometrial cancer than women who had never smoked regularly (Table 3.1). Past smokers and current smokers had comparable risk [relative risk (RR) = 0.7] compared to lifetime non-smokers, but neither risk was statistically significant. A somewhat different picture emerges when exploring smoking habits at the time of the last menstrual period. Women smoking at that time had one-half the risk of endometrial cancer compared to lifetime non-smokers (RR = 0.5; 95 per cent CI = 0.3, 0.98), whereas there was no evidence of a reduced risk among women who had smoked during

Table 3.1. Cigarette smoking and risk of endometrial cancer in Leisure World

Risk factor	Person-years‡	Number of cases‡	Age-adjusted rate/1000	Age-adjusted relative risk
Smoking at last menstrual period				
Never	15734	34	2.3	1.0
Ex	3285	10	2.7	1.3
Current	9037	11	1.1	0.5†
Smoking at study entry				
Never	15734	34	2.3	1.0
Ex	8729	14	1.5	0.7
Current	3759	7	2.0	0.7
Number of cigarettes/day				
None	15734	34	2.3	1.0
1–10	6318	12	1.8	0.8
11–20	3604	8	2.0	0.9
21+	2149	1	0.3	0.2
Duration of smoking				
None*	15780	34	2.3	1.0
1–10 years	962	2	1.9	0.9
11–30 years	3657	5	1.1	0.6
31+ years	7316	13	1.8	0.7§

* Includes eight women who smoked for only a few months.
† 95% confidence interval excludes 1.0.
‡ Person-years do not always sum to 28222 or number of endometrial cancer cases to 55 due to exclusion of persons with missing information.
§ $P<0.05$, test for trend.

their premenstrual years but had stopped before menopause. All five cases of endometrial cancer occurring among women with no history of past ORT use occurred among lifetime non-smokers. There was no clear evidence of a dose–response relationship based on risk assessment by number of cigarettes smoked daily either at the time of study entry or at the time of menopause. Women whose lifetime average cigarette consumption was more than a pack-a-day were at very low risk (RR = 0.2) but this result was not statistically significant. There was some indication that risk decreased with increased duration of smoking (trend test, $P < 0.05$).

Based especially on smoking habits at menopause, 'current' smokers appeared to be at lower risk whether or not they were oestrogen users (Table 3.2). Dose information was available for women taking oestrogens, and, as used in Table 3.2, is the dose of conjugated oral oestrogens taken for the longest period. As predicted (Jensen *et al.* 1985), at any given dose of oestrogen replacement, smokers were at lower risk than non-smokers. At each category of age at menopause, smokers had lower risk of endometrial cancer than non-smokers. Thus it appears that the protective effect of smoking was not mediated by an early age at menopause. However, the number of cases in each category is very small and the confidence intervals around the risk estimates are correspondingly wide. Adjustment for age and weight at last menstrual period and dose and duration of oestrogen use did not substantially alter the risk of endometrial cancer in smokers.

Breast cancer

Most factors thought to be related to breast cancer risk in post-menopausal women were risk factors in this cohort. High weight was associated with some increased risk; weight at last menstrual period was more consistently associated with risk than weight at entry into the study. As with endometrial cancer, late menopause was significantly associated with increased risk ($P < 0.05$, test for trend), and women with artificial menopause were at reduced risk compared to women with spontaneous menopause (RR = 0.7). Alcohol consumption was not consistently related to risk, although women in the most extreme category of alcohol consumption (four or more alcoholic drinks per day) had a 60 per cent increased risk compared to abstainers.

This study provides no evidence that cigarette smokers have a reduced risk of breast cancer (Table 3.3). In fact, based on smoking habits at the time of menopause, risk of breast cancer in smokers was increased (RR = 1.3, $P = 0.06$). There was no clear evidence that risk of breast cancer was related to either amount or duration of smoking, although the highest risk was observed in those individuals smoking more than a pack-a-day. Cigarette smokers had a higher breast cancer risk than non-smokers within each age at menopause category.

The risk of breast cancer by smoking status at menopause adjusting for weight at last menstrual period, age at and type of menopause, lifetime

Table 3.2. Risk of endometrial cancer by smoking history stratified by and adjusted for selected risk factors

	Smoking status at last menstrual period					
	Never		Ex		Current	
	Number of cases	Age-adjusted relative risk	Number of cases	Age-adjusted relative risk	Number of cases	Age-adjusted relative risk
Weight at last menstrual period						
<55 kg	12	1.0	0	—	4	0.4
55–59	7	0.7	7	2.5	5	0.7
60+	14	0.9	3	0.8	2	0.2
Adjusted relative risk*		1.0		1.2		0.5†
Age at last menstrual period						
≤45	8	1.0	0	—	2	0.3
46–49	6	0.9	1	0.7	2	0.4
50–52	9	0.7	4	1.4	5	0.6
53+	10	1.0	5	1.6	2	0.4
Adjusted relative risk*		1.0		1.2		0.5

* Relative risk adjusted for variable above and age.
† 95% confidence intervals excludes 1.0, for these adjusted relative risks.

Table 3.2. (*cont.*) Risk of endometrial cancer by smoking history stratified by and adjusted for selected risk factors

	Smoking status at last menstrual period					
	Never		Ex		Current	
	Number of cases	Age-adjusted relative risk	Number of cases	Age-adjusted relative risk	Number of cases	Age-adjusted relative risk
Duration of oestrogen use †						
≤8 years	13	1.0	2	0.5	2	0.2
>8 years	16	2.2	8	3.8	9	1.5
Adjusted relative risk*		1.0		1.2		0.5‡
Dose of oral conjugated oestrogen†						
None	8	1.0	0	—	1	0.2
Low (≤0.625 mg)	12	6.7	5	9.8	5	4.0
High (>0.625 mg)	9	6.4	2	5.1	4	3.1
Adjusted relative risk*		1.0		0.9		0.5‡

* Relative risk adjusted for variable above and age.
† Analyses restricted to women who had ever used oestrogens.
‡ 95% confidence intervals excludes 1.0, for these adjusted relative risks.

Table 3.3. Cigarette smoking and risk of female breast cancer in Leisure World

Risk factor	Person-years†	Number of cases†	Age-adjusted rate/1000	Age-adjusted relative risk
Smoking at last menstrual period				
Never	25111	91	3.5	1.0
Ex	5263	24	4.7	1.4
Current	14681	64	4.5	1.3
Smoking at study entry				
Never	25111	91	3.5	1.0
Ex	14440	66	4.6	1.3
Current	5747	22	4.1	1.2
Number of cigarettes/day				
None	25111	91	3.5	1.0
1–10	10448	46	4.4	1.3
11–20	5696	21	3.6	1.1
21 +	3378	15	5.4	1.4
Duration of smoking				
None*	25211	91	3.5	1.0
1–10 years	1700	9	5.6	1.6
11–30 years	6237	26	4.2	1.2
31 + years	11367	47	4.2	1.3

* Includes 16 women who smoked only a few months.
† Person-years do not always sum to 45298 or number of breast cancer cases to 179 due to exclusion of persons with missing information.

oestrogen use, and amount of alcoholic beverages regularly consumed in addition to age was examined, and none of these factors substantially altered the age-adjusted risk estimates (Table 3.4).

Hip fracture

Clearly, women who smoke cigarettes are at increased risk of hip fracture (Table 3.5). Unlike the situation for breast cancer and endometrial cancer, smoking status at study entry was a better predictor of risk than smoking status at menopause. Women smoking at the time they completed the health survey had an 80 per cent higher risk of sustaining a hip fracture than women who were lifetime non-smokers (RR = 1.8, 95 per cent CI = 1.3, 2.5); past smokers had intermediate risk, about 20 per cent higher than never smokers. As with breast cancer and endometrial cancer, there was no consistent relationship between number of years or usual amount smoked and hip fracture risk.

Other hip fracture risk factors in this study included low weight at study entry, regular intake of large amounts of alcohol, no use or short duration use of ORT, and early menopause. After adjustment for these factors, the relative risk of hip fractures in current smokers was essentially unchanged. When the confounding effect of each of these variables was explored in bivariate analysis, smokers had a higher risk of fractures than non-smokers in nearly every category of alcohol use, oral oestrogen use, weight at entry, and age at menopause (Table 3.6).

Prostate cancer

Cigarette smokers had a slightly reduced risk of prostate cancer compared to lifetime non-smokers, although this reduction in risk was not statistically significant (Table 3.7). There was some evidence to suggest that risk decreased with increasing number of cigarettes regularly smoked. Men who smoked for more than 30 years had a significantly reduced risk of prostate cancer compared to lifetime non-smokers (RR = 0.6; 95 per cent CI = 0.4, 0.97), but risk in short duration smokers was actually significantly increased (RR = 2.2, 95 per cent CI = 1.2, 3.9). Additional adjustment for weight and exercise patterns had no major impact on these age-adjusted risk estimates, either for smoking in general or by dose and duration of smoking. Additional adjustment for alcohol consumption caused each of the unadjusted risk estimates to be reduced further, but the patterns of risk were essentially unchanged.

Benign prostatic hypertrophy

Smoking habits had little overall effect on risk of having surgical treatment for benign prostatic hypertrophy (BPH) (Table 3.8). The age-adjusted relative risk for current smokers was 0.8 and for past smokers was 1.1, compared to lifetime non-smokers. Diagnosis with BPH may be partially a function of

Table 3.4. Risk of female breast cancer by smoking history stratified by and adjusted for selected risk factors

	Smoking status at last menstrual period					
	Never		Ex		Current	
	Number of cases	Age-adjusted relative risk	Number of cases	Age-adjusted relative risk	Number of cases	Age-adjusted relative risk
Weight at last menstrual period						
<55 kg	18	1.0	8	2.3	19	1.6
55–60	19	1.3	8	2.4	23	2.6
61+	45	2.1	7	1.7	18	1.8
Adjusted relative risk †		1.0		1.4		1.3
Age at last menstrual period						
≤45	24	1.0	7	1.9	21	1.4
46–49	15	1.2	4	1.8	9	1.3
50–52	24	1.4	4	1.1	18	2.0
53+	22	1.7	9	2.6	15	2.7
Adjusted relative risk †		1.0		1.4		1.4

* Hyst, hysterectomy; BSO, bilateral salpingo-oophorectomy.
† Relative risk adjusted for variable above and age.

Table 3.4. (*cont.*) Risk of female breast cancer by smoking history stratified by and adjusted for selected risk factors

	Smoking status at last menstrual period					
	Never		Ex		Current	
	Number of cases	Age-adjusted relative risk	Number of cases	Age-adjusted relative risk	Number of cases	Age-adjusted relative risk
Oestrogen use						
Never	48	1.0	2	0.3	30	1.3
Ever	43	0.8	22	1.8	33	1.0
Adjusted relative risk †		1.0		1.4		1.3
Type of menopause*						
Natural	69	1.0	19	1.4	48	1.3
Hyst Only	9	0.6	2	0.8	9	1.1
Hyst + BSO	8	1.0	2	1.0	3	0.5
Adjusted relative risk †		1.0		1.4		1.3

* Hyst, hysterectomy; BSO, bilateral salpingo-oophorectomy.
† Relative risk adjusted for variable above and age.

Table 3.5. Cigarette smoking and risk of hip fractures in women in Leisure World

Risk factor	Person-years‡	Number of cases‡	Age-adjusted rate/1000	Age-adjusted relative risk
Smoking at last menstrual period				
Never	25611	187	6.1	1.0
Ex	5498	23	5.6	0.9
Current	15007	99	8.2	1.4†
Smoking at study entry				
Never	25611	187	6.1	1.0
Ex	14904	87	7.0	1.2
Current	5816	40	10.1	1.8†
Number of cigarettes/day				
None	25611	187	6.1	1.0
1–10	10685	59	6.4	1.1
11–20	5848	43	9.7	1.7†
21+	3492	19	7.3	1.6§
Duration of smoking				
None*	25706	189	6.1	1.0
1–10 years	1796	10	6.4	1.0
11–30 years	6424	32	6.7	1.0
31+ years	11599	75	7.9	1.4§

* Includes 16 women who smoked only for a few months.
† 95% confidence interval excludes 1.0.
‡ Person years do not always sum to 46331 or number of hip fracture patients to 309 due to exclusion of persons with missing information.
§ $P<0.03$, test for trend.

Table 3.6. Risk of hip fracture by smoking history stratified by and adjusted for selected risk factors

	Smoking status at entry					
	Never		Ex		Current	
	Number of cases	Age-adjusted relative risk	Number of cases	Age-adjusted relative risk	Number of cases	Age-adjusted relative risk
Weight at entry						
<55 kg	90	1.0	33	1.0	19	1.5
55–60	46	0.7	23	0.9	11	1.6
61+	50	0.5	30	0.7	10	0.9
Adjusted relative risk*		1.0		1.2		1.7†
Age at last menstrual period						
≤45	67	1.0	38	1.3	18	2.0
46–49	37	1.1	11	0.8	6	1.4
50–52	48	1.0	19	1.0	9	1.6
53+	25	0.7	17	1.1	6	1.8
Adjusted relative risk*		1.0		1.2		1.8†

* Relative risk adjusted for variable above and age.
† 95% confidence interval excludes 1.0, for these adjusted relative risks.

Table 3.6. (*cont.*) Risk of hip fracture by smoking history stratified by and adjusted for selected risk factors

	Smoking status at entry					
	Never		Ex		Current	
	Number of cases	Age-adjusted relative risk	Number of cases	Age-adjusted relative risk	Number of cases	Age-adjusted relative risk
Oestrogen use						
Never	98	1.0	42	1.1	17	2.0
Ever	85	0.9	45	1.3	23	1.5
Adjusted relative risk*		1.0		1.2		1.8†
Alcohol use						
None	64	1.0	16	1.3	6	1.9
≤1/day	74	1.1	32	1.2	11	1.4
2+/day	49	1.3	39	1.9	23	2.0
Adjusted relative risk*		1.0		1.1		1.7†

* Relative risk adjusted for variable above and age.
† 95% confidence interval excludes 1.0, for these adjusted relative risks.

Table 3.7. Cigarette smoking and risk of prostate cancer in Leisure World

Risk factor	Person-years‡	Number of cases‡	Age-adjusted rate/1000	Age-adjusted relative risk
Smoking status				
Never	8341	56	6.5	1.0
Ex	14056	73	5.1	0.8
Current	2010	9	5.4	0.9
Cigarettes/day				
None	8341	56	6.5	1.0
1–10	4601	30	5.9	0.9
11–20	5513	24	4.4	0.7
21+	5310	22	4.8	0.7
Duration smoked				
Never*	8364	56	6.4	1.0
1–10 years	1022	14	14.3	2.2†
11–30 years	5301	26	5.1	0.8
31+ years	9204	38	4.1	0.6†§

* Includes four men who smoked for only a few months.
† 95% confidence interval excludes 1.0.
‡ Person years do not always sum to 24407 or number of prostate cancer cases to 138 due to exclusion of persons with missing information.
§ $P<0.02$, test for trend.

Table 3.8. Cigarette smoking and risk of benign prostatic hypertrophy in Leisure World

Risk factor	Person-years †	Number of cases †	Age-adjusted rate/1000	Age-adjusted relative risk
Smoking status				
Never	8389	129	15.4	1.0
Ex	13884	227	16.3	1.1
Current	2017	25	14.6	0.8
Cigarettes/day				
None	8389	129	15.4	1.0
1–10	4552	71	15.5	1.0
11–20	5464	90	16.4	1.1
21 +	5281	72	14.1	0.9
Duration smoked				
Never*	8412	131	15.6	1.0
1–10 years	1028	21	20.7	1.3
11–30 years	5237	76	14.5	1.0
31 + years	9114	141	15.4	1.0

* Includes four men who smoked for only a few months.

† Person-years do not always sum to 24290 or number of benign prostatic hypertrophy patients to 381 due to exclusion of persons with missing information.

frequency of contact with the health care system. Although smokers reported visiting their doctor somewhat less frequently than non-smokers, when adjusted for differences in reported annual frequency of doctor visits, risk estimates were not substantially changed.

Other factors, such as weight and alcohol use, which might confound the association between smoking and risk of BPH because of their independent effects on circulatory testosterone levels (Gordon *et al.* 1976; Dai *et al.* 1981) were also not strong predictors of risk. Controlling for these factors had no effect on the age-adjusted risk estimates for smoking. There was no strong, consistent or statistically significant association between duration of smoking or usual amount smoked and risk of BPH.

3.4. Discussion

Consistent with results of numerous previous case-control studies (Williams and Horm 1977; Weiss *et al.* 1980; Kelsey *et al.* 1982; Lesko *et al.* 1985; Tyler *et al.* 1985; Baron *et al.* 1986b; Franks *et al.* 1987; Lawrence *et al.* 1987; Levi *et al.* 1987; Stockwell and Lyman 1987) this cohort study found a marked reduction in risk of developing endometrial cancer among cigarette smokers. Among residents of this elderly retirement community, the strongest association existed for smoking habits at the time of menopause rather than later in life. Smokers in this cohort tended to weigh less than non-smokers and to undergo menopause at an earlier age. Although both of these factors are themselves associated with a reduced risk of endometrial cancer (Weiss *et al.* 1980; Kelsey *et al.* 1982), and might therefore explain the protective effect observed for smoking in the cohort, smokers were at reduced risk in all weight and age at menopause categories and adjustment for these variables had no effect on the protective effect of smoking. Since smokers who use oral ORT achieve lower circulating levels of oestrogens than non-smokers (Jensen *et al.* 1985), one would expect that carcinogenicity of oral ORT would be attenuated by smoking, and this appeared to be the case in these data.

Case-control studies have not consistently found the reduction in risk of endometrial cancer in smokers to be related to dose or duration of smoking (Williams and Horm 1977; Weiss *et al.* 1980; Lesko *et al.* 1985; Baron *et al.* 1986b; Franks *et al.* 1987; Lawrence *et al.* 1987; Levi *et al.* 1987; Stockwell and Lyman 1987). The Leisure World data are also inconsistent, but compatible with a lower risk in long versus short duration smokers. In fact, the lowest risk observed among any of the subgroups studied was for smokers of more than one pack-a-day.

The mechanism for the beneficial effect of smoking on endometrial cancer risk has not yet been elucidated. There are few data on circulating oestrogen levels in post-menopausal smokers, but in Chapter 17 Barrett-Connor presents data suggesting that levels are not greatly different from those in non-smokers. Based on the relationship between circulating oestrogen levels and endometrial mitotic activity (Key and Pike 1988), such differences appear insufficient to 'explain' an approximately 50 per cent reduction in endometrial cancer risk in smokers. Michnovicz *et al.* (1986) have hypothesized that smokers have increased 2-hydroxylation of oestradiol to inactive metabolites compared to non-smokers. Jensen *et al.* (1985) have similarly proposed that smoking alters the metabolic clearance of oestradiol. The possible contribution of such a mechanism to endometrial cancer risk is unstudied.

Baron (1984), previously, and MacMahon (Chapter 15) have reviewed the epidemiologic evidence relating smoking to breast cancer risk. Overall these data provide no strong evidence that risk is reduced by cigarette smoking. In fact, the data from the Leisure World cohort study suggest that risk may be slightly increased. This observation is surprising and appears incompatible with the considerable epidemiologic and experimental evidence that oestrogens 'cause' breast cancer (Henderson *et al.* 1988), and the growing body of evidence that smoking is 'anti-oestrogenic'. However, as noted above, the exact mechanism for the anti-oestrogenic effect of smoking is unclear; there is no strong evidence that post-menopausal smokers have lower circulating oestrogen levels than non-smokers (Barrett-Connor, Chapter 17).

It may be noteworthy that cigarette smoking has potent acute stimulatory effects on the pituitary, causing marked increases in, among other hormones, circulating prolactin levels (Seyler *et al.* 1986). Prolactin is an important factor in the development of mammary tumours in rodents (Welsch and Meites 1978) and there is some evidence of a comparable role in man (Pike *et al.* 1979). However, despite these strong acute effects, the chronic impact of cigarette smoking may be to reduce slightly circulating prolactin (Baron *et al.* 1986a).

The study provides strong support for the growing evidence that smoking increases risk of post-menopausal osteoporotic fractures. The effects of smoking were not explained by the lower weight or earlier menopause of smokers or their higher prevalence of regular alcohol use. Post-menopausal smokers experience greater bone loss than non-smokers (Daniell 1976). Bone loss in the peri-menopausal period and beyond is strongly related to oestrogen deficiency and can be totally negated by ORT (Lindsay *et al.* 1976). It seems reasonable to conclude that the adverse effects of smoking on bone are mediated via oestrogen-related routes, but again the exact mechanism has yet to be elucidated.

The growth and development of the prostate is under the control of testosterone and its metabolite dihydrotestosterone (Ross *et al.* 1983). Experimental studies (Noble 1982) and epidemiologic studies comparing hormone levels in men with and without prostate cancer (Ghanadian *et al.* 1979; Drafta *et al.* 1982) and in high risk vs. low risk populations (Ross *et al.* 1986) provide some support for the hypothesis that these hormones are involved in the etiology of prostate cancer. The larger and better designed studies find higher testosterone levels in smokers compared to non-smokers (Dai *et al.* 1981; Deslypere and Vermeulen 1984) although these differences are not large and, based on data presented by Barrett-Connor (Chapter 17), are not dose-related.

A number of previous studies including three large well-designed cohort studies have reported on the relationship between prostate cancer and smoking. Doll and Peto (1976) followed 34 000 male British physicians for approximately 20 years and observed 186 deaths from prostate cancer; smokers had a 23 per cent reduction in risk which was not statistically significant. Hammond (1966), in the large American Cancer Society cohort study with 319 men who died of prostate cancer, found no alteration in risk among smokers. In the Dorn study of 250 000 military veterans followed for 16 years, there were 1020 prostate cancer deaths; smokers had a 31 per cent increase and ex-smokers an 18 per cent increase in risk of dying of prostate cancer compared to non-smokers (Rogot and Murray 1980). Most of the case-control studies have been hospital-based (Wynder *et al.* 1971; Armenian *et al.* 1975) and therefore difficult to interpret. Mandel (1981) examined smoking habits of prostate cancer cases and of both hospital and neighbourhood controls. The relative risks were 0.7 and 1.1 in smokers compared to non-smokers, respectively, supporting the idea that hospital controls might bias somewhat studies of this association. In a recent population-based case-control study conducted in Los Angeles males aged 60 or less, prostate cancer risk was found to be significantly related to smoking (RR = 1.9 for ever vs. never smoked regularly; 95 per cent CI = 1.2, 3.0) (Honda *et al.* 1988). There was a positive relationship between prostate cancer risk and smoking duration ($P = 0.001$, test for trend); men who had smoked at least 40 years had 2.6 times the risk of men who had never smoked.

Honda *et al.* (1988) hypothesized that socio-cultural determinants of smoking in the US might be age-related and that this might explain both an association between smoking and prostate cancer that is limited to young men and an association between smoking and testosterone level that is non-causal. In younger cohorts, in which the overall prevalence of cigarette smoking is low, regular use of cigarettes may be more closely linked with risk-taking tendencies and, perhaps, elevated testosterone levels.

As with prostate cancer, hormonal studies suggest a relationship between male steroid hormone levels, especially dihydrotestosterone, and risk of developing BPH (Bartsch *et al.* 1979; Drafta *et al.* 1982). Several studies have suggested a possible inverse association between cigarette smoking and surgically treated BPH. Most of these studies have been population-based case-control studies and have reported risk estimates for smokers compared to non-smokers between 0.4 and 0.7 (Greenwald *et al.* 1974; Armenian *et al.* 1975; Morrison 1978). While a small reduction in risk was observed, this result was statistically non-significant. Although the number of cases was large, the lower 95 per cent confidence limit on the risk estimate of BPH among smokers was still 0.55, so the results may not be totally incompatible with these previous studies.

Acknowledgement

Supported by Grants CA 17054 and CA 32197 of the National Institutes of Health, USA.

References

Armenian, H. K., Lilienfeld, A. M., Diamond, E. L., and Bross, I. D. J. (1975). Epidemiologic characteristics of patients with prostatic neoplasms. *American Journal of Epidemiology*, **102**, 47–54.

Baron, J. A. (1984). Smoking and estrogen-related disease. *American Journal of Epidemiology*, **119**, 9–22,

Baron, J. A., Bulbrook, E. R., Wang, D. Y., and Kwa, H. G. (1986a). Cigarette smoking and prolactin in women. *British Medical Journal*, **293**, 482–3.

Baron, J. A., Byers, T., Greenberg, E. R., Cummings, K. M., and Swanson, M. (1986b). Cigarette smoking in women with cancer of the breast and reproductive organs. *Journal of the National Cancer Institute*, **77**, 677–80.

Bartsch, W., Becker, H., Pinkenberg, F. A., and Krieg, M. (1979). Hormone blood levels and their inter-relationships in normal men and men with benign prostatic hyperplasia (BPH). *Acta Endocrinologica*, **90**, 727–37.

Breslow, N. E., Lubin, J. H., Marek, P., and Langholtz, B. (1983). Multiplicative models and cohort analysis. *Journal of the American Statistical Association*, **78**, 1–12.

Briggs, M. H. (1973). Cigarette smoking and infertility. *Medical Journal of Australia*, **1**, 616–7.

Dai, W. S., Kuller, L. H., LaPorte, R. E., Gutai, J. P., Falvo-Gerad, L., and Caggiula, A. (1981). The epidemiology of plasma testosterone levels in middle-aged men. *American Journal of Epidemiology*, **114**, 804–16.

Daniell, H. W. (1976). Osteoporosis of the slender smoker. *Archives of Internal Medicine*, **136**, 298–304.

Deslypere, J. P. and Vermeulen, A. (1984). Leydig cell function in normal men: Effect of age, lifestyle, residence, diet, and activity. *Journal of Clinical Endocrinology and Metabolism*, **59**, 955–62.

Doll, R. and Peto, R. (1976). Mortality in relation to smoking: 20 year's observations on male British doctors. *British Medical Journal*, **2**, 1525–36.

Drafta, D., Proca, E., Zamfir, V., Schindler, A. E., Neacsu, E., and Stroe, E. (1982). Plasma steroids in benign prostatic hypertrophy and carcinoma of the prostate. *Journal of Steroid Biochemistry*, **17**, 689–93.

Franks, A. L., *et al.* (1987). Postmenopausal smoking, estrogen replacement therapy, and the risk of endometrial cancer. *American Journal of Obstetrics and Gynecology*, **156**, 20–3.

Ghanadian, R., Puah, C. M., and O'Donoghue, E. P. (1979). Serum testosterone and dihydrotestosterone in carcinoma of the prostate. *British Journal of Cancer*, 39, 696–9.

Gordon, G. G., Altman, K., Southern, A. L., Rubin, E., and Lieber, C. S. (1976). Effect of alcohol (ethanol) administration on sex-hormone metabolism in normal men. *New England Journal of Medicine*, 295, 793–7.

Greenwald, P., Kirmss, V., Polan, A. K., and Dick, V. S. (1974). Cancer of the prostate among men with benign prostatic hyperplasia. *Journal of the National Cancer Institute*, 53, 335–40.

Hammond, E. C. (1966). Smoking in relation to the death rates of one million men and women. *National Cancer Institute Monograph*, 19, 127–204.

Henderson, B. E., Ross, R. K., and Bernstein, L. (1988). Estrogens as a cause of human cancer: The Richard and Hinda Rosenthal Foundation Award Lecture. *Cancer Research*, 48, 246–53.

Honda, G. D., Bernstein, L., Ross, R. K., Greenland, S., and Henderson, B. E. (1988). Vasectomy, cigarette smoking, and age at first sexual intercourse as risk factors for prostate cancer in middle-aged men. *British Journal of Cancer*, 57, 326–31.

Jensen, J., Christiansen, C., and Rodbro, P. (1985). Cigarette smoking, serum estrogens, and bone loss during hormone-replacement therapy early after menopause. *New England Journal of Medicine*, 313, 973–5.

Kelsey, J. L., *et al.* (1982). A case-control study of cancer of the endometrium. *American Journal of Epidemiology*, 116, 333–42.

Key, T. J. A. and Pike, M. C. (1988). The dose-effect relationship between unopposed oestrogens and endometrial mitotic rate: Its central role in explaining and predicting endometrial cancer risk. *British Journal of Cancer*, 57, 205–12.

Lawrence, C., *et al.* (1987). Smoking, body weight, and early-stage endometrial cancer. *Cancer*, 59, 1665–9.

Lesko, S. M., *et al.* (1985). Cigarette smoking and the risk of endometrial cancer. *New England Journal of Medicine*, 313, 593–6.

Levi, F., LaVecchia, C., and Decarli, A. (1987). Cigarette smoking and the risk of endometrial cancer. *European Journal of Cancer and Clinical Oncology*, 23, 1025–9.

Lindsay, R., Hart, D. M., Aitken, J. M., MacDonald, E. B., Anderson, J. B., and Clarke, A. C. (1976). Long-term prevention of postmenopausal osteoporosis by oestrogens. *Lancet*, i, 1038–41.

Lobo, R. A. (1987). Prevention of postmenopausal osteoporosis. In *Menopause* (ed D. R. Mishell), p. 165. Yearbook Medical Publishers, Chicago.

Mandel, J. S. (1981). Epidemiologic study of etiology factors in prostatic cancer. Dissertation. University of Minnesota.

Michnovicz, J. J., Hershcopf, R. J., Naganuma, H., Bradlow, H. L., and Fishman, J. (1986). Increased 2-hydroxylation of estradiol as a possible mechanism for the anti-estrogenic effect of cigarette smoking. *New England Journal of Medicine*, 815, 1305–9.

Morrison, A. S. (1978). Prostatic hypertrophy in greater Boston. *Journal of Chronic Diseases*, 31, 357–62.

Noble, R. L. (1982). Prostate carcinoma of the Nb rat in relation to hormones. *International Review of Experimental Pathology*, 23, 113–57.

Paffenbarger, R. S., Kampert, J. B., and Chang, H. G. (1979). Oral contraceptives and breast cancer risk. *Institut National de La Sante Et de La Recherche Medicale*, **83**, 93–114.

Paganini-Hill, A., Ross, R. K., and Henderson, B. E. (1989). Endometrial cancer and patterns of use of estrogen replacement therapy: A cohort study. *British Journal of Cancer*, **59**, 445–7.

Pike, M. C., Gerkins, V. R., Casagrande, J. T., Gray, G. E., Brown, J., and Henderson, B. E. (1979). The hormonal basis of breast cancer. *National Cancer Institute Monograph*, **53**, 187–94.

Rogot, E. M. and Murray, J. L. (1980). Smoking and causes of death among US veterans: 16 years of observation. *Public Health Reports*, **95**, 213–22.

Ross, R. K., Paganini-Hill, A., Henderson, B. E. (1983). Etiology of prostate cancer: What does the epidemiology suggest? *Prostate*, **4**, 333–44.

Ross, R. K., Bernstein, L., Judd, H., Hanisch, R., Pike, M. C., and Henderson, B. E. (1986). Serum testosterone levels in healthy young black and white men. *Journal of the National Cancer Institute*, **76**, 45–8.

Royal Statistical Society (1978). *Generalized linear interactive modeling. The GLIM system, Release 3.* Numerical Algorithm Group, Oxford.

Seyler, L. E., Pomerleau, O. F., Fertig, J. B., Hunt, D., and Parker, K. (1986). Pituitary hormone response to cigarette smoking. *Pharmacology Biochemistry Behavior*, **24**, 159–62.

Stockwell, H. G. and Lyman, G. H. (1987). Cigarette smoking and the risk of female reproductive cancer. *American Journal of Obstetrics and Gynecology*, **157**, 35–40.

Tsitouras, P. D., Martin, C. E., and Harman, S. M. (1982). Relationship of serum testosterone to sexual activity in healthy elderly men. *Journal of Gerontology*, **37**, 288–93.

Tyler, C. W., Webster, L. A., Ory, H. W., and Rubin, G. L. (1985). Endometrial cancer: How does cigarette smoking influence the risk of women under age 55 years having this tumor? *American Journal of Obstetrics and Gynecology*, **151**, 899–905.

Vessey, M., Baron, J., Doll, R., McPherson, K., and Yeates, D. (1983). Oral contraceptives and breast cancer. Final report of an epidemiological study. *British Journal of Cancer*, **47**, 455–62.

Weiss, N. S., Farewell, V. T., Szekely, D. R., English, D. R., and Kiviat, N. (1980). Oestrogens and endometrial cancer: effect of other risk factors on the association. *Maturitas*, **2**, 185–90.

Welsch, C. W. and Mietes, J. (1978). Prolactin and mammary carcinogenesis. In *Endocrine control in neoplasia* (ed. R. Sharma and W. Criss), pp. 71–92. Raven Press, New York.

Williams, R. R. and Horm, J. W. (1977). Association of cancer sites with tobacco and alcohol consumption and socioeconomic status of patients. Interview study from the Third National Cancer Survey. *Journal of the National Cancer Institute*, **58**, 525–47.

Wynder, E. L., Mabuchi, K., and Whitmore, W. F. (1971). Epidemiology of cancer of the prostate. *Cancer*, **28**, 344–60.

II

Smoking, the Menopause, and Benign Reproductive Disorders

4. Cigarette smoking and age at natural menopause

John A. Baron

Abstract

Women who smoke cigarettes have consistently been found to have a natural menopause at an earlier age than women who do not smoke. Expressed as a difference of median menopausal ages, currently smoking women have a menopause one to two years earlier than never smokers. Expressed as prevalence odds ratios, currently smoking women have a relative risk of 1.6 to 2.0 of being menopausal. Ex-smokers appear to have only a small excess risk of menopause, suggesting that the effect of smoking is reversible. Possible mechanisms for these associations include direct toxic effects on the ovaries, interference in gonadotropin release, and alteration in metabolism of sex steroids.

4.1. Introduction

The association between cigarette smoking and an early natural menopause was one of the first recognized indications that smoking might affect events related to sex hormones in women. This relationship, which was apparently first noticed by Jick and Porter (1977), may have relevance for other topics considered in these proceedings. An early menopause, by hastening the onset of the relatively oestrogen-deficient post-menopausal state, may alter the risk of oestrogen-related processes in post-menopausal women.

Published studies of the association between smoking and age of natural menopause have tended *not* to report relative risks as is common in most epidemiological investigations. Instead, comparison of the mean or median age of menopause in smokers and non-smokers has typically been used. In populations containing both pre-menopausal and post-menopausal women, use of the mean age at menopause is subject to follow-up fallacies (Colton 1974), and studies employing this technique on such populations have not been included in this survey. Comparison of median menopausal ages may also not be the analysis of choice.

The effect measure is not on a familiar scale such as relative risk, and investigation of variation in the strength of the effect with age is impossible.

Table 4.1. Cigarette smoking and age at natural menopause

Study	Source and number of subjects studied	Covariates considered	Difference in median menopausal ages* (years)
Jick and Porter (1977)	2143 hospital patients	Parity, marital status, coffee/tea/alcohol, hospital service, diagnosis	1.7 †
	1391 hospital patients	As above	1.3 †
Bailey *et al.* (1977)	475 health screenees	None	1.3 †
McNamara *et al.* (1978)	1553 general population subjects	None	0.8 ‡
Lindquist & Bengtsson (1979)	873 general population subjects	Weight	1.2 †
Kaufman *et al.* (1980)	656 hospital patients	Parity, ponderal index, age first smoked, geographic region	1.7 ‡
Adena and Gallagher (1982)	10 995 health screenees	Weight, alcohol intake drug taking	1.0
Willett *et al.* (1983)	66 663 nurses	Height, weight, diabetes, hypertension, age of menarche, nulliparity	1.4
McKinlay *et al.* (1985)	5350 general population subjects	None	1.7
Everson *et al.* (1986)	261 population subjects	Passive smoking	1.1
Hiatt and Fireman (1986)	5346 HMO health screenees	None	0.95 †
Stanford *et al.* (1987)	1472 breast cancer screenees	None	0.3

* Median menopausal age in non-smokers minus median menopausal age in smokers.
† Computed by Adena and Gallagher (1982).
‡ Difference of mean menopausal ages.

Moreover, consideration of covariates is difficult without strong parametric assumptions about the relationship between age, smoking, the covariates, and age of menopause. A traditional epidemiological analysis can avoid many of these problems, and will be included here.

The censoring effect of surgical menopause has been dealt with in each of the published reports through the exclusion of women with an operative menopause. Underlying this practice is the assumption that were the ages of natural menopause among women who had hysterectomy actually observed, they would have followed the same pattern as that of the women who did not have an operative menopause. There are no data to confirm (or refute) this assumption, but a competing risk analysis suggests that censoring women with an operative menopause probably does not distort results very much (Krailo and Pike 1983).

4.2. Epidemiological summary

The available data regarding cigarette smoking and age at natural menopause are summarized in Table 4.1. All studies except one reported that women currently smoking cigarettes had a menopause between one and two years earlier than non-smokers, though studies of hospitalized patients tended to show larger differences than those based on well subjects. Indications of a trend of an earlier menopause with increasing amounts smoked was found in most studies that presented data relevant to that issue, although often this was not formally tested (Jick and Porter 1977; McNamara *et al.* 1978; Lindquist and Bengtsson 1979; Kaufman *et al.* 1980; Adena and Gallagher 1982; Andersen *et al.* 1982; Willett *et al.* 1983; Hiatt and Fireman 1986). Two studies that did not report median ages of menopause also noted a tendency for smoking women to have an early natural menopause (Andersen *et al.* 1982; Kato *et al.* 1988).

Although relative risks were presented in only one study, sufficient data are presented in several others to permit these to be computed (Table 4.2). The relative risks (odds ratios) vary with age and amount smoked from just over 1.0 to 3.0 or more, typically in the range of 1.5 to 2.0. These exhibit no consistent pattern with increasing age: Willett *et al.* (1983) reported decreasing odds ratios, in the data reported by Jick and Porter (1977) there were increasing odds ratios, and in other studies there was no particular pattern.

Several of the studies controlled for potential confounding variables. Because of the associations of nulliparity and low body weight with an early natural menopause, parity and body habitus are probably the most important to consider, though a low body weight could be part of a mechanism by which smoking causes menopause to occur sooner. However, control for these (or other) covariates did not seem to alter greatly the magnitude of the smoking/menopause association.

Table 4.2. Cigarette smoking and age at natural menopause: odds ratio analysis

Study	Number of subjects	Evidence for heterogeneity*	Summary odds ratio†
Jick and Porter (1977)	1842	MAYBE ($P=0.10$) trend of increasing ORs with age	2.1 (1.7–2.6)
	1253	NO ($P=0.76$)	1.8 (1.4–2.3)
Bailey *et al.* (1977)	733	NO ($P=0.95$)	2.0 (1.2–3.3)
Lindquist and Bengtsson (1979)	873	MAYBE ($P=0.07$) no particular trend with age	2.1 (1.4–3.0)
Adena and Gallagher (1982)	2983	NO ($P=0.51$)	1.7 (1.4–2.1)
Andersen *et al.* (1982)	11 809	NO ($P=0.36$)	1.6 (1.4–1.8)
Willett *et al.* (1983)	66 663	YES (?) trend of decreasing ORs with age	Not reported; age-specific ORs 1.9, 2.2, 1.5, 1.2

* Over age groups, using Breslow-Day x^2.
† Mantel-Haenszel summary odds ratio, with age strata as defined in the data available.

The menopause risks of women who have stopped smoking cigarettes have been described in several investigations (Jick and Porter 1977; Lindquist and Bengtsson 1979; Kaufman *et al.* 1980; Adena and Gallagher 1982; Willett *et al.* 1983; Hiatt and Fireman 1986). In general, the risks for ex-smokers have been found to be intermediate between those of light smokers and never smokers (Table 4.3). Only Willett *et al.* (1983) considered the effect of time since last smoked. Those who ceased smoking in the two years previously retained a somewhat elevated risk of menopause (OR = 1.4). Beyond that, there was no measurable impact of previous smoking.

4.3. Discussion

With the exception of one study (Stanford *et al.* 1987), the data are quite consistent in showing currently smoking women to have an earlier age at natural menopause than never smoking women. Expressed as a difference in median age of menopause, current smokers have a menopause which is one

Table 4.3. Age of natural menopause in former smokers

Study	Number of ex-smokers	Covariates considered	
Jick and Porter (1977)	439	None	Ex-smokers had median menopausal age between current light smokers and never smokers
Lindquist and Bengtsson (1979)	30	None	Odds ratio of being menopausal for ex-smokers vs. never smokers was 1.8
Kaufman *et al.* (1980)	10	Parity, region Quetelet's Index	Mean age at menopause was 0.2 years earlier in ex-smokers than in never smokers
Adena and Gallagher (1982)	Not reported	None	In 2 populations, median age at menopause was 0.3 and 0.4 years earlier in ex-smokers than in never smokers
Willett *et al.* (1983)	16 034	Age, weight nulliparity	Odds ratio of being menopausal for current smokers vs. never smokers was 1.10
Hiatt and Fireman (1986)	576	None	Mean age at menopause 0.5 years earlier in ex-smokers than in never smokers

to two years earlier than never smokers. Expressed as a prevalence odds ratio, smokers have a relative risk of 1.6 to 2.0 of being menopausal. The consistency of the results, the presence of dose–response trends, and the persistence of the effect after control for covariates suggests that the relationship is causal.

Ex-smokers appear to have a menopause risk close to that of never smokers, though there are inconsistent indications of a modest residual effect. This could be due to misclassification of some current smokers as 'ex' smokers, or could reflect an effect of smoking that persists for a period of time. In the data presented by Willett *et al.* (1983), any association of ex-smoking with an early menopause was confined to the first two years (at most) after cessation of smoking. Thus, in aggregate, the data suggest that the effect of cigarette smoking on menopause is reversible. Unfortunately there are no published data regarding the menopause risks of ex-smokers categorized by lifetime history of smoking. If the ex-smokers studied had little cumulative lifetime exposure, then the analysis really cannot say much meaningful either way.

Three basic explanations for how smoking might advance the age of natural menopause have been proposed. First, there is evidence that polycyclic aromatic hydrocarbons of the sort found in cigarette smoke are directly toxic to ovarian follicles (Mattison and Thorgeirsson 1978). Indeed, early uncontrolled studies in rodents showed that cigarette smoke exposure is associated with ovarian atresia (Essenberg *et al.* 1951). This mechanism would seem to cause a permanent alteration in the risk of menopause, in contrast to the epidemiological results which suggest a reversible process, as discussed above. Secondly it is clear that, at least in rodents, cigarette smoking or nicotine can affect the secretion of pituitary hormones including luteinizing hormone, which has an important role in the regulation of the menstrual cycle (Blake *et al.* 1972; McLean *et al.* 1977; Eneroth *et al.* 1977). It is possible that an interference in the pituitary–ovarian axis might contribute to the association of cigarette smoking with an early menopause. This would certainly be more reversible than a direct toxic effect on ovarian follicles. Finally, as discussed elsewhere in this symposium, cigarette smoking may well affect the metabolism of sex hormones, and these effects could contribute to an early cessation of menses.

References

Adena, M. A. and Gallagher, H. G. (1982). Cigarette smoking and the age at menopause. *Annals of Human Biology*, 9, 121–30.

Andersen, F. S., Transbol, I., and Christiansen, C. (1982). Is cigarette smoking a promotor of the menopause? *Acta Medica Scandinavica*, **212**, 137–9.

Bailey, A., Robinson, D., and Vessey, M. (1977). Smoking and age of natural menopause. *Lancet*, ii, 722.

Blake, C. A., *et al.* (1972). Nicotine delays the ovulatory surge of luteinizing hormone in the rat. *Proceedings of the Society for Experimental Biology and Medicine*, 141, 1014–16.

Colton, T. (1974). *Statistics in medicine*, pp. 299–301. Little, Brown, Boston.

Eneroth, P., *et al.* (1977). The effect of nicotine on central catecholamine neurons and gonadotropin secretion. II. Inhibitory influence of nicotine on LH, FSH, and prolactin secretion in the ovariectomized female rat and its relation to regional changes in dopamine and noradrenaline levels and turnover. *Medicine and Biology*, 55, 158–66.

Essenberg, J. M., Fagan, L., and Malerstein, A. J. (1951). Chronic poisoning of the ovaries and testes of albino rats and mice by nicotine and cigarette smoke. *Western Journal of Surgery Obstetrics and Gynecology*, 59, 27–32.

Everson, R. B., Sandler, D. P., Wilcox, A. J., Schreinemachers, D., Shore, D. L., and Weinberg, C. (1986). Effect of passive exposure to smoking on age at natural menopause. *British Medical Journal*, **293**, 792.

Hiatt, R. A. and Fireman, B. H. (1986). Smoking, menopause and breast cancer. *Journal of the National Cancer Institute*, 76, 833–8.

Jick, H. and Porter, J. (1977). *Lancet*, **i**, 1354–5.

Kato, I., Tominaga, S., and Suzuki, T. (1988). Factors related to late menopause and early menarche as risk factors for breast cancer. *Japanese Journal of Cancer Research*, 79, 165–72.

Kaufman, D. W., Slone, D., Rosenberg, L., Mietteninen, O. S., and Shapiro, S. (1980). Cigarette smoking and age at natural menopause. *American Journal of Public Health*, **70**, 420–2.

Krailo, M. D. and Pike, M. C. (1983). Estimation of the distribution of age at natural menopause from prevalence data. *American Journal of Epidemiology*, 117, 356–61.

Lindquist, O. and Bengtsson, C. (1979). Menopausal age in relation to smoking. *Acta Medica Scandinavica*, **205**, 73–7.

McKinlay, S. M., Bifano, N. L., and McKinlay, J. B. (1985). Smoking and age at menopause in women. *Annals of Internal Medicine*, **103**, 350–6.

McLean, B. K., Rubel, A., and Nikitovitch-Winer, M. B. (1977). The differential effects of exposure to tobacco smoke on the secretion of luteinizing hormone and prolactin in the proestrous rat. *Endocrinology*, **100**, 1566–70.

McNamara, P. M., Hjortland, M. C., Gordon, T., and Kannel, W. B. (1978). Natural history of menopause: the Framingham Study. *Journal of Continuing Education in Obstetrics and Gynecology*, **20**, 27–35.

Mattison, D. R. and Thorgeirsson, S. S. (1978). Smoking and industrial pollution, and their effects on menopause and ovarian cancer. *Lancet*, **i**, 187–8.

Stanford, J. L., Hartge, P., Brinton, L. A., Hoover, R. N., and Brookmeyer, R. (1987). Factors influencing the age at natural menopause. *Journal of Chronic Diseases*, **40**, 995–1002.

Willett, W. *et al.* (1983). Cigarette smoking, relative weight and menopause. *American Journal of Epidemiology*, 117, 651–8.

5. Hyperemesis gravidarum, uterine fibroids, and endometriosis: effects of cigarette smoking on risk

Ronald K. Ross, Leslie Bernstein, Martin P. Vessey, and Brian E. Henderson

Abstract

Vomiting of pregnancy, uterine fibroids, and endometriosis are relatively common problems of pre-menopausal women that are thought to be oestrogen-related. Although the available evidence regarding the relationship of these conditions to cigarette smoking is not extensive, there are indications that women who smoke have a lowered risk of each of these, consistent with an 'anti-oestrogenic' effect.

5.1. Introduction

There is substantial evidence that smoking produces an 'anti-oestrogen' effect (Baron 1984). This important consequence of smoking appears to be the end result of a number of metabolic pathways: altered hepatic metabolism of endogenously-derived oestrogens (Michnovicz *et al.* 1986), early ovarian failure (Willett *et al.* 1983), reduced circulating levels of orally ingested exogenous oestrogens (Jensen *et al.* 1985), and, possibly, reduced ovarian oestrogen production (MacMahon *et al.* 1982). The anti-oestrogenic effect of smoking has led to a series of reports on the association of cigarette smoking with diseases caused by oestrogen deficiency or oestrogen excess. These reports have focused particularly on diseases which are major causes of mortality in post-menopausal women, such as hip fracture, endometrial cancer, and breast cancer (Baron 1984). This chapter summarizes the available data on the relationship of cigarette-smoking with three other diseases in women thought to have a hormonal aetiology: hyperemesis gravidarum (Depue *et al.* 1987), uterine fibroids (Ross *et al.* 1986), and endometriosis (Dizerega *et al.* 1980). While none of these diseases are associated with significant mortality, all are important sources of morbidity and hospitalization in pre-menopausal women.

5.2. Hyperemesis gravidarum

To identify factors that are related to hyperemesis gravidarum, a case-control study was conducted using data obtained prospectively during pregnancy (Depue *et al.* 1987). The data were obtained from the Collaborative Perinatal Project of the National Institute of Neurological and Communicative Disorders and Stroke. This large prospective study was conducted between 1958 and 1965 and included the collection of medical histories and serum samples from 55 000 pregnancies registered at 12 university-affiliated medical centres in the United States. The study focused especially on oestrogen-related factors, such as body weight and parity, as well as on smoking habits. Hyperemesis is defined as a condition of pregnant women with vomiting severe enough to cause weight loss, dehydration or acidosis, but the Perinatal Project did not set rigorous diagnostic criteria, which could therefore be expected to vary between centres. To address these possible differences in diagnostic criteria between centres and over time, control subjects were matched to patients with hyperemesis by participating centre and date of registration. Controls, like cases, were white and in the same lunar month of pregnancy as the patient at registration. Four-hundred and seventeen white women with hyperemesis were each matched with two control women who reported no vomiting during the index pregnancy. Relative risks (RR) were calculated by conditional logistic regression for matched case-control studies.

Forty-one per cent of cases vs. 54 per cent of controls were cigarette smokers at the time of registration into the study. Current smokers had a 40 per cent reduction in risk of hyperemesis gravidarum compared to non-smokers ($P<0.0001$) (Table 5.1). Other factors studied supported the hypothesis that hyperemesis gravidarum is caused by elevated oestrogen levels.

Table 5.1. 'Oestrogen related' risk factors for hyperemesis gravidarum

Factor	Number of cases/ number of controls	Relative risk	*P*
Cigarette smoker			
No	242/381	1.0	
Yes	170/448	0.6	<0.0001
Parity			
Parous	263/602	1.0	
Nulliparous	156/234	1.6	0.0007
Quetelet's Index (kg/m^2)			
<24	259/571	1.0	
≥24	106/162	1.5	0.006

Nulliparous women were at high risk (RR = 1.6, $P = 0.0007$); Bernstein *et al.* (1985) have demonstrated previously that nulliparous women have higher circulating and urinary oestrogen levels than parous women and that women in their first pregnancies have higher first trimester oestrogen levels than in subsequent pregnancies (Bernstein *et al.* 1986). Another maternal risk factor for hyperemesis was high body weight. Women with a Quetelet's index greater than 24kg/m^2 had a 50 per cent increase in risk ($P = 0.006$). Increased weight is associated with increased circulating oestrogen levels and with reduced levels of sex-hormone binding globulin and, thus, presumably with increased levels of bioavailable oestradiol (Siiteri *et al.* 1981).

Furthermore, in a subset of women with hyperemesis and their matched controls the serum levels of oestradiol and of non-protein bound oestradiol were found to be significantly higher in the women with vomiting (Table 5.2); and women who smoke during pregnancy have a reduction in circulating oestrogen levels that is dependent on the number of cigarettes smoked (Bernstein *et al.* 1989). Based on these observations, it seems reasonable to conclude that the reduction in risk of hyperemesis associated with cigarette smoking is mediated by an anti-oestrogenic mechanism.

Other researchers have also found that women who vomit in pregnancy are less likely to smoke. Klebanoff (1985) used the data from the Collaborative Perinatal Project to study the epidemiology of vomiting in early pregnancy (in the absence of hyperemesis) and found that smokers had a 30 per cent reduction in risk after adjustment for age, race, educational level, pre-pregnancy weight, pregnancy outcome, and previous pregnancies. Weigel and Weigel (1988) evaluated cigarette smoking as a part of a study on the role of maternal risk factors in the development of nausea and vomiting in pregnancy, using an historical cohort of 825 women who gave birth at the University of California, Los Angeles Medical Center during a one year period. Heavy cigarette smoking (more than a pack-a-day) was associated with an approximately one-third reduction in risk of nausea with or without vomiting, but neither reduction was statistically significant. However, in a multivariate analysis including age, ethnicity, occupation, reproductive history, and alcohol use, the reduction in risk associated with cigarette

Table 5.2. Geometric mean hormone levels in women with hyperemesis gravidarum and controls

Hormone	Cases ($n = 35$)	Controls ($n = 35$)	P
Oestradiol			
Total (ng/dl)	179	142	0.05
Non-protein bound (ng/dl)	1.5	1.2	0.05
SHBG-binding capacity (gm/dl)	7.5	5.5	0.03

Table 5.3. Studies of smoking as a risk factor for vomiting in pregnancy

Author	Year	Number with vomiting	Percentage smokers	RR
Little and Hook	1979	150	21	0.3 ($P<0.01$)
Klebanoff *et al.*	1985	5095	34	0.7 ($P<0.001$)
Depue *et al.*	1987	417*	41	0.6 ($P<0.0001$)
Weigel and Weigel	1988	390	7†	0.9 (NS)

* Hyperemesis gravidarum.
† Defined as 1+ packs-per-day.

smoking was substantially attenuated (RR = 0.9). Finally, Little and Hook (1979) reported on risk factors for nausea and vomiting during pregnancy in 210 members of a health maintenance organization on the west coast of the United States. Based on pre-pregnancy smoking habits, 31 of 150 women with nausea and vomiting of pregnancy were smokers vs. 26 of 60 women with no nausea and vomiting (RR = 0.3, $P<0.01$). The various studies which have evaluated smoking as a risk factor for nausea and vomiting in pregnancy are summarized in Table 5.3. No data were found on risk by amount smoked. The reduced risk of vomiting in pregnancy among smokers appears to be pre-existing and not a response to either the pregnancy or the vomiting. A less easily verifiable but plausible alternative explanation for the observed association is that women with a low threshold for nausea and vomiting never become regular cigarette smokers.

5.3. Fibroids

Uterine leiomyomas are the most common pelvic neoplasm and may be the most common of all female tumours (Novak and Woodruff 1979). They are benign tumours of smooth muscle but in common usage have become known as fibroids. They are most commonly diagnosed during reproductive life, usually in the fourth to fifth decade, and they tend to shrink or fibrose after the menopause.

Risk factors for fibroids were studied recently using data from the Oxford Family Planning Association Cohort Study (Ross *et al.* 1986). Evidence that fibroids share risk factors with endometrial cancer led to the conclusion that fibroids, like endometrial cancer, are caused by 'unopposed' oestrogen. Consistent with this hypothesis, and also with epidemiologic studies of endometrial cancer, cigarette smoking was associated with a substantial reduction in risk.

The Oxford Family Planning Association study is a long-term follow-up study of married white women using various methods of contraception.

Between 1968 and 1974, 17 032 women were recruited at 17 Family Planning Clinics in England and Scotland. At the time of recruitment, all women were aged 25–39 and were either using oral contraceptives and had done so for at least 5 months, or were using the diaphragm or an IUD (and had done so for at least 5 months) without previous use of oral contraceptives. All women have been subsequently contacted at least annually with an annual loss to follow-up averaging 0.3 per cent. As of July 1985, 538 women in the cohort had had a pathologically confirmed fibroid during follow-up. For each of these women, an individual control was selected matched on date of entry into the study, age at entry, and clinic. The controls had to have an intact uterus and had to have been followed to the date of surgical diagnosis of the case. Relative risks were calculated by multivariate logistic regression for individually matched studies.

The major risk factors identified by this study were number of term pregnancies and weight. Women with five term pregnancies had only one-quarter the risk of women who had none and risk decreased consistently with increasing number of pregnancies. Risk increased consistently with increasing weight, which was a slightly better predictor of risk than Quetelet's index or other measures of obesity; risk of fibroids increased about 21 per cent for each 10 kg increment in weight. Both oral contraceptive use and cigarette smoking reduced risk. There was about 30 per cent reduction in risk for each 10 years of oral contraceptive use. There was a dose-dependent relationship between amount smoked and risk of fibroids (Table 5.4). A one pack-a-day smoker had two-thirds the risk of a lifetime non-smoker. The risk reduction with increasing cigarette consumption was statistically significant ($P = 0.02$, test for trend) and independent of the other observed risk factors in this study.

Since each of these risk factors has been linked previously to endometrial cancer, a disease known to be caused by 'unopposed' oestrogen, it seems reasonable to conclude that this might also be the cause of fibroids and that the protective effect of cigarette smoking is oestrogen-mediated.

There have been other investigations of fibroid risk factors (Ratech and Stewart 1982) but there is no other specific study on the association between

Table 5.4. Cigarette smoking and risk of fibroids: results of Oxford Family Planning Association Study

Cigarettes/day	Cases	Controls	RR
0	395	354	1.0
1–14	90	110	0.7
15+	50	71	0.6*

* $P = 0.02$, based on test for linear trend.

cigarette smoking and occurrence of fibroids. Matsunaga and Shiota (1980) compared maternal smoking histories from 97 myomatous pregnancies and from 3473 normally implanted pregnancies, all of which ended artificially. These pregnancies were part of a Japanese study conducted from 1962–74 to determine the relationship of ectopic implantation and leiomyomas to the prevalence of localized malformations of the embryo. Smoking histories were available from 64 (66 per cent) of the myomatous pregnancies and from 2772 (80 per cent) of the normal pregnancies. Of the former, 9.4 per cent were smokers compared with 15.1 per cent of the latter (OR = 0.6, $P > 0.05$).

In an interim summary of findings from the Walnut Creek prospective study of the side-effects of oral contraceptives, Ramcharan *et al.* (1981) reported that heavy smokers had a slightly decreased risk of uterine fibroids, but no specific data were provided. Finally, in a prevalence survey of nearly 5400 female former college athletes and non-athletes, Wyshak *et al.* (1986) reported a 24 per cent reduction of uterine fibroids among smokers, a result which approached statistical significance ($P = 0.07$).

5.4. Endometriosis

Endometriosis is defined as the presence of functioning endometrial tissue outside the endometrium. Adequate prevalence data are few, but the condition appears to affect at least 10 per cent of all pre-menopausal women (Ranney 1980). The major aetiologic hypothesis proposes that endometriosis is caused by pelvic implantation of endometrial cells, transported through the fallopian tubes during menstruation. In support of this hypothesis, short cycles and lengthy menses have been shown to be risk factors (Cramer *et al.* 1986). In primate models, maintenance of pelvic endometriosis is dependent on ovarian steroids (Dizerega *et al.* 1980).

Only two published reports contain data relevant to the possible association of cigarette smoking with risk of endometriosis. In the most definitive report to date, Cramer *et al.* (1986) in a multicentre study compared smoking habits in 268 women presenting with infertility, who on laparotomy had a diagnosis of endometriosis, with 3794 women admitted for delivery of a liveborn child. There was no significant reduction in risk of endometriosis among either current (RR = 0.9) or former (RR = 0.9) smokers, compared to lifetime non-smokers. Heavy smokers (≥ 1 pack per day) who started smoking during adolescence had a significant reduction in risk (RR = 0.6, $P = 0.02$), but no reduction in risk was observed among smokers starting later in life, regardless of amount smoked. While these risks were maintained in multivariate analysis including centre, age, education, and religion, it is unclear whether parous women represent an appropriate comparison group for evaluating smoking effects in infertile nulliparous patients. Hiller *et al.* (1987) presented data on a case-control study of endometriosis at a recent meeting of the American Fertility Society. Details of the control selection were not provided. Past smokers had a substantial reduction in risk compared to non-smokers (RR = 0.6), and risk was reduced even more among current smokers (RR = 0.4). Therefore, although available data suggest that, as with uterine fibroids and hyperemesis gravidarum, risk of endometriosis may be reduced in smokers, further, more definitive, studies of this association are needed.

References

Baron, J. A. (1984). Smoking and estrogen-related disease. *American Journal of Epidemiology*, 119, 9–22.

Bernstein, L., Pike, M. C., Ross, R. K., Judd, H. L., Brown, J. B., and Henderson, B. E. (1985). Estrogen and sex hormone binding globulin levels in nulliparous and parous women. *Journal of the National Cancer Institute*, 74, 741–5.

Bernstein, L., Depue, R. H., Ross, R. K., Judd, H. L., Pike, M. C., and Henderson, B. E. (1986). Higher maternal levels of free estradiol in first compared to second pregnancy: a study of early gestational difference. *Journal of the National Cancer Institute*, 76, 1035–9.

Bernstein, L., Pike, M. C., Lobo, R. A., DePue, R. H., Ross, R. K., and Henderson, B. E. (1989) Cigarette smoking in pregnancy results in marked decrease in maternal hCG and oestradiol levels. *British Journal of Obstetrics and Gynaecology*, 96, 92–6.

Cramer, D. W., *et al.* (1986). The relation of endometriosis to menstrual characteristics, smoking and exercise. *Journal of the American Medical Association*, 255, 1904–8.

Depue, R. H., Bernstein, L., Ross, R. K., Judd, H. L., and Henderson, B. E. (1987). Hyperemesis gravidarum in relation to estradiol levels, pregnancy outcome, and other maternal factors: a sero-epidemiologic study. *American Journal of Obstetrics and Gynecology*, 156, 1137–41.

Dizerega, G. S., Barber, D. L., and Hodgen, G. D. (1980). Endometriosis: role of ovarian steroids in initiation, maintenance, and suppression. *Fertility and Sterility*, 33, 649–53.

Hiller, J. E., Liang, K. Y., Polk, B. F., Rock, J. A., and Stillman, R. J. (1987). The protective effect of smoking on endometriosis. Program Supplement of the 43rd Annual Meeting of the American Fertility Society. *Fertility and Sterility Abstract*, 56, 137.

Jensen, J., Christiansen, C., and Rodbro, P. (1985). Cigarette smoking, serum estrogens, and bone loss during hormone-replacement therapy early after menopause. *New England Journal of Medicine*, 313, 973–5.

Klebanoff, M. A., Kaslow, P. A., Kaslow, R., and Rhoads, G. C. (1985). Epidemiology of vomiting in early pregnancy. *Obstetrics and Gynecology*, 66, 612–16.

Little, E. L. and Hook, E. B. (1979). Maternal alcohol and tobacco consumption and their association with nausea and vomiting during pregnancy. *Acta Obstetrica et Gynecologica Scandinavica*, 58, 15–17.

MacMahon, B., Trichopoulos, D., Cole, P., and Brown, J. (1982). Cigarette smoking and urinary estrogens. *New England Journal of Medicine*, 307, 1062–5.

Matsunaga, E. and Shiota, K. (1980). Ectopic pregnancy and myoma uteri: teratogenic effects and maternal characteristics. *Teratology*, **21**, 61–9.

Michnovicz, J. J., Hershcopf, R. J., Naganama, H., Bradlow, H. L., and Fishman, J. (1986). Increased 2-hydroxylation of estradiol as a possible mechanism for the anti-estrogenic effect of cigarette smoking. *New England Journal of Medicine*, **315**, 1305–9.

Novak, E. R. and Woodruff, J. D. (1979). In *Novak's gynecologic and obstetric pathology* (8th edn), (ed. W. B. Saunders), p. 260. Philadelphia, London.

Ramcharan, S., Pellegrin, F. A., Ray, R., and Hsu, J. P. (1981). The Walnut Creek contraceptive drug study: A prospective study of the side effects of oral contraceptives. Volume III, an interim report. A comparison of disease occurrence leading to hospitalization or death in users and nonusers of oral contraceptives. Center for Population Research Monograph, NIH Publication No. 81-564.

Ranney, B. (1980). Etiology, prevention and inhibition of endometriosis. *Clinical Obstetrics and Gynecology*, **23**, 875–81.

Ratech, H. and Stewart, M. E. (1982). Uterine leiomyomas, serum cholesterol, and oral contraceptives. *Diagnostic Gynecology and Obstetrics*, **4**, 21–4.

Ross, R. K., Pike, M. C., Vessey, M. P., Yeates, D., Bull, D., and Casagrande, J. T. (1986). Risk factors for uterine fibroids: reduced risk associated with oral contraceptives. *British Medical Journal*, **293**, 359–62.

Siiteri, P. K., Hammond, G. L., and Nisker, J. A. (1981). Increased availability of serum estrogens in breast cancer: A new hypothesis. In *Hormones and breast cancer*, (ed. M. C. Pike, P. K. Siiteri, and C. W. Welsch), p. 87. Banbury Report 8. Cold Spring Harbor, New York.

Weigel, M. M. and Weigel, R. M. (1988). The association of reproductive history, demographic factors, and alcohol and tobacco consumption with the risk of developing nausea and vomiting in early pregnancy. *American Journal of Epidemiology*, 127, 562–70.

Willett, W., *et al.* (1983). Cigarette smoking, relative weight, and menopause. *American Journal of Epidemiology*, **117**, 651–8.

Wyshak, G., Frisch, R. E., Albright, N. L., Albright, T. E., and Schiff, I. (1986). Lower prevalence of benign diseases of the breast and benign tumours of the reproductive system among former college athletes compared to non-athletes. *British Journal of Cancer*, **54**, 841–5.

6. Cigarette smoking and benign breast disease

Thomas E. Rohan and John A. Baron

Abstract

Benign breast 'disease' (BBD) represents a heterogeneous group of processes which appear sensitive to endogenous oestrogens. Data regarding their relationship with cigarette smoking are not extensive. A few studies have found an inverse association, particularly among older women. However, other investigations have shown no substantial relationship between smoking and BBD. These conflicting results may be due to confounding and biases associated with studying a process which is often not brought to medical attention.

6.1. Introduction

The rubric 'benign breast disease' (BBD) encompasses a wide range of histological conditions, many of which may not actually be diseases (Love *et al.* 1982). The histological heterogeneity of the process, together with the lack of a universally accepted classification scheme for it, complicate study of its aetiology. Commonly, however, these conditions are either examined collectively as BBD, or the major subcomponents of BBD (fibrocystic disease, itself a collective term, and fibroadenoma) are identified for separate study. For the purposes of the discussion which follows, the term BBD is used, unless reference to a specific study permits use of an alternative.

A number of clinical and epidemiological features of BBD suggest that ovarian hormones play an important role in its aetiology. The process is relatively common in young pre-menopausal women (Cole *et al.* 1978) and symptoms vary with the menstrual cycle (Preece *et al.* 1976). Oestrogen replacement therapy is associated with increased risk of BBD (Trapido *et al.* 1984; Berkowitz *et al.* 1985a; Jick *et al.* 1986), while use of oral contraceptives is associated with reduced risk (Ernster 1981). In one report, risk of BBD was inversely associated with the strength of the progestational component of combined oral contraceptives (Royal College of General Practitioners 1977).

Studies investigating the relationship between BBD and sex hormone levels have been conflicting, and no widely accepted patterns have emerged

(Wang and Fentiman 1985). However, some endocrinological studies in which women with BBD have been compared with controls have shown them to have higher levels of oestradiol in their breast fluid (Ernster *et al.* 1987), higher plasma levels of unbound (biologically active) oestradiol (Reed *et al.* 1983), higher levels of serum (England *et al.* 1974) and plasma (Sitruk-Ware *et al.* 1979) oestradiol during the luteal phase of the menstrual cycle, and lower levels of luteal phase plasma progesterone (Sitruk-Ware *et al.* 1979). This last observation led Sitruk-Ware *et al.* (1979) to suggest that benign breast disease might arise as a result of an imbalance between oestrogenic and progestational influences; a relative excess of oestrogen would result in the stimulation of breast tissue without the counterbalancing effect of progesterone. If these suggestions are correct, factors which affect these sex hormones might be associated with altered risk of BBD. If smoking has an 'anti-oestrogenic' effect then one might expect a lowered risk of BBD among women who smoke cigarettes.

6.2. Epidemiological summary

Studies in which the association between cigarette smoking and BBD has been examined are summarized in Table 6.1. The data are quite mixed. One study (Nomura *et al.* 1977) found elevated risks of cystic disease among women who ever smoked. However, several investigations have shown an inverse association. Two hospital-based case-control studies found reduced risk of fibrocystic disease among post-menopausal smokers, although there was no similar association among pre-menopausal women (Berkowitz *et al.* 1985b; Pastides *et al.* 1987; Pastides, personal communication). One of these studies also noted decreased risks for fibroadenoma among post-menopausal smokers (Berkowitz *et al.* 1985b). A cohort analysis reported by Wyshak *et al.* (1988) disclosed a reduced risk of fibrocystic disease among smokers, but not of 'benign tumours'. Another cohort study reported 'slightly decreased' risks of fibroadenoma among heavy smokers (Ramachandran *et al.* 1981).

Other investigations have not confirmed the patterns reported by these studies. In the study of Berkowitz *et al.* (1985b) the reduction in risk was confined largely to current smokers. However in separate data sets analysed by Mant *et al.* (1986), Rohan *et al.* (1989), and Brinton (personal communication) current smokers were not at reduced risk. Additionally, in data from Roswell Park, there was no variation in risk of fibrocystic disease or fibroadenoma with pack-years of cigarette use (Byers, personal communication). Nor were there differences between pre-menopausal and post-menopausal women with regard to the effect of smoking in the analyses conducted by Byers and colleagues (personal communication) and Brinton and colleagues (personal communication) and Rohan *et al.* (1989).

In aggregate, therefore, studies to date provide hints of an association

Table 6.1. Cigarette smoking and benign breast disease (BBD): A summary of case-control and cohort studies

Reference	Study design; subjects; location	Case definition	Confounding variables considered	Comparison	Point estimate of effect* (95% confidence interval)
Nomura *et al.* (1977)	Case-control; 320 prevalent cases (275 with cystic disease, 45 with fibroadenoma), 320 population controls; Maryland, USA	Biopsy for BBD—cases included women with cystic disease	Age, education, income, area of residence, age at first pregnancy, parity, oestrogen use	Ever smoked vs. never:	
				Cystic disease	1.6†
				Fibroadenoma	0.8†
Berkowitz *et al.* (1985b)	Case-control; 633 incident cases of fibrocystic disease, 251 incident cases of fibroadenoma, and 1062 hospital controls; Connecticut, USA	Biopsy-confirmed fibrocystic breast disease (defined as presence of microcysts and gross cysts)	Age, Quetelet's index	Fibrocystic disease:	
				Ever smoked vs. never	0.8 (0.7–1.0)
				Current smoker vs. never	0.6 (0.5–0.8)
				Ex-smoker vs. never	1.0 (0.8–1.3)
				Fibroadenoma:	
				Ever smoked vs. never	0.6 (0.5–0.8)
				Current smoker vs. never	0.7 (0.5–0.9)
				Ex-smoker vs. never	0.7 (0.6–1.2)

Table 6.1. (*cont.*)

Reference	Study design; subjects; location	Case definition	Confounding variables considered	Comparison	Point estimate of effect* (95% confidence interval)
Mant *et al.* (1986)	Cohort; 570 cases, 17 032 women; Oxford, UK	First episode of hospitalization for BBD (includes chronic cystic disease and benign neoplasms)	Age, oral contraceptive use, social class, Quetelet's index	Ex-smoker vs. never	1.1 †
				Current smokers:	
				1–14 cigs/day vs. never	1.2 †
				≥15 cigs/day vs. never	1.1 †
Pastides *et al.* (1987)	Case-control; 255 incident cases, 787 hospital controls; Connecticut, USA	Biopsy-confirmed fibrocystic disease		Ever smoked vs. never	0.5 (0.2–0.8)
Wyshak *et al.* (1988)	Cohort; 520 cases, 5398 women; college alumnae, Massachusetts, USA	BBD defined as report of at least one benign breast tumour or at least one breast biopsy	Age, family history of cancer, relative fatness, endometrial biopsy, replacement hormones, age at menarche, history of pregnancy, athlete or non-athlete	Ever smoked vs. never:	
				Fibrocystic disease	0.47 (0.29–0.76)
				Benign tumour	no association

* Odds ratio for case-control studies, rate ratio for cohort studies.
† Confidence intervals not available.

Table 6.1. (*cont.*) Cigarette smoking and benign breast disease (BBD): A summary of case-control and cohort studies

Reference	Study design; subjects; location	Case definition	Confounding variables considered	Comparison	Point estimate of effect* (95% confidence interval)
Rohan *et al.* (1989, in press)	Case-control; 383 cases, 192 biopsy controls (no evidence of epithelial proliferative disorder), 383 community controls; South Australia	Histologically-confirmed first diagnosis of benign proliferative epithelial disorder	Income, number of medical examinations per year, frequency of practice of breast self-examination, Quetelet's index, and ever use of oral contraceptives	Cases vs. community controls:	
				Ever smoked vs never	0.9 (0.6–1.4)
				Current smoker vs. never	1.2 (0.7–1.9)
				Ex-smoker vs. never	0.6 (0.3–1.0)
				Cases vs. biopsy controls:	
				Ever smoked vs. never	0.9 (0.6–1.3)
				Current smoker vs. never	1.1 (0.7–1.6)
				Ex-smoker vs. never	0.8 (0.5–1.3)
Byers (unpublished data)	Case-control; 718 cases, 2734 hospital controls; New York State, USA	Chronic cystic breast disease and benign neoplasms of the the breast	Age	Ever smoked vs. never	1.0 (0.7–1.5)
				1–14 pack-years of cigarette use vs. none	1.0 (0.7–1.5)
				≥15 pack-years of cigarette use vs. none	0.9 (0.5–1.7)

Table 6.1. (*cont.*) Cigarette smoking and benign breast disease (BBD): A summary of case-control and cohort studies

Reference	Study design; subjects; location	Case definition	Confounding variables considered	Comparison	Point estimate of effect* (95% confidence interval)
Brinton (unpublished data)	Case-control (within screening programme—see Brinton *et al.* 1979); 1780 cases; multicentre study, USA	Not available	Age, menopausal status	Ever smoked vs. never Current smoker vs. never Ex-smoker vs. never	1.1 † 1.2 † 1.0 †

* Odds ratio for case-control studies, rate ratio for cohort studies.
† Confidence intervals not available.

between cigarette smoking and BBD. However, the discrepant results do not permit a confident general conclusion regarding this association.

6.3 Discussion

The majority of the studies summarized in Table 6.1 are case-control in design, and one reason for the discrepant findings may be the selection biases inherent in this approach to the study of BBD. Since some (perhaps most) women with BBD do not have their disease confirmed by biopsy, women who are biopsied represent an unknown proportion of all women with BBD. Therefore the target population for any generalizations which can be made from most studies of BBD is limited to women with biopsy-determined BBD. This renders the choice of the appropriate control group problematic, as reflected in the use of three different types of controls in the studies reported in Table 1. Community controls may be inappropriate since the case series may not represent all cases; hospital controls may be inappropriate since smokers may be over-represented amongst them; and controls who have undergone the same diagnostic procedure as the cases may be inappropriate as their use may result in 'overmatching' (Vessey 1979). However, in relation to a somewhat analogous problem, namely study of the association between oestrogen replacement therapy and risk of endometrial cancer, it has been shown that in the absence of estimates of exposure-specific detection rates and exposure-specific rates of special treatment (e.g. biopsy), it is not possible to determine *a priori* which control group will give the correct result (Greenland and Neutra 1981). These considerations suggest the need for further cohort studies of the association between cigarette smoking and BBD, and for further case-control studies in which more than one control group is employed. Most valuable would be studies in which women are surveyed for BBD, rather than detected through routine care.

Nicotine has been identified in breast fluid from non-lactating women (Petrakis *et al.* 1978), and it is possible that substances contained in cigarette smoke may adversely affect the breast epithelium to produce BBD. Thus an indirect protective hormonal effect might be counterbalanced by a direct causative influence. This mixture of effects would obviously complicate the conclusions that could be drawn about an anti-oestrogenic effect of smoking from the relationship between BBD and smoking.

In conclusion, it is clear that the data regarding cigarette smoking and BBD are conflicting. Unfortunately, there are methodological difficulties associated with the study of these conditions which may hamper clarification of the issue.

References

Berkowitz, G. S., *et al.* (1985a). Cigarette smoking and benign breast disease. *Journal of Epidemiology and Community Health*, **39**, 308–13.

Berkowitz, G. S., *et al.* (1985b). Estrogen replacement therapy and fibrocystic disease in postmenopausal women. *American Journal of Epidemiology*, **121**, 238–45.

Brinton, L. A., *et al.* (1979). Breast cancer risk factors among screening program participants. *Journal of the National Cancer Institute*, **62**, 37–43.

Cole, P., Elwood, J. M., and Kaplan, S. D. (1978). Incidence rates and risk factors of benign breast neoplasms. *American Journal of Epidemiology*, **108**, 112–20.

England, P. C. *et al.* (1974). Serum oestradiol-17β, in women with benign and malignant breast disease. *British Journal of Cancer*, **30**, 571–6.

Ernster, V. L. (1981). The epidemiology of benign breast disease. *Epidemiologic Reviews*, **3**, 184–202.

Ernster, V. L., *et al.* (1987). Benign and malignant breast disease: initial study results of serum and breast fluid analyses of endogenous estrogens. *Journal of the National Cancer Institute*, 79, 949–60.

Greenland, S. and Neutra, R. (1981). An analysis of detection bias and proposed corrections in the study of estrogens and endometrial cancer. *Journal of Chronic Diseases*, **34**, 433–8.

Jick, S. S., Walker, A. M., and Jick, H. (1986). Conjugated estrogens and fibrocystic breast disease. *American Journal of Epidemiology*, **124**, 746–51.

Love, S. M., Gelman, R. S., and Silen, W. (1982). Fibrocystic 'disease' of the breast—a nondisease? *New England Journal of Medicine*, **307**, 1010–14.

Mant, D., *et al.* (1986). Cigarette smoking and benign breast disease. *Journal of Epidemiology and Community Health*, **40**, 277–8.

Nomura, A., Comstock, G. W., and Tonascia, J. A. (1977). Epidemiologic characteristics of benign breast disease. *American Journal of Epidemiology*, **105**, 505–12.

Pastides, H., Najjar, M. A., and Kelsey, J. L. (1987). Estrogen replacement therapy and fibrocystic breast disease. *American Journal of Preventive Medicine*, **3**, 282–6.

Petrakis, N. L., *et al.* (1978). Nicotine in breast fluid of non-lactating women. *Science*, **199**, 303–5.

Preece, P. E., *et al.* (1976). Clinical syndromes of mastalgia. *Lancet*, **ii**, 670–3.

Ramachandran, S., *et al.* (1981). *The Walnut Creek Contraceptive Drug Study*, Vol. III. Department of Health and Human Services, Washington.

Reed, M. J., *et al.* (1983). Plasma levels of estrone, estrone sulfate, and estradiol and the percentage of unbound estradiol in postmenopausal women with and without breast disease. *Cancer Research*, **43**, 3940–3.

Rohan, T. E., Cook, M. J., and Baron, J. A. (1989). Cigarette smoking and benign proliferative epithelial disorders of the breast in women; a case-control study. *Journal of Epidemiology and Community Health*, **43**, 362–8.

Royal College of General Practitioners (1973). Oral Contraception Study. Effect on hypertension and benign breast disease of progestogen component in combined oral contraceptives. *Lancet*, **i**, 624.

Sitruk-Ware, R., Sterkers, N., and Mauvais-Jarvis, P. (1979). Benign breast disease I: hormonal investigation. *Obstetrics and Gynecology*, 53, 457–60.
Trapido, E. J., *et al.* (1984). Estrogen replacement therapy and benign breast disease. *Journal of the National Cancer Institute*, 73, 1101–5.
Vessey, M. P. (1979). Comment. *Journal of Chronic Diseases*, 32, 64–6.
Wang, D. Y. and Fentiman, I. S. (1985). Epidemiology and endocrinology of benign breast disease. *Breast Cancer: Advances in Research and Treatment*, 6, 5–36.
Wyshak, G., *et al.* (1988). Cigarette smoking and benign breast disease. *New England Journal of Medicine*, 319, 1736–7.

III

Smoking and Osteoporosis

7. Smoking and osteoporosis

Malcolm Law

Abstract

The mineral density of bone is a useful simple index of its propensity to fracture. This chapter reviews 13 studies that have compared bone mineral density in cigarette smokers and non-smokers. In women who are 8 years or more post-menopausal, and in older men, bone density is lower in smokers than non-smokers, by about half a standard deviation (i.e. about one-eighth of the range of bone density in the population). In women who are pre-menopausal or less than 5 years post-menopausal, bone density is similar in smokers and non-smokers. These observations, and measures of the rate of bone loss in one study, indicate that smoking does not have an important influence on peak bone density but is associated with an increased rate of subsequent bone loss. It is likely that smoking directly causes this faster bone loss, as confounding with other determinants of bone density, or other sources of bias, appear unlikely. Of the possible mechanisms for this effect of smoking, the lower body weight of smokers is partly responsible, but an important action independent of body weight is likely. In women, the earlier menopause of smokers can be no more than a minor factor, and the effects of smoking in inhibiting oestrogen synthesis and inducing the selective production of inert metabolites appears irrelevant to the effect of smoking on the rate of bone loss, as the former action seems confined to pre-menopausal women, and the latter to post-menopausal women. The effects of smoking on other hormones, notably androstenedione and cortisol, could be important.

Cigarette smoking, one of several known potential determinants of bone mineral density, may be important in terms of prevention of osteoporotic fractures. This chapter discusses the association between smoking and bone density.

7.1. Bone mineral density and osteoporosis

Bone mineral density attains a peak at about the age of 25 years, and declines from age 35–40. At any age there is a wide range between individuals. Bone density is higher on average in men than women at all ages, and in women there is a period of rapid bone loss after the menopause. The term 'osteoporosis' generally refers to an unspecified lower end of the range of bone density, and implies an increased risk of age-related fracture. Bone mineral density is indeed the best simple index of bone strength. For cortical (compact) bone, susceptibility to experimental mechanical fracture varies approximately in proportion to density, although with loss of trabecular bone the decreased number and density of trabecular elements and their interconnections increases the risk of fracture disproportionately to the amount of bone lost. Nonetheless, measurements of bone density do provide a useful index of the risk of age-related fractures.

7.2. Bone density and risk of fracture

An association between fracture risk and low bone density has been clearly shown for crush fractures of the vertebral body; most fractures affect individuals in the lowest quartile or so of the distribution of bone mineral density (Riggs and Melton 1986). For hip fracture in the elderly, bone density is also lower on average in cases than controls, although the difference is smaller and the distributions overlap considerably. Other factors besides bone density are also important, especially propensity to fall and the loss (through neurological disease or senility) of the protective reflexes that normally prevent or reduce the impact of falls (Cummings 1985; Cooper *et al.* 1987). Riggs and Melton (1986) showed that age-related fractures of the hip and vertebral body occur only below a threshold of bone density of about 1 g/cm^2, and that as bone density falls below this threshold, fracture risk increases. Therefore, either a low peak bone density or a rapid subsequent rate of bone loss will increase the risk of osteoporosis and hip fracture in old age. With increasing age and continuing bone loss, more and more people fall below the bone density threshold, and risk of hip fracture increases. The two- to threefold higher age-specific incidence of hip fracture in women than men is consistent with their lower average bone mineral density.

7.3. Determinants of bone density other than smoking

Lifestyle determinants of peak bone density have not been clearly established, although exercise probably has an influence and dietary calcium may. Factors that influence bone loss are better recognized (Cummings *et al.* 1985). Endogenous oestrogens are a well-established determinant, and in older women, bone density correlates directly with circulating oestrogen levels and with factors that influence them such as age at menopause and history of bilateral oophrectomy before the natural menopause. Trials show that oestrogens halt the rapid post-menopausal bone loss in women and that calcium supplementation also has some effect. Exercise reduces rate of bone loss and immobilization increases it. Obese people have higher bone density and a lower risk of hip fracture than thin people. Heavy alcohol consumption is associated with low bone density. Certain drugs and diseases also reduce bone density, but can account for only a small proportion of cases of hip fracture.

7.4. Cigarette smoking and bone mineral density

The results of studies that have compared bone density in smokers and never-smokers are summarized in Tables 7.1 and 7.2. Different studies have measured the density of different bones, but none have measured the neck of femur, the fracture site of greatest public health importance. However, one would expect an effect of cigarette smoking on one bone to reflect that on the entire skeleton: it is implausible that this effect of smoking should be localized. None the less smoking may affect the density of some bones more than others, and in particular may affect trabecular bone more than cortical since the former is generally more metabolically active. In Tables 7.1 and 7.2 the measures of density vary between studies, both because different measurement techniques are used and because different bones are measured. To allow a comparison between the studies, the difference in density between smokers and non-smokers in each study has been expressed as a proportion of the standard deviation of the distribution of bone density in that study. This is not entirely valid because the different measurements are unlikely to be linearly related, but it does allow a convenient approximation.

In all but one of the studies of post-menopausal women (eight or more years since the menopause), smokers have lower bone density than non-smokers (Table 7.1). Rundgren and Mellstrom (1984) studied ex-smokers and found their bone density to be on average between that of current smokers and non-smokers. Lindsay (1981) also found the annual rate of bone loss to be greater in smokers than in non-smokers. However, in peri-menopausal women (0–5 years since the menopause) and in pre-menopausal women the bone density of smokers was no lower than that of non-smokers (Table 7.1).

These studies indicate, therefore, that smoking is not a determinant of peak bone density, but that post-menopausal bone loss is greater in smokers than non-smokers so that several years after the menopause there is a detectable difference.

In men (Table 7.2) all studies are consistent in showing bone density to be lower in smokers above the age of about 50. Sparrow *et al.* (1982) also found the rate of bone loss to be greater in smokers. In younger men the data are too limited to allow a conclusion; Suominen *et al.* (1984) found smokers aged 31–35 to have lower bone density than non-smokers of the same age, but the difference was not statistically significant ($P = 0.09$).

Table 7.1. Bone density in smokers and non-smokers—women

Study	Age (years)	Measurement technique	Bone density units	Current smokers		Never smokers		Difference (expressed in standard deviations)
				Number	Bone density	Number	Bone density	
Post-menopausal								
Rundgren and Mellstrom (1984)	70–79	d.p.a. (calcaneus)	μm calcium phosphate	(111)	730	(825)	872	−0.5 sd ($P<0.001$)
Hollo *et al.* (1979)	61–75	s.p.a. (forearm)	g/cm	(41)	0.68	(125)	0.72	−0.4 sd ($P=0.03$)
G. F. Jensen (1986)	70	s.p.a. (forearm)	g/cm	(77)	31.3	(103)	33.0	−0.3 sd ($P=0.08$)
Daniell (1976)	60–69	X-ray (metacarpal)	% cortical area	(45)	72.0	(84)	79.5	−1.1 sd ($P<0.001$)
Lindquist *et al.* (1981)	54 and 62	d.p.a. (lumbar spine)	g/cm	(26)	3.41	(46)	3.53	−0.2 sd ($P>0.1$)
Lindsay (1981)	45–50 (oophorectomy)	s.p.a. (metacarpal)	mg/mm	(29)	39.7	(252)	42.9	−0.5 sd ($P=0.04$)
Sowers *et al.* (1985)	55–80 (mean 67)	s.p.a. (forearm)	mg/cm^2	(72)	0.635	(252)	0.625	+0.1 sd

Table 7.1. (*cont.*) Bone density in smokers and non-smokers—women

Study	Age (years)	Measurement technique	Bone density units	Current smokers		Never smokers		Difference (expressed in standard deviations)
				Number	Bone density	Number	Bone density	
Peri-menopausal								
J. Jensen *et al.* (1985)	44-56	s.p.a. (forearm)	g/cm	(67)	38.2	(69)	38.0	0.0 sd
Friedman *et al.* (1987)	(mean 52)	s.p.a. (forearm)	g/cm^2	(9)	0.72	(16)	0.66	+1.0 sd ($P=0.02$)
Johnell and Nilsson (1984)	49	s.p.a. (forearm)	mg/cm^2	(186)	320	(185)	318	0.0 sd
Pre-menopausal								
Lindquist *et al.* (1981)	46 and 54	s.p.a. (lumbar spine)	g/cm	(16)	3.84	(42)	3.90	0.1 sd
Daniell (1976)	40–49	X-ray (metacarpal)	% cortical area	(36)	89.3	(48)	88.4	0.0 sd

s.p.a. and d.p.a., single and dual photon absorptiometry.

Table 7.2. Bone density in smokers and non-smokers—men

Study	Age (years)	Measurement technique	Bone density units	Current smokers		Never smokers		Difference (expressed in standard deviations)
				Number	Bone density	Number	Bone density	
Hollo *et al.* (1979)	61–90	s.p.a. (forearm)	g/cm	(73)	1.05	(71)	1.14	−0.6 sd ($P<0.001$)
Rundgren and Mellstrom (1984)	70–79	d.p.a. (calcaneus)	μm calcium phosphate	(280)	1239	(206)	1431	−0.5 sd ($P<0.001$)
Suominen *et al.* (1984)	71–75	s.p.a. (calcaneus)	g/cm³	(8)	0.129	(23)	0.136	−0.3 sd ($P>0.1$)
	51–55			(18)	0.132	(34)	0.155	−0.8 sd ($P=0.007$)
	31–35			(21)	0.155	(38)	0.166	−0.5 sd ($P=0.09$)
Sparrow *et al.* (1982)	48–80 (mean 51)	X-ray (metacarpal)	%cortical area	(139)	79	(202)	80.5	−0.2 sd ($P=0.09$)
McNair *et al.* (1980) (diabetics, 32% female)	21–70 (mean 42)	s.p.a. (forearm)	% of controls	(114)	89.4	(49)	94.6	−0.3 sd ($P=0.05$)

s.p.a. and d.p.a., single and dual photon absorptiometry.

It can be concluded that smoking increases the rate of bone loss in both sexes.

7.5. Is the association of smoking with low bone density causal?

The association is consistent in the studies of older subjects, and is statistically significant in individual studies. No evidence for confounding by the other determinants of bone density discussed above has emerged. The association of smoking with low bone density could not be explained by smokers being more likely to take post-menopausal oestrogens (Daniell 1976; G. F. Jensen 1986). Dietary calcium was similar in smokers and non-smokers (Mellstrom *et al.* 1982), and exercise did not confound the association between smoking and bone density (Lindquist *et al.* 1981; Suominen *et al.* 1984; Rundgren and Mellstrom 1984). Heavy alcohol consumption and partial gastric resection both reduce bone density, but Mellstrom *et al.* (1982) reported that the lower bone density of smokers persisted after adjustment for these two factors. Finally, the age of smokers and non-smokers was similar in each study.

The lower bone density of smokers is likely to be causal. The magnitude of the difference between older smokers and non-smokers is of the order of half a standard deviation (Tables 7.1 and 7.2). This difference might be expected to produce a moderately large relative risk for vertebral body fracture in smokers, since fractures tend to affect individuals at the extreme of the bone density distribution and a difference of half a standard deviation in non-smokers should prevent many fractures. For hip fracture one would expect smoking to be associated with a smaller relative risk, as there is a smaller average difference in the bone density of cases and controls, with considerable overlap. These expectations correspond with the results of case-control studies of fracture patients (Cooper and Wickham, Chapter 8).

7.6. Possible mechanisms for the faster bone loss of smokers

Smokers are thinner

The lower average body weight of smokers must be a partial explanation for their lower bone density. Five of the studies that show older smokers to have lower bone density have used various statistical techniques to examine the question of whether the difference is entirely attributable to lower body weight, although none have used multiple regression. Rundgren and Mellstrom (1984) reported that the lower body weight of smokers did not influence the statistical significance of the association between smoking and bone mineral density. G. F. Jensen (1986) found the association of smoking with low bone density to be attenuated after adjustment for body weight, but some difference persisted. Daniell (1976) found that the difference in bone density persisted when 'normal weight' smokers and non-smokers were compared, but that there was no difference in the bone density of smokers and non-smokers who were more than 10 per cent overweight. Lindsay (1981) selected from his study a subset of smokers and non-smokers individually matched for height and weight, and found that the absolute difference in bone mineral density was unaffected, but that the rate of bone loss was much attenuated. McNair *et al.* (1980) found that body weight was only minimally lower in smokers than non-smokers in their study, and so could not explain the lower bone density of smokers.

Two case-control studies have shown that smoking and low body weight added independently to the risk of fracture—Williams *et al.* (1982) studying hip and Colles' fracture in women, and Seeman *et al.* (1983) studying vertebral fractures in men. Thus there is consistent evidence from diverse sources that the lower bone density of post-menopausal smokers is only partly due to their lower body weight; there appears to be an important independent association as well.

Menopause is earlier in smokers

Smokers have an earlier menopause (Baron, Chapter 4), and there is a rapid period of bone loss in the years after the menopause, so that on this basis alone post-menopausal smokers would have lower bone density than non-smokers of the same age. None of the studies examined whether the lower bone density for smokers persisted after adjustment for age at menopause, but one would expect a persistent difference, because the effect of smoking on age at menopause is relatively small, and because smoking lowers bone density in both sexes.

Effects of smoking on oestrogen synthesis and metabolism

Oestrogens prevent bone loss, and smoking inhibits oestrogen synthesis (Canick and Barbieri, Chapter 19) and stimulates the production of inactive rather than active oestrogen metabolites (Michnovicz and Fishman, Chapter 18). However, these effects have been demonstrated only in pre-menopausal women, and serum levels of active oestrogens in post-menopausal women are similar in smokers and non-smokers (J. Jensen *et al.* 1985; Friedman *et al.* 1987). If these effects of smoking are indeed confined to pre-menopausal women they cannot explain the effect of smoking on bone density, which is confined to post-menopausal women. An effect of smoking in reducing active oestrogen availability in the tissues but not the blood in post-menopausal women can be proposed as a hypothesis, no evidence is available to examine it.

Effects of smoking on other hormones

In men, plasma concentration of androstenedione was greater in smokers than in non-smokers (Barrett-Connor and Khaw 1987) but the effect that this difference might have on bone density is difficult to estimate. Smoking (and probably nicotine) increases adrenocortical secretion; Kershbaum *et al.* (1968) reported that, in nine men and women aged 22–30, plasma 11-hydroxysteroid concentration was on average 47 per cent higher during a one week smoking period than in the same subjects during a one week non-smoking period. In post-menopausal women, Freidman *et al.* (1987) found serum cortisol concentration to be greater in smokers (mean 169.2 mg/ml, $n=9$) than non-smokers (mean 115.3 mg/ml, $n=16$), $P<0.001$. Diseases causing over-production of cortisol, and treatment with corticosteroid hormones, cause osteoporosis; the effect of smoking on serum cortisol is much smaller, but none the less may contribute to the lower bone density of smokers.

7.7. Conclusions

Low bone mineral density (or osteoporosis) increases the risk of hip fracture and other age-related fractures, and smoking increases the rate of bone loss in post-menopausal women and in older men. This effect of smoking appears to be causal; it cannot be attributed to confounding. It must partly reflect the fact that smokers are thinner on average, but there seems also to be an effect of smoking on bone density that is independent of body weight. Influences of smoking on the synthesis or metabolism of various hormones, including oestrogens, androstenedione and cortisol, are possible mechanisms, but the evidence is limited.

References

Barrett-Connor, E. and Khaw, K. T. (1987). Cigarette smoking and increased endogenous estrogen levels in men. *American Journal of Epidemiology*, 126, 187–92.

Cooper, C., Barker, D. J. P., Morris, J., and Briggs, R. S. J. (1987). Osteoporosis, falls and age in fracture of the proximal femur. *British Medical Journal*, 295, 13–15.

Cummings, S. R. (1985) Are patients with hip fractures more osteoporotic? Review of the evidence. *American Journal of Medicine*, 78, 487–94.

Cummings, S. R., Kelsey, J. L., Nevitt, M. C., and O'Dowd, K. J. (1985). Epidemiology of osteoporosis and osteoporotic fractures. *Epidemiologic Reviews*, 7, 178–208.

Daniell, H. W. (1976). Osteoporosis of the slender smoker. *Archives of Internal Medicine*, 136, 298–304.

Friedman, A. J., Ravnikar, V. A., and Barbieri, R. L. (1987). Serum steroid hormone profiles in post-menopausal smokers and non-smokers. *Fertility and Sterility*, 47, 398–401.

Hollo, I., Gergely, I., and Boross, M. (1979). Influence of heavy smoking upon the bone mineral content of the radius of the aged and effect of tobacco smoke on the sensitivity to calcitonin of rats. *Aktuelle Gerontologica*, 9, 365–8.

Jensen, G. F. (1986). Osteoporosis of the slender smoker revisited by epidemiologic approach. *European Journal of Clinical Investigation*, **16**, 239–42.

Jensen, J., Christiansen, C., and Rodbro, P. (1985). Cigarette smoking, serum estrogens and bone loss during hormone-replacement therapy early after menopause. *New England Journal of Medicine*, **313**, 973–5.

Johnell, O. and Nilsson, B. E. (1984). Life-style and bone mineral mass in perimenopausal women. *Calcified Tissue International*, **35**, 354–6.

Kershbaum, A., Pappajohn, D. J., Bellet, S., Hirabayashi, M., and Shafiha, H. (1968). Effect of smoking and nicotine on adrenocortical secretion. *Journal of the American Medical Association*, **203**, 275–8.

Lindsay, R. (1981). The influence of cigarette smoking on bone mass and bone loss. In: *Osteoporosis: recent advances in pathogenesis and treatment* (ed. H. F. Deluca, *et al.*). University Park Press, Baltimore.

Lindquist, O., *et al.* (1981). Bone mineral content in relation to age and menopause in middle-aged women. *Scandinavian Journal of Clinical and Laboratory Investigation*, **41**, 215–23.

McNair, P., *et al.* (1980). Bone loss in patients with diabetes mellitus: effects of smoking. *Mineral and Electrolyte Metabolism*, **3**, 94–7.

Mellstrom, D., Rundgren, A., Jagenburg, R., Steen, B., and Svanborg, A. (1982). Tobacco smoking, aging and health among the elderly: A longitudinal population study of 70-year-old men and an age cohort comparison. *Age and Ageing*, **11**, 45–58.

Riggs, B. L. and Melton, L. J. (1986). Involutional osteoporosis. *New England Journal of Medicine*, **314**, 1676–86.

Rundgren, A. and Mellstrom, D. (1984). The effect of tobacco smoking on the bone mineral content of the ageing skeleton. *Mechanisms of Ageing and Development*, **28**, 272–7.

Seeman, E., Melton, L. J., O'Fallon, W. M., and Riggs, B. L. (1983). Risk factors for spinal osteoporosis in men. *American Journal of Medicine*, **75**, 977–83.

Sowers, M. R., Wallace, R. B., and Lemke, J. H. (1985). Correlates of mid-radius bone density among postmenopausal women: a community study. *American Journal of Clinical Nutrition*, **41**, 1045–53.

Sparrow, D., *et al.* (1982). The influence of cigarette smoking and age on bone loss in men. *Archives of Environmental Health*, **37**, 246–9.

Suominen, H., *et al.* (1984). Mineral density of calcaneous in men at different ages: a population study with special reference to life-style factors. *Age and Ageing*, **13**, 273–81.

Williams, A. R., Weiss, N. S., and Ure, C. L. (1982). Effect of weight, smoking and oestrogen use on the risk of hip and forearm fracture in postmenopausal women. *Obstetrics and Gynaecology*, **60**, 695–9.

8. Cigarette smoking and the risk of age-related fractures

Cyrus Cooper and Carol Wickham

Abstract

Age-related fractures constitute a major public health problem. Their incidence depends on osteoporosis and the risk of falling. Evidence exists to support an association between cigarette smoking and fracture risk. The strength of this association, however, varies with type of fracture, being stronger for vertebral than hip fracture. A clear understanding of the relationship between smoking and these fractures is fundamental to the design of preventive strategies.

8.1. Introduction

Fractures of the proximal femur, vertebrae, and distal radius are an important cause of ill health and death in the elderly. A reduction in bone mass (i.e. osteoporosis) is thought to have a role in causing these age-related fractures, but this has not been clearly proven. This review outlines the epidemiology of age-related fractures, their relationship to osteoporosis, and the role of cigarette smoking as a risk factor for fracture.

8.2. The epidemiology of age-related fractures

More information is available on the epidemiology of hip fractures than of vertebral or distal radial fractures, as they require hospitalization.

The incidence of hip fractures in Caucasian populations rises exponentially with age, and above the age of 50 years there is a female to male incidence ratio of 2.5 to 1 (Cummings *et al.* 1985). Hip fractures are much less frequent in Negroid populations (Solomon 1968). Most large studies in the United Kingdom have reported a winter peak in incidence, possibly explained by impaired neuromuscular co-ordination in cold weather (Bastow *et al.* 1983), or by vitamin D deficiency (Aaron *et al.* 1974). Recent evidence suggests a secular increase in hip fracture incidence in this country (Boyce and Vessey 1985) and the USA (Melton *et al.* 1987) over the last three decades, the reason for which remains unknown.

Vertebral fractures may be classified as partial (or wedge) deformities and complete (or crush) fractures. Although they may cause back pain, many are asymptomatic. The prevalence of vertebral crush fractures in Caucasian women rises from 2.5 per cent at age 60 years to 7.5 per cent at age 80 years (Nordin *et al.* 1980). Wedge fractures are considerably more frequent with a prevalence of around 70 per cent in women aged over 75 years.

Distal radial fractures are the most common fractures in Caucasian women below 75 years of age (Miller and Evans 1985). In these women, the incidence increases linearly from age 40 to age 70 years, with rates stabilizing thereafter. In men, the incidence remains constant between age 20 and 80 years. As with hip fractures, there is a winter peak in incidence.

8.3. The relationship between bone mass and fracture

The advent of non-invasive methods for measuring bone mass has led to greater understanding of the relationship between osteoporosis and fracture risk. Reduced spinal trabecular bone mass has consistently been found in patients with vertebral crush fractures when compared with non-fracture controls (Cann *et al.* 1984). Furthermore, a threshold value can be defined below which crush fractures occur, but above which they are rarely found. The prevalence of fracture increases the further bone mass falls below this threshold.

The relationship between bone mass and hip fracture is less clear. Stochastic models can wholly explain the variation of hip fracture incidence with age and sex on the basis of changes in bone mass with ageing (Horsman *et al.* 1985). Early histological and radiological studies suggested that osteoporosis is an important determinant of hip fracture (Nordin 1971). Case-control studies, however, have not shown large differences in bone mass between fracture cases and controls of similar age (Cummings 1985), and the independent contributions of osteoporosis, the risk of falling, and other age-related factors to the risk of hip fracture remain unknown (Cooper *et al.* 1987).

8.4. Cigarette smoking and the risk of age-related fractures

There is evidence for a role of cigarette smoking as a risk factor for all three age-related fractures. The strength of the association, however, varies with fracture type.

Hip fracture

Six case-control studies (Baker 1980; Paganini-Hill *et al.* 1981; Williams *et al.* 1982; Kreiger *et al.* 1982; Boyce 1985; Alderman *et al.* 1986) have examined the relationship between cigarette smoking and the risk of hip fracture (Table 8.1). In the two English studies (Baker 1980; Boyce 1985)

Table 8.1. Cigarette smoking and the risk of hip fracture

Study	Subjects	Contrast	Findings
Baker (1980)	189 cases 95 community controls	Ever smoker vs. never	No difference reported
Paganini-Hill *et al*. (1981)	91 cases (<80 years) 182 community controls	>10 cigarettes daily after menopause vs. none	OR = 1.5 (0.8–3.0)*
Williams *et al*. (1982)	160 cases (50–74 years) 567 community controls	Ever smoker vs. never in thin, non-oestrogen users	OR = 2.2 (0.6–8.2)*
Kreiger *et al*. (1982)	98 cases 884 hospital controls	Ever smoker vs. never	OR = 1.3 (0.8–2.1)
Boyce (1985)	139 cases (MTS passed) 139 controls	Ever smoker vs. never	OR = 1.2
Alderman *et al*. (1986)	160 cases (50–74 years) 567 community controls	>1 cigarette daily vs. never smoker	OR = 1.2 (0.9–1.6)

OR, odds ratio, with 95 per cent confidence intervals in parentheses where available.
* 95 per cent confidence intervals estimated from data provided assumed no matching.
MTS = mental test score.

there was no difference between the proportions of cases and controls reporting ever having smoked. In that of Baker, cases and controls were not matched by age and adjustment for this variable was not mentioned in the analysis. Paganini-Hill *et al.* (1981) found an increased risk of hip fracture among women who smoked, with a suggested dose–response relationship, although this trend was not statistically significant. In the King County study (Williams *et al.* 1982), an increased fracture risk was found among ever smoking women who were thin, particularly if they were not taking oestrogens. A re-analysis of the data (Alderman *et al.* 1986), however, to examine an overall smoking effect, suggested that this was not statistically significant, although this again was not adjusted for age.

There are several potential sources of bias in these studies. In many, selection criteria limited the choice of cases to people who were relatively young (less than 80 years) or who were able to pass a mental test score. These criteria are necessary to improve the validity of the information recalled but might lead to bias in the risk estimates obtained. The use of hospital controls in one study (Kreiger *et al.* 1982) might also have conservatively biased the observed odds ratio. Finally, several environmental factors are thought to influence both peak bone mass and its subsequent rate of loss (Cummings 1985). These include oestrogen deficiency, body weight, dietary calcium and protein intake, alcohol consumption, physical activity, diseases, and certain drugs. Many of these factors might confound an association between cigarette smoking and the risk of hip fracture. Yet the possible confounding effects of many of these variables remain unexplored.

Table 8.2. Cigarette smoking and the risk of hip fracture in the Southampton case-control study

	Cases	Controls
Women		
Ever smoked	100	142
Never smoked	140	338
OR = 1.7 (95% CI 1.2–2.4)		
1.5 (95% CI 1.0–2.3)*		
Men		
Ever smoked	45	81
Never smoked	15	39
OR = 1.5 (95% CI 0.7–3.1)		
0.7 (95% CI 0.3–1.8)†		

* Odds ratio after adjusting for alcohol, body mass, activity, and calcium intake.
† Odds ratio after adjusting for alcohol.

The Southampton case-control study of hip fracture provided an opportunity to examine some of these factors. In this study, 240 elderly women and 60 elderly men presenting with hip fractures to Southampton General Hospital, were compared with 600 randomly selected community controls matched for sex and age within four years. All the cases and controls were able to pass a ten point Hodkinson abbreviated mental test score. Information on exposure to risk factors was obtained by an interview-administered questionnaire. This included a history of current and previous smoking. Table 8.2 shows that the risk of hip fracture in women who had ever smoked was 1.7 times greater than in those who had never smoked. This increase in risk was statistically significant. A similar increase in risk was found in men, but this was not significant due to the smaller number of men in the study. In men, the increased risk associated with smoking did not remain after allowance for alcohol consumption. In women, the increased risk of fracture in ever smokers remained significantly elevated even after adjustment for alcohol consumption, body mass index, physical activity, and calcium intake. These findings suggest that in men, other risk factors for hip fracture, particularly alcohol consumption, might confound the effect of smoking on fracture risk. This would not appear to be the case in women, in whom a potential oestrogenic mechanism exists for the association between smoking and fracture.

In a second study, the risk factors for falls in the elderly were examined using data from a Department of Health and Social Security survey of health and nutrition in the elderly. Detailed information was obtained in 1973–4 from 983 elderly people resident in eight places in Britain. This included a smoking history as well as a record of previous falls. No association was detected between cigarette smoking and a history of one or more falls in the previous year, after adjusting for age and sex (OR = 1.2 [0.8–1.7]).

In summary, the evidence to associate cigarette smoking with the risk of hip fracture is consistent with a weak association. Although smokers have lower bone mass than non-smokers, smoking does not appear to be a risk factor for falls in the elderly. As hip fracture risk depends not only upon osteoporosis, but also on the risk of falling, it is perhaps reasonable to expect the smoking–hip fracture relationship to be weaker than that between smoking and bone mass.

Vertebral fracture

Three studies (Daniell 1976; Aloia *et al.* 1985; Seeman *et al.* 1983) have examined the relationship between cigarette smoking and the risk of vertebral fractures (Table 8.3). Daniell (1976) reported that 76 per cent of a series of 38 women with one or more vertebral crush fractures following minor trauma had smoked at least 10 cigarettes daily for five or more years, as compared with 43 per cent of 572 female controls. This difference was statistically significant. Aloia *et al.* (1985) compared 58 post-menopausal Caucasian

Table 8.3. Cigarette smoking and the risk of vertebral fracture

Study	Subjects	Contrast	Findings
Daniell (1976)	38 women (<70 years) with crush fracture 572 clinic attenders	Smoker (10 cigarettes daily, <5 years)	OR = 4.3 (2.0–9.2)*
Aloia *et al.* (1985)	58 women with crush fracture 58 age-matched controls	Current smoker vs. non-smoker	OR = 3.4 (1.6–7.4)*
Seeman *et al.* (1983)	105 men with crush fracture 105 men with Paget's disease	Current smoker vs. non-smoker	OR = 2.3 (1.2–4.1)*

* 95% confidence intervals estimated from data provided assumed no matching.

women with vertebral crush fractures and 58 age-matched controls. Approximately twice as many cases as controls reported current smoking. Cigarette smoking is also a risk factor for vertebral crush fractures in men, with a study from the Mayo Clinic (Seeman *et al.* 1983) reporting an odds ratio for fracture of 2.3 in men who were current smokers. In this study, cigarette smoking and alcohol consumption independently influenced vertebral fracture risk and the effect of smoking became more pronounced with increasing age.

Distal radial fracture

In the only study to examine the association between smoking and distal radial fracture (Williams *et al.* 1982), a significantly greater risk of fracture was found in thin smokers, when compared with thin non-smokers, who were not taking oestrogens. The effects of smoking, body weight, and oestrogen use on the risk of distal radial fracture in this study were less marked than their effects on the risk of hip fracture.

8.5. Conclusion

There is evidence to suggest an association between cigarette smoking and the risk of sustaining hip, vertebral and distal radial fractures. The strength of the association, however, varies with fracture type. It appears to be stronger for vertebral than for hip fractures. This might reflect variation in the contribution made by osteoporosis to the incidence of these fractures.

The reasons for the dramatic secular increase in hip fracture incidence observed over the last three decades in the USA, Scandinavia, and Britain remain unknown. Cigarette smoking has been proposed as a factor which might have contributed to this increase. In Rochester, Minnesota, however, hip fracture incidence rates increased most steeply prior to the general acceptability of smoking among women (Melton *et al.* 1987). Rates have, if anything, levelled off over the period when smoking became more widespread among older women.

Population-based preventive strategies to reduce the incidence of age-related fractures are urgently required. A clear understanding of the relation between cigarette smoking and fracture risk is fundamental to the design of these strategies.

References

Aaron, J. E., *et al.* (1974). Frequency of osteomalacia and osteoporosis in fractures of the proximal femur. *Lancet*, i, 229–33.

Alderman, B. W., Weiss, N. S., Daling, J. R., Ure, C. L., and Ballard, J. H. (1986). Reproductive history and postmenopausal risk of hip and forearm fracture. *American Journal of Epidemiology*, 124, 262–7.

Aloia, J. F., Cohn, S. H., Vaswani, A., Yeh, J. K., Yuen, K., and Ellis, K. (1985). Risk factors for postmenopausal osteoporosis. *American Journal of Medicine,* **78**, 95–100.

Baker, M. R. (1980). The epidemiology and aetiology of femoral neck fracture. M.D. Thesis. University of Newcastle-upon-Tyne.

Bastow, M. D., Rawlings, J., and Allison, S. P. (1983). Undernutrition, hypothermia and injury in elderly women with fractured femur: an injury response to altered metabolism? *Lancet*, **i**, 143–6.

Boyce, W. J. (1985). Fracture of the proximal femur: studies of the distribution, risk factors, care and outcome in Oxford, 1983–1984. MFCM Thesis. Royal College of Physicians, London.

Boyce, W. J. and Vessey, M. P. (1985). Rising incidence of fracture of the proximal femur. *Lancet*, **i**, 150–1.

Cann, C. E., Genant, H. K., Kolb, F. O., and Ettinger, B. (1984). Quantitative computed tomography for prediction of vertebral fracture risk. *Metabolic Bone Disease and Related Research*, **5**, 1–7.

Cooper, C., Barker, D. J. P., Morris, J., and Briggs, R. S. J. (1987). Osteoporosis, falls and age in fracture of the proximal femur. *British Medical Journal*, **295**, 13–15.

Cummings, S. R. (1985). Are patients with hip fractures more osteoporotic? Review of the evidence. *American Journal of Medicine*, **78**, 487–94.

Cummings, S. R., Kelsey, J. L., Nevitt, M. C., and O'Dowd, K. J. (1985). Epidemiology of osteoporotic fractures. *Epidemiologic Reviews*, **7b**, 178–208.

Daniell, H. W. (1976). Osteoporosis of the slender smoker. *Archives of Internal Medicine*, **136**, 298–304.

Horsman, A., Marshall, D. H., and Peacock, M. A. (1985). A stochastic model of age-related bone loss and fractures. *Clinical Orthopaedics and Related Research*, **195**, 207–15.

Kreiger, N., Kelsey, J. L., Holford, T. R., and O'Connor, T. (1982). An epidemiologic study of hip fracture in postmenopausal women. *American Journal of Epidemiology*, **116**, 141–8.

Melton, L. J., O'Fallon, W. M., and Riggs, B. L. (1987). Secular trends in the incidence of hip fractures. *Calcified Tissue International*, **41**, 57–64.

Miller, S. W. M. and Evans, J. G. (1985). Fractures of the distal forearm in Newcastle: an epidemiological survey. *Age and Ageing*, **14**, 155–8.

Nordin, B. E. C. (1971). Clinical significance and pathogenesis of osteoporosis. *British Medical Journal*, **1**, 571–6.

Nordin, B. E. C., *et al.* (1980). Osteoporosis and osteomalacia. *Clinics in Endocrinology and Metabolism*, **9**, 177–204.

Paganini-Hill, A., Ross, R. K., Gerkins, V. R., Henderson, B. E., Arthur, M., and Mack, T. M. (1981). Menopausal estrogen therapy and hip fractures. *Annals of Internal Medicine*, **95**, 28–31.

Seeman, E., Melton, L. J., O'Fallon, W. M., and Riggs, B. L. (1983). Risk factors for spinal osteoporosis in men. *American Journal of Medicine*, **75**, 977–83.

Solomon, L. (1968). Osteoporosis and fracture of the femoral neck in the South African Bantu. *Journal of Bone and Joint Surgery*, **50b**, 2–13.

Williams, A. R., Weiss, N. S., Ure, C. L., Ballard, J., and Daling, J. R. (1982). Effect of weight, smoking and estrogen use on the risk of hip and forearm fractures in postmenopausal women. *Obstetrics and Gynaecology*, **60**, 695–9.

IV

Smoking and Other Benign Disorders

9. Smoking and gallstones

John A. Baron and Richard F. A. Logan

Abstract

The formation of gallstones is an oestrogen-related process. Exogenous oestrogen increases biliary cholesterol saturation and epidemiological studies have shown that the formation of gallstones is associated with endogenous oestrogen excretion and with the therapeutic administration of oestrogen. Any anti-oestrogenic effect of smoking might therefore be expected to reduce the frequency of gallstones and clinical gall-bladder disease (GBD). Few studies have examined the relationship between smoking and gallstones. Until recently these studies were only concerned with clinical disease and found no reduction in the frequency of clinical GBD in smokers. In fact three of these studies found an approximately twofold increase in clinical GBD in smokers. Recently, two large ultrasound surveys have reported that smoking was associated with all GBD (clinical and asymptomatic combined) in men and to a lesser extent in women.

Contrary to expectations, available data indicate that smoking, rather than protecting from GBD may promote GBD, particularly in men.

9.1. Introduction

Gallstones and cholecystitis are commonly considered to be oestrogen-related processes. Women have a higher risk than men of gallstones (Brett and Barker 1976), and pregnancy, menopausal oestrogens, and oral contraceptives (OCs) all increase their risk of clinical gall-bladder disease (GBD) (Scragg *et al.* 1984a). Exogenous oestrogens increase the lithogenicity of bile (Bennion *et al.* 1976; Davis and Kern 1976), and, moreover, urinary excretion of oestrone has been found to be higher in women with GBD than in similar women without (Scragg *et al.* 1984a). Oestrogens given to men increase the risk of clinical GBD (Bennion *et al.* 1976).

Despite apparent consistency of the data, the position is not completely straightforward. The oestrogenic link with GBD seems stronger in the young than the old; several studies have found higher relative risks for oral contraceptives, pregnancy, or obesity among younger women than among older women (Bernstein *et al.* 1977; Scragg *et al.* 1984b; Strom *et al.* 1986).

Table 9.1. Cigarette smoking and clinical gall-bladder disease

Authors	Study design and size	Confounding considered	Conclusion re: smoking
Friedman *et al.* (1966)	Population cohort 427 incidence and past cases	Age, sex	Among women, smokers had a lower risk of clinical GBD than non-smokers ($0.05 < P < 0.1$)
Boston Collaborative Drug Surveillance Program (1973)	Hospital case-control, 212 cases	Age	No relationship between clinical GBD and smoking
Diehl *et al.* (1980)	Clinical case-control, 107 cases	Age, sex, ethnic group, adiposity, diabetes	No relationship between clinical GBD and smoking
Petitti *et al.* (1981)	Population case-control (female twins), 65 cases	Age, adiposity, alcohol use, OC or oestrogen use	Cigarette smokers had an increased risk of clinical GBD OR = 2.1 (1.2–3.7)
Ramcharon *et al.* (1981)	Cohort	Not reported	No relationship between clinical GBD and smoking
Layde *et al.* (1982)	Cohort (17 000 women attending family planning clinics), 227 incident cases	Age, parity, OC use, adiposity, social class	Cigarette smokers had increased risk of clinical GBD OR = 1.63 ($P = 0.004$)
Diehl *et al.* (1987)	Cross-sectional survey, 2990 subjects	Age, sex adiposity	No relationship between GBD and smoking in women, positive relationship in men OR = 2.1 (0.8–5.4)

Some studies of oral contraceptives and GBD noted that while short-term use of OCs was associated with an increased risk, longer use may be associated with a decreased risk (Wingrave and Kay 1982)—a result that is difficult to interpret. Some investigators have failed to find any relationship at all between OCs or menopausal oestrogen therapy and the risk of clinical GBD (Smith and Gee 1979; Diehl *et al.* 1980; Williams and Johnston 1980; Layde *et al.* 1982; Kakar *et al.* 1988). In one study, oestrogens were found to predispose to cholecystectomy but not to gallstones (Everson *et al.* 1982). These results indicate that the relationship between oestrogens and GBD is complex.

To the extent that oestrogens do increase the risk of GBD, one might expect that any effect of smoking which renders a woman relatively oestrogen-deficient would decrease the risk of these problems. However, the complicated relationship between oestrogens and GBD suggests that the relationship between cigarette smoking and GBD may also be complex.

9.2. Epidemiological summary

Clinical GBD

Several studies have reported on the relationship between cigarette smoking and the risk of clinical GBD (Table 9.1). Early data from the Framingham study suggested a decreased risk of GBD in female smokers, but subsequent investigation has not confirmed this result (Friedman *et al.* 1966). In fact, one case-control study (Pettiti *et al.* 1981) has suggested an increased risk among smoking women. Using data prospectively collected during the Oxford Family Planning Association contraceptive study, Layde and colleagues also found a significant excess of clinical GBD in those smoking at study entry compared to non-smokers (Layde *et al.* 1982). Data on men with clinical GBD is even more fragmentary. A recent survey of a mixed population of Caucasian and Mexican American men and women found a twofold increase in clinical GBD in heavy smoking men but no increase in lighter smokers or in women smokers (Diehl *et al.* 1987).

Gallstone surveys

In recent years several large population surveys of GBD have been performed using ultrasonography and three of these surveys have related the presence of GBD to smoking habit. In a study of the prevalence of GBD in vegetarian women and meat-eating general practice controls, Pixley *et al.* (1985) found no association between smoking and GBD. In contrast, a survey of Italian civil servants (GREPCO 1988) found GBD to be significantly more common in men who smoked but not in women civil servants who smoked. However, the relationship with smoking was not evident from a logistic regression analysis (Table 9.2). Jorgensen's (1989) large population survey in Copenhagen has also found moderately increased risks of

Table 9.2. Cigarette smoking and the prevalence of gallstones

Authors	Study design and size	Confounding considered	Conclusion re: smoking
Pixley *et al*. (1985)	Cross-sectional survey, 130 vegetarian women 632 control women	Not reported	No relationship between gallstones and smoking
Jorgensen (1989)	Cross-sectional survey, 3418 subjects	Age, sex, education, adiposity, parity, OC use, age at menarche	Significant relationship in men (OR = 3.0), weak and insignificant relationship in women (OR = 1.2)
GREPCO (1988)	Cross-sectional survey, 2320 Italian civil servants age 20–69	Age, sex, adiposity, parity, OC use, alcohol use, blood lipids	Significant relationship in men (OR = 1.5) after age adjustment which disappeared in multivariate analyses, no relationship in women

Table 9.3. Prevalence (%) of asymptomatic and symptomatic gallstone disease according to smoking habits in Glostrup, Western Copenhagen (adapted from Jorgensen 1989)

Sex and age (years)	Never smoked		Ex smokers		Current smokers (g)					
					<14.9 g		15–24 g		>25 g	
	%	N	%	N	%	N	%	N	%	N
Men ($n = 1737$)										
30—	0.0	103	1.8	57	3.2	94	2.9	136	0.0	40
40—	0.0	94	3.5	85	2.0	101	0.0	112	4.2	48
50—	4.1	49	7.9	101	6.4	110	6.6	137	11.1	45
60—	11.4	35	14.6	137	8.8	113	11.1	113	11.1	27
Age-adjusted relative risk	1.0		2.0		1.6		2.0		2.1	
95% confidence limits	—		0.9–4.2		0.7–3.6		0.9–4.4		0.8–5.3	
Women ($n = 1681$)										
30—	2.5	121	1.7	58	4.9	123	8.7	126	6.3	16
40—	3.5	173	11.1	45	11.2	107	3.1	98	20.0	10
50—	12.1	116	10.0	70	16.9	124	18.9	106	30.0	10
60—	27.4	124	23.6	89	20.4	108	22.6	53	0.0	4
Age-adjusted relative risk	1.0		1.0		1.2		1.3		1.9	
95% confidence limits	—		0.7–1.14		0.9–1.7		0.9–1.9		0.9–4.3	

Note: Age-adjusted relative risks for ever vs. never smoking:
Men: RR—2.0, 95% CL 0.96–4.3, M-H $\chi^2 = 2.8$;
Women: RR—1.2, 95% CL 0.90–1.6, M-H$\chi^2 = 1.2$.

GBD for both men and women who smoke (Table 9.3). Using univariate analysis, neither increased risk was conventionally significant but using logistic regression to allow for the effects of age, family history, education, and marital status, the odds ratio for men who had ever smoked increased from 2 to 3 ($P = 0.02$).

Gall-bladder cancer

A related issue is that of cancer of the gall-bladder or biliary passages, both of which are associated with gallstones. There are very little published data regarding these uncommon malignancies. The large American Cancer Society prospective study found essentially no relationship between cigarette smoking and either cancer (Garfinkel and Boffetta, Chapter 1). However, Yen and colleagues (1987), in a case-control study of 67 patients with extra-hepatic bile-duct cancer and 2/3 controls with other cancers found a marked reduction in risk with smoking (OR = 0.4).

9.3. Discussion

The epidemiological data regarding cigarette smoking and GBD are mixed. Among women only one study has suggested an inverse relationship, several have found no association, and two have found a positive relationship. Of the three surveys performed, two have reported no association and the other has suggested a weak positive effect. There certainly is no strong evidence for a 'protective' effect of cigarette smoking. Among men the available data are a little more consistent in that three studies have shown an approximately two-fold increased risk of clinical GBD, or all GBD.

There are several limitations to studies of cigarette smoking and clinical GBD. Since a substantial proportion of gallstones are probably silent (Jorgensen 1987; Gracie and Ransohoff 1982), in many cases what is being studied is the relationship between cigarette smoking, on the one hand, and a combination of gallstones, precipitating factors, and health care seeking behaviour on the other (Bennion and Grundy 1978). Only population surveys using ultrasonography can overcome this problem. Studying acute cholecystitis avoids the issues of health care seeking behaviour, but leaves unresolved the possible distorting effects of factors which convert silent gallstones into the acute event.

Secondly, since there are limitations to the association between oestrogenic exposures and GBD, there are naturally limitations to the extent to which smoking could be expected to influence the risk of GBD through any influence on this aspect of hormonal milieu. From the age and duration effects evident in the relationship between OC use or pregnancy and GBD, it is possible that smoking might influence the risk of GBD only if a woman is smoking during the first years she is taking OCs, or only during early pregnancy. There are no data available relevant to these issues, but in any case, clarification must await more precise specification of the relationship between oestrogens and GBD.

Finally, of course, the studies are subject to the usual issues of bias and confounding. Since both the risk of GBD and cigarette smoking are related to reproductive behaviour, it is desirable for these factors to be controlled for in any analysis. Alcohol intake may similarly confound the smoking/gall-stone relationship (Scragg *et al.* 1984b; Diehl *et al.* 1987). Weight is a more complicated issue, as changes in weight may be part of the causal chain by which smoking could alter the risk of hormone related processes. These factors, with the limited data available, mean that, while cigarette smoking is in general associated with GBD (more so in men than women) the position is still inconclusive.

References

Bennion, L. J. and Grundy, S. M. (1978). Risk factors for the development of cholelithiasis in man. *New England Journal of Medicine*, **299**, 1161–6, 1221–6.

Bennion, L. J., Ginsberg, R. L., Garnick, M. B., and Bennett, P. H. (1976). Effects of oral contraceptives on the gallbladder bile of normal women. *New England Journal of Medicine*, **294**, 189–92.

Bernstein, R. A., *et al.* (1977). Gallbladder disease—II. Utilization of the life table method in obtaining clinically useful information. *Journal of Chronic Disease*, **30**, 529–41.

Boston Collaborative Drug Surveillance Programme (1973). Oral contraceptives and venous thromboembolic disease, surgically confirmed gallbladder disease, and breast tumours. *Lancet*, **i**, 1399–404.

Brett, M. and Barker, D. J. P. (1976). The world distribution of gallstones. *International Journal of Epidemiology*, **5**, 335–41.

Davis, R. A. and Kern, F. Jr. (1976). Effects of ethinyl estradiol and phenobarbital on bile acide synthesis and biliary bile acide and cholesterol excretion. *Gastroenterology*, **70**, 1130–5.

Diehl, A. K., Stern, M. P., Ostrower, W. S., and Friedman, P. C. (1980). Prevalence of clinical gallbladder disease in Mexican-American, Anglo and black women. *Southern Medical Journal*, **73**, 438–42.

Diehl, A. K., Hafner, S. M., Hazada, H. P., and Stern, M. P. (1987). Coronary risk factors and clinical gallbladder disease: an approach to the prevention of gallstones? *American Journal of Public Health*, **77**, 841–5.

Everson, R. B., Byar, D. P., and Bischoff, A. J. (1982). Estrogen predisposes to cholecystectomy but not to stones. *Gastroenterology*, **82**, 4–8.

Friedman, D. B., Friedman, G. D., and Klatsky, A. L. (1966). The epidemiology of gallbladder disease: observations in the Framingham Study. *Journal of Chronic Disease*, **19**, 273–92.

Gracie, W. A. and Ransohoff, D. F. (1982). The natural history of silent gallstones. The innocent gallstone is not a myth. *New England Journal of Medicine*, **307**, 798–800.

GREPCO (Rome Group for Epidemiology and Prevention of Chololithiasis) (1984).

Prevalence of gallstone disease in an Italian adult female population. *American Journal of Epidemiology*, **119**, 796–805.
GREPCO (Rome Group for Epidemiology and Prevention of Chololithiasis) (1988). The epidemiology of gallstone disease in Rome Part II. Factors associated with the disease. *Hepatology*, **8**, 907–13.
Jorgensen, T. (1987). Prevalence of gall-stones in a Danish population. *American Journal of Epidemiology*, **126**, 912–21.
Jorgensen, T. (1989). Gallstones in a Danish population. Relation to weight, physical activity, smoking, coffee consumption and diabetes mellitus. *Gut*, **30**, 528–34.
Kakar, F., Weiss, N. S., and Strite, S. A. (1988). Non-contraceptive estrogen use and the risk of gallstone disease in women. *American Journal of Public Health*, **78**, 564–6.
Layde, P. M., Vessey, M. P., and Yeates, D. (1982). Risk factors for gall-bladder disease: a cohort study of young women attending family planning clinics. *Journal of Epidemiology and Community Health*, **36**, 274–8.
Petitti, D. B., Friedman, G. D., and Klatsky, A. L. (1981). Association of a history of gallbladder disease with a reduced concentration of high-density lipoprotein cholesterol. *New England Journal of Medicine*, **304**, 1396–8.
Pixley, F., Wilson, D., McPherson, K., and Mann, J. (1985). Effect of vegetarianism on development of gall stones in women. *British Medical Journal*, **291**, 11–12.
Ramcharon, S., *et al.* (1981). *The Walnut Creek Drug Study*, Vol II. Department of Health and Human Services, Washington.
Scragg, R. K. R., MacMichael, A. J., and Seamark, R. F. (1984a). Oral contraceptives, pregnancy, and endogenous oestrogen in gall stone disease—a case-control study. *British Medical Journal*, **288**, 1795–9.
Scragg, R. K. R., MacMichael, A. J., and Baghurst, P. A. (1984b). Diet, alcohol, and relative weight in gall stone disease: a case-control study. *British Medical Journal*, **288**, 1113–9.
Smith, D. A. and Gee, M. J. (1979). A dietary survey to determine the relationship between diet and cholelithiasis. *American Journal of Clinical Nutrition*, **32**, 1519–26.
Strom, B. L., *et al.* (1986). Oral contraceptives and other risk factors for gallbladder disease. *Clinical Pharmacology Therapy*, **39**, 335–41.
Williams, C. N. and Johnston, J. L. (1980). Prevalence of gallstone risk factors in Caucasian women in a rural Canadian community. *Canadian Medical Association Journal*, **120**, 664–8.
Wingrave, S. J. and Kay, C. R. (1982). Oral contraceptives and gallbladder disease. *Lancet*, **ii**, 957–9.
Yen, S., Hsieh, C-C., and MacMahon, B. (1987). Extrahepatic bile duct cancer and smoking, beverage consumption, past medical history, and oral-contraceptive use. *Cancer*, **59**, 2112–16.

10. Cigarette smoking and skin atrophy in women. A possible connection?

Mark Brincat

Abstract

Smokers as a group have a lower serum oestradiol and an earlier menopause. Both these factors have been shown to lead to thinner skin and a lower skin collagen content. Although direct work on smokers has not yet been carried out, the hypothesis that cigarette smoking could affect the skin, especially in women, through a hormonal mechanism is discussed.

10.1. Introduction

Apart from anecdotal observations, no direct work has been carried out linking cigarette smoking with the skin in men or women. This chapter, therefore, must remain hypothetical.

There do exist mechanisms whereby smoking can and probably does affect the skin. Smokers as a group have been shown to have an earlier menopause than non-smokers (Jick *et al.* 1977). In addition, one study has shown that cigarette smoking reduced oestrogen excretion in pre-menopausal women (MacMahon *et al.* 1982), possibly due to liver enzymes induced by cigarette smoke, thereby affecting steroid metabolism (Weg 1987).

Attempts have been made to show that skin collagen content and skin thickness decline with the years since the menopause and that this sharp decline bears no relationship to the chronological age of a woman (Brincat *et al.* 1987a,b).

10.2. Methods

One hundred and forty eight post-menopausal women were studied (Brincat 1987b). They had not been on any form of sex hormone treatment since their menopause. These women had their skin collagen content, their skin thickness, their metacarpal index, and their forearm bone mineral content assessed. Skin collagen content was assessed from 3 mm punch biopsy forceps taken from the right thigh. Hydroxyproline was extracted and collagen content then calculated (Woessner 1960; Neuman and Logan 1950).

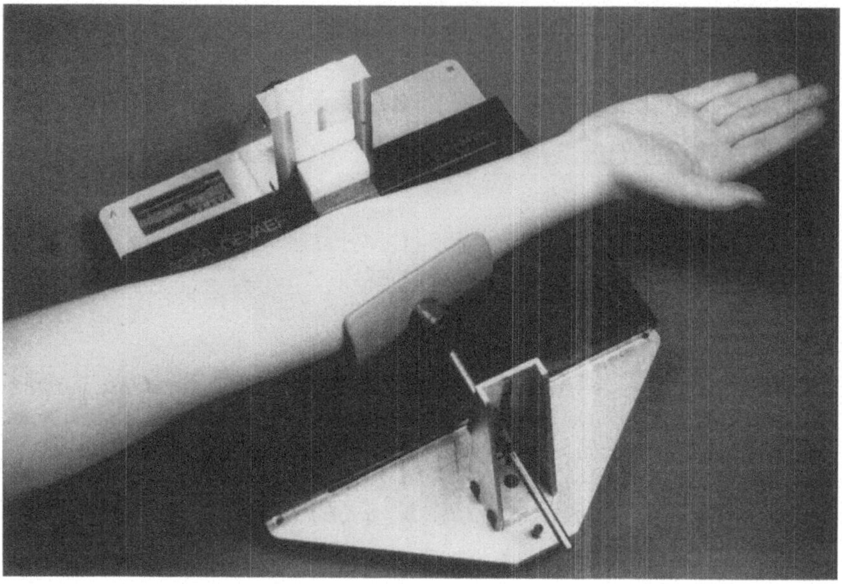

Fig. 10.1. Measurement of skin thickness of the forearm using X-ray frame.

The skin thickness on the ulnar aspect of the forearm was measured using the X-ray frame in Fig. 10.1. Because skin is not radiotranslucent, compression of the skin with a wooden block makes the top of the epidermis and the bottom of the dermis clearly visible and it is this portion of the skin, which is predominantly the dermis, that was of interest.

Using the same equipment, a second exposure over the second metacarpal enabled measurement of the metacarpal index. This is a ratio of the cortical area of the metacarpal to the total area. This method was described by Gallagher (1983).

A single beam photon absorptiometer was used to measure the bone mineral content of the radius and ulna of the left forearm at 3 cm and at 8 cm from the epicondyles.

10.3. Results

All the variables measured, apart from the bone mineral content at 3 cm, showed wide individual variation. A highly significant correlation was found between changes in thigh skin collagen, forearm skin thickness, metacarpal index, and the mean bone mineral content at 8 cm with the years since the menopause (Figs 10.2 and 10.3), with all these variables declining with the duration of time from the menopause (Figs 10.2 and 10.3).

The average linear decline in skin collagen content was calculated to be

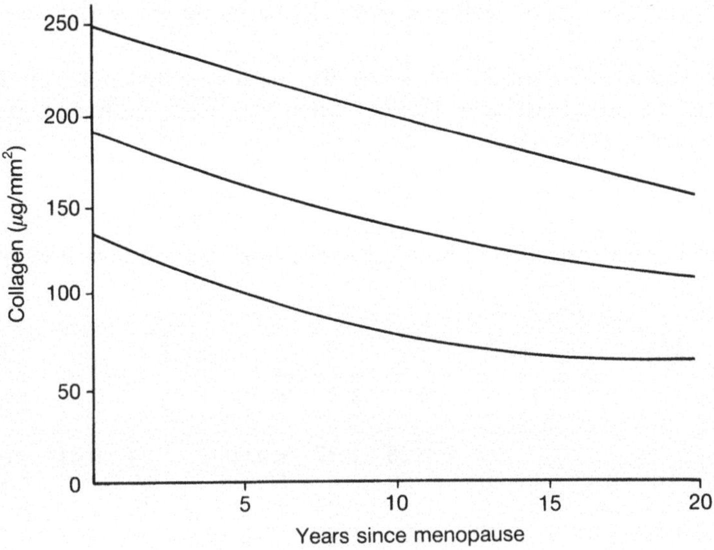

Fig. 10.2. Thigh skin collagen content (Mean ± s.d.) in untreated post-menopausal women.

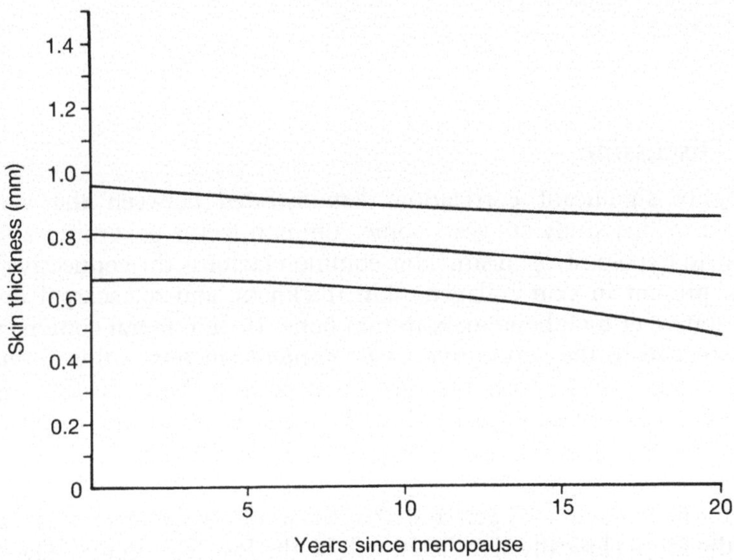

Fig. 10.3. Forearm skin thickness (Mean ± s.d.) in 133 post-menopausal women.

2.1 per cent post-menopausal year and that of skin thickness 1.13 per cent which was virtually identical to the decline in metarcarpal index, 1.22 per cent (Brincat 1987b). The decline in bone mineral content at 8 cm was 0.94 per cent per post-menopausal year (Brincat 1987b). These declines were in fact not linear; the rate of decline was much sharper in the initial years than in the latter ones.

Highly significant correlations were also demonstrated between all the parameters measured (Brincat 1987b) when sets from individual patients were compared (Table 10.1).

Table 10.1. Correlations between various parameters in post-menopausal women

	MI			SC			ST		
	N	*r*	*P*	*N*	*r*	*P*	*N*	*r*	*P*
MI				128	0.37	<0.0001	124	0.41	<0.0001
BMC 3 cm	59	0.38	<0.001	59		NS	59		NS
BMC 8 cm	63	0.41	<0.001	63	0.24	<0.05	63	0.24	<0.05
ST	124	0.41	<0.0001	109	0.45	<0.0001			

MI, metacarpal index; SC, thigh skin collagen content; ST, forearm skin thickness; BMC 3 cm, bone mineral content 3 cm up the forearm from the styloid process; BMC 8 cm, bone mineral content 8 cm up the forearm from the styloid process.

NS, not significant.

10.4. Discussion

The highly significant correlation demonstrated between the variables measured in this study suggests some common factor governing a similar response to hypo-oestrogenism. This common factor is the connective tissue element present in skin collagen, skin thickness, and metacarpal index, a representative of total bone mass in that bone. Bone mineral content would also be related to the connective tissue content since it is this connective tissue content that supports the mineral content in bone. In fact smokers have been described as having a low bone mass and an increased risk of osteoporotic fractures (Cooper, Chapter 8; Law, Chapter 7; Aloria *et al.* 1985).

The lower the skin collagen and skin thickness at the start of the menopause, the more clinically significant will be the loss that occurs. The earlier menopause experienced by smokers (Jick *et al.* 1977) could further compound the problem and make smokers more at risk of having thin skin with a lower skin collagen content at an earlier age. This thin skin with a low skin collagen content would parallel a more clinically significant decline in a bone mass, since all these parameters would already be on the lower side of normal at the start of the menopause.

10.5. Conclusion

Thin skin containing lower skin collagen content is more likely to occur in women smokers because of the anti-oestrogenic effect of cigarette smoke. Properly conducted studies are, however, needed to verify this hypothesis.

References

Aloria, J. F., Cohn, S. H., Vaswani, A., Yen, J. K., Yuen, K., and Ellis, K. (1985). Risk factors for postmenopausal osteoporosis. *American Journal of Medicine*, **78**, 95–100.

Brincat, M., *et al.* (1987a). Decline in skin collagen content and metacarpal index after the menopause and its prevention with sex hormone replacement. *British Journal of Obstetrics and Gynaecology*, **94**, 126–9.

Brincat, M., *et al.* (1987b). A study of the relationship of skin collagen content, skin thickness and bone mass in the postmenopausal woman. *Obstetrics and Gynaecology*, **70**, 840–5.

Gallagher, J. C. and Nordin, B. E. C. (1983). Estrogens and calcium metabolism. *Frontiers in Hormone Research*, **2**, 98.

Jick, H., Porter, J., and Morrison, A. S. (1977). Relation between smoking and age of natural menopause. *Lancet*, **i**, 1354–5.

MacMahon, B., Trichopoulos, D., Cole, P., and Brown, J. (1982). Cigarette smoking and urinary oestrogens. *New England Journal of Medicine*, **307**, 1062–5.

Neuman, R. E. and Logan, M. A. (1950). The determination of collagen and elastin in tissues. *Journal of Biological Chemistry*, **186**, 549.

Weg, R. B. (1987). Demography. In *The menopause: physiology and pharmacology* (ed. D. R. Mischell Jr), pp. 23–40. Year Book Medical Publishers, Chicago.

Woessner, T. E. Jr (1960). The determination of hydroxyproline in tissue and protein samples containing small proportions of this amino acid. *Archives of Biochemistry and Biophysics*, **93**, 440.

11. Smoking and prostatic hypertrophy

Alan S. Morrison

Abstract

Incidental findings in a few studies suggest an inverse association between cigarette smoking and surgery for prostatic hypertrophy, but little if any association between smoking and prostatic hypertrophy that is not surgically treated. There is no evidence of a relation between intensity of smoking and risk of prostatic hypertrophy. Two studies show a lower risk in current smokers than in ex-smokers. The relation between smoking and prostatic hypertrophy is uncertain. Even if there is an association it may not be causal. There may be characteristics of smokers that result in a reduced frequency of surgery (compared to non-smokers) for a given degree of urinary obstruction. Or, smoking may be an index of other (unidentified) exposures that are the actual causes of severe prostatic hypertrophy.

11.1. Introduction

Hospitalization and surgery for urinary obstruction from prostatic hypertrophy (PH) is a major public health problem. PH ranks among the most common discharge diagnoses for men 65 years of age and older who are admitted to short-stay hospitals. The probability that a 40-year-old man will have an operation for PH, if he lives to age 80, has been estimated as 10 per cent to 30 per cent (Lytton *et al.* 1968; Glynn *et al.* 1985). Furthermore, PH may be a risk factor for prostatic cancer (Hutchison 1976).

The symptoms of PH vary from non-existent or mild, to severe. PH is chronic and progressive in that there is a general, although not absolute, tendency for mild cases to progress and ultimately require surgery (Walsh 1979). However, a substantial proportion of operated cases have not had a diagnosis of PH as a result of symptoms before the current episode (Glynn *et al.* 1985).

Histologically, PH ranges from purely adenomatous to purely fibromuscular hyperplasia. The glandular epithelium may be secretory or non-secretory, and may or may not show evidence of dysplasia or atypia. Additional epithelial changes have also been described (Mostofi and Price 1973;

Franks 1976). Detailed histologic descriptions of surgical specimens are not given routinely, and terminology has been used inconsistently.

Despite the importance of PH, there has been very little study of its relationship to environmental risk factors. A few reports, however, suggest the possibility of an inverse association between cigarette smoking and PH.

11.2. Epidemiological summary

Greenwald *et al.* (1974) carried out a retrospective follow-up study for the primary purpose of comparing the rate of prostatic cancer between 838 men with surgically confirmed PH and 802 control subjects selected from men who had been hospitalized for surgical treatment of a condition other than prostatic disease or cancer. In their report, Greenwald *et al.* summarized the smoking histories of the PH patients and the controls. Fifty-eight per cent of the PH patients were current smokers, compared to 65 per cent of the controls. As computed from the published data, the relative risk of PH in current smokers compared to non-smokers and ex-smokers is 0.74, with an approximate 95 per cent confidence interval (CI) 0.60–0.93. There was little difference in risk between heavier vs. lighter smokers.

Armenian *et al.* (1975) compared the frequencies of several demographic and environmental factors between cases of PH and controls in two overlapping analyses based on patients who had been admitted to Roswell Park Memorial Institute. The first analysis involved PH patients and controls who had been discharged with a diagnosis other than cancer in the period 1957–65. Armenian *et al.* reported 'no major differences' between these groups in smoking patterns, although the data were not presented. The second comparison involved subjects in a retrospective follow-up study of PH and prostatic cancer based on patients admitted in the period 1945–65 (Armenian *et al.* 1974). From data in the 1975 paper, the relative risk of PH in smokers compared to non-smokers can be estimated as 0.4. No data were presented on risk in relation to frequency of smoking, or quitting.

Morrison (1978) evaluated the association of cigarette smoking and PH in data collected by the Boston Collaborative Drug Surveillance Program. The subjects were identified at 24 Boston-area hospitals in 1972 and included 219 patients who had been surgically treated for PH, 97 patients with a discharge diagnosis of PH that had not been surgically treated, and 4669 controls who did not have prostatitis or cancer of any site. Compared to non-smokers, the relative risk of surgically treated PH was estimated as 0.5 (0.3–0.7, 95 per cent CI) in current smokers, 0.7 (0.5–1.0) in ex-smokers, and 1.0 (0.6–1.6) in smokers of tobacco other than cigarettes. Among current smokers, there was very little variation in risk with amount smoked. For PH that had not been surgically treated, the relative risk was estimated as 0.9 (0.5–1.5) in current smokers compared with non-smokers.

Risk factors for PH were investigated in the Normative Aging Study, a prospective follow-up study of 2280 male volunteers who were 21–81 years old at entry who had no history of serious chronic diseases such as heart disease, cancer, or diabetes, and no clinical evidence of hypertension or glucose intolerance (Glynn *et al.* 1985). The intake period was 1961–70. Subjects were re-examined at intervals that depended on age. A smoking history was obtained at the second examination. Of the 1937 men with no history of PH at entry, 336 had a subsequent diagnosis of the condition, whether or not surgically treated. A history of cigarette smoking was only slightly (although inversely) associated with this outcome. There were, however, 57 men who developed PH that was surgically treated, and cigarette smoking was inversely associated with surgically treated PH.

In a study described by Ross *et al.* in Chapter 3 the relative risk of surgical treatment for PH was found to be 0.8 in current smokers, and 1.1 in ex-smokers, compared to non-smokers.

In contrast to most of the findings described above, Araki *et al.* (1983) reported, 'No statistically significant difference (in PH) was observed with regard to consumption of alcohol, Japanese tea, coffee, tobacco . . .'. This was a small study, however (100 cases, 100 controls), and it appears that some, and perhaps most, of the cases had not been treated surgically. Moreover, data were not given in support of the statement quoted.

11.3. Discussion

Taken together, these studies suggest an inverse association between cigarette smoking and PH that is surgically treated, but little if any association between smoking and PH that is not surgically treated. The studies described, however, were not designed specifically to evaluate a possible smoking–PH association, and data on the relation of risk to the intensity, duration, and timing of the exposure are quite limited. The studies of Greenwald *et al.* and of Morrison do not show a relation between frequency of smoking and risk of PH. The Greenwald data, however, were obtained from hospital records, which are unlikely to yield smoking histories of high quality. As far as current vs. past smoking is concerned, the results of Greenwald *et al.*, Morrison, and Ross *et al.* suggest that the protective effect is conveyed at least by current smoking. Only the reports by Morrison and by Ross *et al.* give data on ex-smokers, and no information is available on change in risk with time since quitting.

Because surgery for PH may be done electively, there is a question as to whether an association of PH with an environmental agent such as smoking reflects determinants of a decision to operate rather than determinants of the development or progression of PH itself. A decision to operate might depend on the presence or absence of other diseases, or on social class. Although smoking history by itself probably does not influence the likelihood of an operation, it might do so through one of these other factors. For example, an operation would be less likely to be done in someone with PH who also has a smoking-related condition such as heart or lung disease, than in someone who is otherwise well. However, confounding of this type is not likely to explain a smoking–PH association. Thus, Morrison's analysis was restricted to subjects who did not have cardiovascular disease or chronic lung disease as a primary diagnosis. Moreover, only a small proportion of men are disqualified from operation for medical reasons (Grayhack and Sadlowski 1976). Therefore, the amount of distortion that relationships between smoking and heart or lung disease can introduce into an observed association of smoking and surgically treated PH also is small.

There is additional evidence against the idea that aspects of the provision of medical care explain the smoking–PH link: Glynn *et al.* (1985) observed an association between *low* social class and surgery for PH, whereas the reverse would be expected if economic conditions were an important determinant of prostatic surgery. The inverse association of smoking and PH as reported by Glynn *et al.* included control of social class. Finally, the reports of Greenwald *et al.* (1974), Armenian *et al.* (1974, 1975) and Morrison (1978) utilized hospital controls, whose level of access to medical care presumably was similar to that of the corresponding cases.

It is possible that an association of smoking and PH is the result of unidentified causes of the disease that are associated with smoking, or of a greater tendency of non-smokers than of smokers to seek medical attention for a given level of symptoms. Little information on either of these possibilities is now available.

An inverse association between smoking and PH would not have immediate disease-control implications, but this relationship, if confirmed, would offer an important opportunity to better understand the aetiology of the disease, with the possibility of developing preventive measures or non-surgical treatments. Although the endocrinologic chain of events has not been worked out, several lines of evidence indicate that the occurrence and progression of PH is hormonally mediated. Early castration prevents PH, and castration in the mature male leads to atrophy of the epithelial component of the prostate (Lee and Jesik 1983). In several clinical investigations, plasma or serum hormone levels have been compared between PH cases and controls (Vermeulen and deSy 1976; Hammond *et al.* 1978; Ortega *et al.* 1979; Bartsch *et al.* 1979; Drafta *et al.* 1982; Rannikko and Adlercreutz 1983; Wright *et al.* 1985). These studies are not strong individually, but as a group they suggest an association of PH with the blood level of dihydrotestosterone (DHT). A few of the studies also suggest case-control differences in testosterone or oestradiol, but these differences were smaller than those in DHT, and not as consistent.

Smoking also appears to cause endocrine changes that may lead to detectable health effects. In women, luteal phase oestrogen excretion has been found to be lower in current smokers compared to ex-smokers (MacMahon *et al.* 1982), and a mechanism has been suggested for the anti-oestrogenic effect of smoking (Michnovicz *et al.* 1986). Women who smoke tend to have an earlier menopause (Jick *et al.* 1977) and higher frequency of osteoporosis (Baron 1984) than non-smokers do, and smoking has been reported to be inversely related to endometrial cancer and benign breast disease (Baron 1984; Lesko *et al.* 1985; Berkowitz *et al.* 1985), diseases that are believed to have hormonal causes. Studies of the relation of smoking to hormone levels in men have been stimulated primarily by interest in the causes of cardiovascular disease. The findings suggest that smoking results in increased oestrogen levels in men. The relation of smoking to the level of DHT does not yet appear to have been evaluated. If smoking is a protective factor for PH, then smoking history might serve to identify patterns of hormonal change that would be useful to investigate further, with respect to the development of PH.

Acknowledgement

Supported by PHS grant DK 35402.

References

Araki, H., Watanabe, H., Mishina, T., and Nakao, M. (1983). High-risk group for benign prostatic hypertrophy. *Prostate*, **4**, 253–64.

Armenian, H. K., Lilienfeld, A. M., Diamond, E. L., and Bross, I. D. J. (1974). Relation between benign prostatic hyperplasia and cancer of the prostate. *Lancet*, **2**, 115–7.

Armenian, H. K., Lilienfeld, A. M., Diamond, E. L., and Bross, I. D. J. (1975). Epidemiologic characteristics of patients with prostatic neoplasms. *American Journal of Epidemiology*, **102**, 47–54.

Baron, J. A. (1984). Smoking and estrogen-related disease. *American Journal of Epidemiology*, **119**, 9–22.

Bartsch, W., Becker, H., Pinkenburg, F.-A., and Krieg, M. (1979). Hormone blood levels and their inter-relationships in normal men and men with benign prostatic hyperplasia (BPH). *Acta Endocrinologia*, **90**, 727–36.

Berkowitz, G. S., Canny, P. F., LiVolsi, V. A., Merino, M. J., O'Connor, T. Z., and Kelsey, J. L. (1985). Cigarette smoking and benign breast disease. *Journal of Epidemiology and Community Health*, **39**, 308–13.

Drafta, D., Proca, E., Zamfir, V., Schlindler, A. E., Neascu, E., and Stroe, E. (1982). Plasma steroids in benign prostatic hypertrophy and carcinoma of the prostate. *Journal of Steroid Biochemistry*, **17**, 689–93.

Franks, L. M. (1976). Gross and microscopic anatomy. In *Benign prostatic hyperplasia* (ed. J. T. Grayhack, J. D. Wilson, and M. J. Scherbenske), pp. 63–89. DHEW Publications No. (NIH) 76–1113, National Institutes of Health, Bethesda.

Glynn, R. J., Campion, E. W., Bouchard, G. R., and Silbert, J. E. (1985). The development of benign prostatic hyperplasia among volunteers in the Normative Aging Study. *American Journal of Epidemiology*, **121**, 78–90.

Grayhack, J. T. and Sadlowski, R. W. (1976). Results of surgical treatment of benign prostatic hyperplasia. In *Benign prostatic hyperplasia* (ed. J. T. Grayhack, J. D. Wilson, and M. J. Scherbenske), pp. 125–34. DHEW Publication No. (NIH) 76–1113, National Institutes of Health, Bethesda.

Greenwald, P., Kirmss, V., Polan, A. K., and Dick, V. S. (1974). Cancer of the prostate among men with benign prostatic hyperplasia. *Journal of the National Cancer Institute*, 53, 335–40.

Hammond, G. L., Kintturi, M., Vihko, P., and Vihko, R. (1978). Serum steroids in normal males and patients with prostatic diseases. *Clinical Endocrinology*, 9, 113–22.

Hutchison, G. B. (1976). Etiology of prostatic cancer. *Seminars in Oncology*, 3, 151–9.

Jick, H., Porter, J., and Morrison, A. S. (1977). Relation between smoking and age of natural menopause. *Lancet*, i, 1354–5.

Lee, C. and Jesik, C. (1983). Effects of castration, estrogen, and androgen administration. In *Benign prostatic hypertrophy* (ed. F. H. Hinman, Jr.), pp. 229–34. Springer-Verlag, New York.

Lesko, S. M., Rosenberg, L., Kaufman, D. W., Helmrich, S. P., Miller, D. R., and Strom, B. (1985). Cigarette smoking and the risk of endometrial cancer. *New England Journal of Medicine*, 313, 593–6.

Lytton, B., Emery, J. M., and Harvard, B. M. (1968). The incidence of benign prostatic obstruction. *Journal of Urology*, 99, 639–45.

MacMahon, B., Trichopoulos, D., Cole, P., and Brown, J. (1982). Cigarette smoking and urinary estrogens. *New England Journal of Medicine*, 307, 1062–5.

Michnovicz, J. J., Herschcopf, R. J., Naganuma, H., Bradlow, H. L., and Fishman, J. (1986). Increased 2-hydroxylation of estradiol as a possible mechanism for the anti-estrogenic effect of cigarette smoking. *New England Journal of Medicine*, 315, 1305–9.

Morrison, A. S. (1978). Prostatic hypertrophy in greater Boston. *Journal of Chronic Disease*, 31, 357–62.

Mostofi, F. K. and Price, E. B. (1973). Tumors of the male genital system. *Atlas of tumor pathology second series*, Number 8. Armed Forces Institute of Pathology, Washington.

Ortega, E., Ruiz, E., Mendoza, M. C., Martin-Andres, A., and Osorio, C. (1979). Plasma steroid and protein hormone concentrations in patients with benign prostatic hypertrophy and in normal men. *Experientia*, 35, 844–5.

Rannikko, S. and Adlercreutz, H. (1983). Plasma estradiol, free testosterone, sex hormone binding globulin binding capacity, and prolactin in benign prostatic hyperplasia and prostatic cancer. *Prostate*, 4, 223–9.

Vermeulen, A. and deSy, W. (1976). Androgens in patients with benign prostatic hyperplasia before and after prostatectomy. *Journal of Clinical Endocrinology and Metabolism*, 43, 1250–4.

Walsh, P. C. (1979). Benign prostatic hyperplasia. In *Campbell's Urology* (4th edn), Vol. 2 (ed. J. H. Harrison, *et al.*), pp. 949–64. W. B. Saunders, Philadelphia.

Wright, F., Poizat, R., Bongini, M., Bozzolan, F., Doukani, A., and Mauvais-Jarvis, P. (1985). Decreased urinary 5a-androstane-3a, 17b-diol glucuroxide excretion in patients with benign prostatic hyperplasia. *Journal of Clinical Endocrinology and Metabolism*, 60, 294–8.

12. Smoking and inflammatory bowel disease

Richard F. A. Logan

Abstract

In 1982 attention was drawn to the relationship between smoking and inflammatory bowel disease by the observation that patients with ulcerative colitis (UC) were predominantly non-smokers. Subsequent studies have confirmed this finding, but the association has been variable and mainly accounted for by an increased risk of UC in ex-smokers. After pooling the results of eight case-control studies, smokers at time of symptom onset or diagnosis, when compared to never smokers, had a relative risk (RR, 95 per cent confidence limits) of UC of 0.47 (0.39, 0.56) and ex-smokers a RR of 1.9 (1.6, 2.2). In contrast a positive *association between smoking and Crohn's disease (CD) has been demonstrated in the same studies with smokers having a RR of CD of 2.4 (2.0, 2.9) and ex-smokers a RR of 1.5 (1.1, 1.9). It is still unclear whether the increased risks of both diseases in ex-smokers are due to recall bias. In only two studies have prospectively collected smoking data been available; both have confirmed the positive association between smoking and CD and the negative association with UC.*

The mechanism by which smoking influences either disease is obscure. Current evidence could indicate two effects but, assuming a common pathogenesis, a single effect—either the promotion of CD or protection from UC—could explain the contrasting associations demonstrated in epidemiological studies.

12.1. Introduction

Despite considerable research, the aetiology of inflammatory bowel disease (IBD) remains disappointingly obscure. For both diseases, the most widely accepted hypothesis broadly involves an infective agent(s) which triggers an abnormal immune response (Kirsner and Shorter 1982). Until recently the only environmental factor that had been demonstrated with any consistency was increased refined sugar consumption by patients with Crohn's disease (Persson *et al.* 1987). The suggestion that cigarette smoking might be another factor arose from the serendipitous finding of Harries *et al.* (1982) that only 8 per cent of patients with ulcerative colitis (UC) were currently smokers, compared to 44 per cent of their controls. In retrospect a similar relationship had been noted earlier in Sweden but had been overlooked (Samuelsson 1976). A positive association between smoking and CD was subsequently reported (Logan *et al.* 1983) and many studies since have confirmed one or both associations.

12.2. Epidemiological summary

Data on the relationship of smoking to IBD have been obtained mainly from case-control studies and clinical case series without controls. The only studies in which smoking data have been collected prospectively are two cohort studies of oral contraceptive users in which smoking habit was ascertained at recruitment (Vessey *et al.* 1986; Logan and Kay 1989). This review concentrates on eight case-control studies, all of which have used

(1) a series of hospital-diagnosed prevalent cases with;
(2) a community based or 'suitable' hospital control series; and
(3) have approached cases and controls in a similar way (Table 12.1).

Each study has been treated as a separate stratum in an extended Mantel–Haenszel analysis with those reporting being never-smokers at the time of the case's disease onset being the referrent level [relative risk estimate (RR) = 1.0]. The results for UC and CD are shown in Tables 12.2 and 12.3 respectively.

Primary or secondary associations?

Initially it was unclear whether non-smoking by UC patients preceded diagnosis or disease onset (Jick and Walker 1983). The eight case-control studies in Table 12.1 have all enquired about habits at diagnosis and/or symptom onset and all have found UC to be associated with non-smoking and CD with smoking. However when smokers have been categorized as current, ex- and never-smokers, the inverse relationship between current smoking and UC becomes inconsistent while a consistently increased risk for ex-smokers is evident (Table 12.2). For CD the results are more homogeneous with CD being fairly consistently two to three times more common in smokers than never-smokers (Table 12.3). CD also appears to be associated with ex-smoking but not as strongly as in UC.

If current and ex-smokers at disease onset are then considered together as 'ever-smokers' (a category probably less prone to recall bias) the association with CD remains significant and consistent while the relationship between ever-smoking and UC is weak and inconsistent.

Ex-smoking—real effect or recall bias?

World-wide, IBD remains uncommon with an annual incidence of less than 20 per 100 000. As a result, all case-control studies so far reported have

Table 12.1. Smoking and inflammatory bowel disease—study methods in eight case-control studies

Study	Centre	Enquiry method	UC*/CD*	Source of controls	Smoking habit at onset of symptoms (S) or diagnosis (D)
Logan *et al.* (1984, 1986)	Nottingham, UK	Postal questionnaire	175/131	Community	S
Tobin *et al.* (1987)	Liverpool, UK	Postal questionnaire	131/127	Community	S
Franceschi *et al.* (1987)	Milan, Italy	Interview (? by doctor)	124/109	Hospital	D&S
Lindberg *et al.* (1988)	Orebro, Sweden	Postal questionnaire	258/144	Community	D
Benoni and Nilsson (1987)	Lund, Sweden	Interview	173/155	Community	D&S
Calkins *et al.* (1984)	Baltimore, US	?	85/132	Community and hospital	?
Boyko *et al.* (1987)	Washington State, US	Telephone interview	212/-	Community	S
Sandler and Holland (1988)	North Carolina, US	Postal questionnaire	170/298	Volunteered by cases	D

* All used prevalent cases.

Table 12.2. Relative risk of ulcerative colitis for current, ex- and ever smokers compared to never smokers at disease onset or diagnosis

Centre	RR current smokers	95% CL	RR ex-smokers	95% CL	RR ever smokers	95% CL
Nottingham	0.23	0.14–0.38	2.1	1.3–3.4	0.67	0.46–0.98
Liverpool	0.18	0.10–0.33	1.5	0.8–2.8	0.46	0.28–0.75
Milan	0.61	0.35–1.0	3.4	2.0–5.9	1.3	0.83–2.0
Orebro, Sweden	0.64	0.45–0.90	2.1	1.4–3.3	0.94	0.69–1.3
Lund, Sweden	0.33	0.21–0.53	1.6	0.9–2.6	0.59	0.41–0.86
Baltimore	0.62	0.29–1.3	1.1	0.5–2.2	0.83	0.45–1.5
Washington State	0.64	0.41–1.0	1.9	1.1–3.3	0.99	0.68–1.5
North Carolina	0.80	0.46–1.4	1.4	0.8–2.5	1.0	0.66–1.6
Combined	0.47*	0.39–0.56	1.9†	1.6–2.3	0.82‡	0.71–0.95

χ^2 for heterogeneity—*27.8, $P<0.001$; †9.5, $P>0.5$; ‡16.1, $P<0.05$.

Table 12.3. Relative risk of Crohn's disease for current, ex- and ever smokers compared to never smokers at disease onset or diagnosis

Centre	RR current smokers	95% CL	RR ex-smokers	95% CL	RR ever smokers	95% CL
Nottingham	4.2	2.5–6.8	1.5	0.7–3.0	3.3	2.0–5.2
Liverpool	3.2	1.9–5.5	1.6	0.5–4.1	2.9	1.7–4.9
Milan	2.9	1.8–4.9	2.4	1.2–5.0	2.8	1.7–4.6
Lund	2.2	1.4–3.3	0.7	0.3–2.0	1.9	1.3–2.9
Orebro, Sweden	2.0	1.3–3.1	1.8	0.8–3.8	2.0	1.3–3.0
Baltimore	2.1	1.2–3.5	0.8	0.4–1.7	1.6	0.99–2.6
North Carolina	1.9	1.3–2.8	1.7	1.0–3.0	2.2	1.3–2.6
Combined	2.4*	2.0–2.9	1.5†	1.1–1.9	2.2‡	1.8–2.6

χ^2 for heterogeneity—*8.8, $P>0.1$; †6.8, $P>0.1$; ‡7.7, $P>0.1$.

used prevalent cases to enquire about smoking habits usually five or more years earlier. If smokers tended to stop smoking close to disease onset or between onset of symptoms and diagnosis, then recall bias would be particularly important. Two clinical case series have found an apparent excess of cases with onset of UC shortly after stopping smoking; neither study reported any comparison data from CD patients (Benoni and Nilsson 1984; Motley *et al.* 1987).

Two studies (Franceschi *et al.* 1987; Benoni and Nilsson 1987) have examined smoking habits at the time of symptom onset and at diagnosis, an interval usually varying from a few weeks to a year. In the Milan study the significant associations of both UC and CD with ex-smoking disappeared if habits at the time of symptom onset were considered, but there was little evidence of such an effect in the study from Lund (Table 12.4). In both studies consideration of smoking habits at symptom onset strengthened the association of current smoking with CD and reduced the inverse association with UC.

Whether stopping smoking is associated with an increased risk of developing UC remains unclear and will be a difficult issue to resolve without prospectively collected smoking data. At present the only prospective data available are from the Oxford FPA contraceptive study (Table 12.5), in which ex-smokers had a small but not significantly increased risk of UC and no increased risk of CD (Vessey *et al.* 1986). However, stronger associations with ex-smoking might have gone undetected as smoking habit was only asked about at recruitment and the number of cases was small.

Table 12.4. Relative risks of IBD for current or ex-smoking compared to never smokers at diagnosis or onset of symptoms

		RR* current smoking		RR* ex-smoking	
		At diagnosis	At symptom onset	At diagnosis	At symptom onset
UC	Milan	0.5	1.0	2.7	1.2
	Lund	0.25	0.33	1.7	1.6
CD	Milan	4.2	5.0	3.5	0.6
	Lund	2.1	2.2	0.92	0.69

* Multiple logistic regression estimates.

Dose–response relationship

An inverse dose–response relationship for UC has been found in several case-control studies but could well be due to patients systematically underestimating the amounts they smoked previously (Tobin *et al.* 1987; Franceschi *et al.* 1987; Boyko *et al.* 1987; Lindberg *et al.* 1988). In these studies there

Table 12.5. Inflammatory bowel disease incidence* in the Oxford FPA and RCGP studies (Vessey *et al.* 1986; Logan *et al.* 1986; Logan and Kay, 1989)

Disease/smoking status	RCGP study			Oxford FPA study		
	Rate*		RR †	Rate*		RR †
Ulcerative colitis	($n=78$)			($n=31$)		
Never smoked	—	22	0.68 (0.41–1.1)	16	17	0.65 (0.25–1.7)
Ex-smoker	—			20		
Light smokers	16	15		16	11	
Heavy smokers	13			4		
Overall	19			15		
Crohn's disease	($n=42$)			($n=18$)		
Never smoked	—	8	1.75 (0.93–3.3)	5	5	3.0 (1.0–9.0)
Ex-smoker	—			4		
Light smokers	13	14		14	15	
Heavy smokers	18			16		
Overall	10			9		

* per 100 000 and standardized for age, social class, and oral contraceptive use.
† RR = relative risk (rate ratio) of disease in current smokers compared to non-smokers and 95% confidence limits.

was no clear-cut dose–response pattern for CD but there was also no evidence that the increased risk was only present in light smokers; again recall bias could be concealing any relationship. In the two cohorts of women contraceptive users, lower rates of UC and higher rates of CD were found in heavy smokers compared to light smokers (Table 12.5). The differences were small but this may reflect the frailty of the smoking data. At present, therefore, the dose–response data can be regarded as no more than suggestive.

Reversibility

The likely significance of either association would be increased if smoking was shown to have some reversible effect on CD or UC, either at an individual level or at a population level. Despite anecdotal reports of improvement of UC after re-starting smoking in the case-control studies there has been no consistent pattern, and most cases report no effect when asked about smoking's effect on their disease (Logan *et al.* 1984; Benoni and Nilsson 1987; Franceschi *et al.* 1987). The only population data available concern the Mormons, in whom smoking is proscribed, and who reported five times more UC than expected but no lack of CD (Penny *et al.* 1983).

Relationship with sugar consumption

The relationship between smoking and increased sugar consumption in CD is not yet clear. It has long been known that smokers tend to take more refined sugar than non-smokers (Bennett *et al.* 1970; Elwood *et al.* 1970). In a small study Thornton *et al.* (1985) found smoking and sugar to have separate effects. In Nottingham both smoking and added sugar were individually associated with CD but exposure to both resulted in no further increase in risk, suggesting that they may operate through a common mechanism (Katschinski *et al.* 1988).

Could smoking's effect be hormone related?

There is some evidence that the development of IBD may be influenced by the hormonal environment. Like most disorders with a presumed 'autoimmune' element the incidence of UC and CD in many studies is about 30 per cent higher in women than men (Calkins and Mendeloff 1986). More direct evidence for the importance of the hormonal milieu comes from the studies of oral contraceptive users in which current users had higher rates of both diseases (Table 12.6). Using a case-control approach Lesko *et al.* (1985) studied CD only and also found a significant increase in the risk of CD for recent users of the pill (RR = 4.3).

In the smoking studies which have reported their results by sex, association of smoking with CD has been notably stronger in women and the negative association with UC slightly weaker (Tobin *et al.* 1987; Franceschi *et al.* 1987; Benoni and Nilsson 1987; Katschinski *et al.* 1988; Sandler and Holland 1988).

Table 12.6. Inflammatory bowel disease incidence* in the Oxford FPA and RCGP studies (Vessey *et al.* 1986; Logan and Kay, 1989)

Disease/oral contraceptive use	RCGP study		Oxford FPA study	
	Rate*	RR†	Rate*	RR†
Ulcerative colitis	(*n* = 78)		(*n* = 31)	
Never and former users	18	—	11	—
Current users	23	1.3 (0.82–2.0)	23	2.1 (0.96–4.5)
Overall	19		15	
Crohn's disease	(*n* = 42)		(*n* = 18)	
Never and former users	9	—	8	—
Current users	15	1.7 (0.88–3.2)	12	1.5 (0.55–4.1)
Overall	10		9	

* per 100 000 and standardized for age, social class, and smoking.
† RR = relative risk (rate ratio) of disease in current pill users compared to non-users and 95% confidence limits.

12.3. Discussion

Some of the variation in relative risk estimates shown in Tables 12.2 and 12.3 are likely to be due to methodological differences. For example, in the studies from Nottingham and Liverpool a postal enquiry was used to determine smoking habits before symptom onset, while in Milan and Lund an interviewer was used. Despite these differences the association of smoking with CD is remarkably consistent with a two- to threefold increased risk, which is similar to the RR estimates obtained from prospective studies of contraceptive users (Vessey *et al.* 1986; Logan and Kay 1989). The picture for UC is less clear cut. Nevertheless, all studies have shown a reduced risk of disease in current smokers. What is unclear is how much this is due to an increased risk of UC in ex-smokers. The contrasting nature of the associations with the two diseases makes it unlikely that both are the consequence of unrecognized biases or confounding.

Current data could be interpreted as indicating that smoking has two separate effects, i.e. an active *disease promoting* effect in CD and a *disease protecting* effect in UC which leaves non-smokers at increased risk, or by withdrawal of protection puts ex-smokers at increased risk (Fig. 12.1).

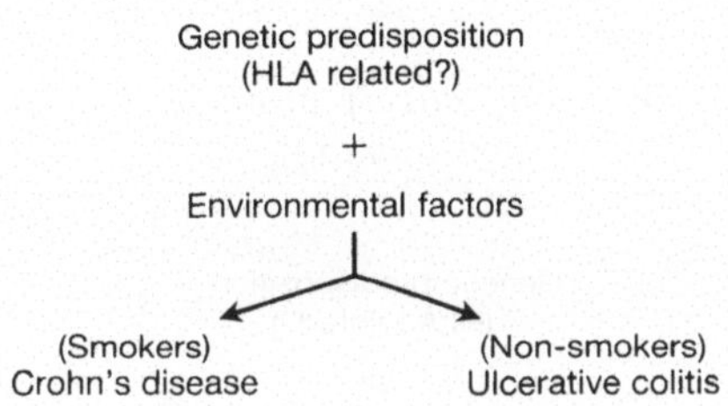

Fig. 12.1. Hypothesis A: smoking both promotes CD and protects from UC (recall bias accounts for ex-smoking).

However, assuming the widely held view of a common genetic predisposition to CD and UC is correct, then the contrasting associations could be explained by a single effect. For example, if the active effect is the promotion of CD, then smokers in the predisposed group would tend to develop CD, leaving a residue of never and ex-smokers who would be available to develop UC (Fig. 12.2). Alternatively, smoking might convert UC to CD. (It should be noted that, in clinical terms, the two diseases are mutually exclusive and the opposite is impossible, i.e. once a diagnosis of CD has been made, all subsequent disease is labelled CD.)

Another possibility is that smoking could actively protect from developing UC with ex-smokers being at increased risk when the protective effect is removed (Fig. 12.3). This hypothesis has the attraction of regarding the

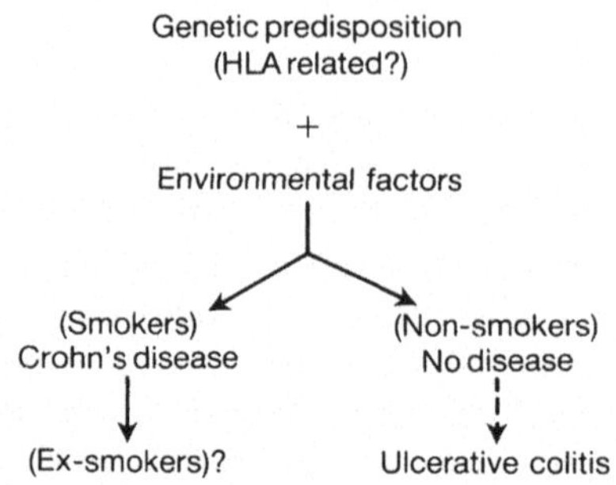

Example:

Assume 1000 people are predisposed to IBD (50% develop UC and 50% develop CD) half are smokers, similar to rest of the population, with RR of CD of 4

Then	CD		UC	
	Case	Controls	Case	Controls
	400	250	100	250
	100	250	400	250
	500	500	50	500
estimated	RR = 4	estimated	RR = 0.25	

Fig. 12.2. Hypothesis B: Smoking *actively* promotes CD (recall bias accounts for ex-smoking).

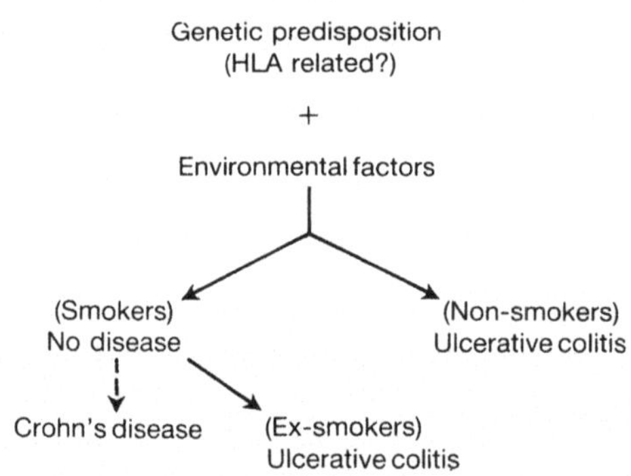

Fig. 12.3. Hypothesis C: smoking *protects* from UC and stopping leads to UC.

increased risk in ex-smokers as a real effect while allowing for an increased risk of UC in never-smokers compared to smokers.

The aetiology and pathogenesis of IBD remains obscure. Indeed, there is still debate as to whether UC and CD should be considered together or separately, despite much clinical evidence for their common origin. It is not surprising therefore that the mechanism through which smoking or non-smoking could exert an effect is equally obscure. Cope *et al.* (1986) have found reduced mucus glycoprotein production from colonic biopsies of non-smoking UC patients. In the small number of colitics who smoked, mucus production was the same as controls. They speculate that smoking improves the quality of mucosal defences but this proposal is difficult to reconcile with the adverse effect of smoking in CD.

12.4. Conclusion

The evidence reviewed here indicates that cigarette smoking has a significant causal role in the aetiology of IBD. The mechanism remains obscure; smoking could be either promoting CD, protecting from UC, or doing both. Current data are arguably most consistent with a disease-promoting effect for CD. If smoking is promoting CD with a two- to threefold increased risk in smokers, and assuming a third of the population currently smoke, then around a third of all CD could be attributed to smoking.

References

Bennett, A. E., Doll, R., and Howell, R. W. (1970). Sugar consumption and cigarette smoking. *Lancet*, **i**, 1011–14.

Benoni, C. and Nilsson, A. (1984). Smoking habits in patients with inflammatory bowel disease. *Scandinavian Journal of Gastroenterology*, **19**, 824–30.

Benoni, C. and Nilsson, A. (1987). Smoking habits in patients with inflammatory bowel disease—a case-control study. *Scandinavian Journal of Gastroenterology*, **22**, 1130–6.

Boyko, E. J., Koepsell, T. D., Perera, D. R., and Inui, T. S. (1987). Risk of ulcerative colitis among former and current cigarette smokers. *New England Journal of Medicine*, **316**, 707–10.

Calkins, B. and Mendeloff, A. I. (1986). Epidemiology of inflammatory bowel disease. *Epidemiology Review*, **8**, 60–91.

Calkins, B., *et al.* (1984). Smoking factors in ulcerative colitis and Crohn's disease in Baltimore. *American Journal of Epidemiology*, **120**, 498A.

Cope, G. F., Heatley, R. V., and Kellner, J. (1986). Smoking and colonic mucus in ulcerative colitis. *British Medical Journal*, **293**, 481.

Elwood, P. C., Waters, W. E., Moore, S., and Sweetnam, P. (1970). Sucrose consumption and ischaemic heart disease. *Lancet*, **i**, 1014–16.

Franceschi, S., Panza, E., La Vecchia, C., Parazzini, F., Decarli, A., and Bianchi Poro, G. (1987). Non-specific inflammatory bowel disease and smoking. *American Journal of Epidemiology*, **125**, 445–52.

Harries, A. D., Baird, A., and Rhodes, J. (1982). Non-smoking: a feature of ulcerative colitis. *British Medical Journal*, **284**, 706.

Jick, H. and Walker, A. M. (1983). Cigarette smoking and ulcerative colitis. *New England Journal of Medicine*, **303**, 261–3.

Katschinski, B., Logan, R. F. A., Edmond, M., and Langman, M. J. S. (1988). Smoking and sugar intake are separate but interactive risk factors in Crohn's disease. *Gut*, **29**, 1202–6.

Kirsner, J. B. and Shorter, R. G. (1982). Recent development in 'non-specific' inflammatory bowel disease. *New England Journal of Medicine*, **306**, 775–85, 837–48.

Lesko, S. M., *et al.* (1985). Evidence for an increased risk of Crohn's disease in oral contraceptive users. *Gastroenterology*, **89**, 1046–9.

Lindberg, E., Tysk, C., Jarnerot, G., and Andersson, K. (1988). Smoking and inflammatory bowel disease. *Gut*, **29**, 352–7.

Logan, R. F. A. and Kay, C. (1989). Oral contraception, smoking and inflammatory bowel disease—findings in the RCGP oral contraception study. *International Journal of Epidemiology*, **18**, 105–7.

Logan, R. F. A., Somerville, K. W., Edmond, M., and Langman, M. J. S. (1983). Is cigarette smoking associated with Crohn's disease? *Gut*, **24**, A940.

Logan, R. F. A., Edmond, M., Somerville, K. W., and Langman, M. J. S. (1984). Smoking and ulcerative colitis. *British Medical Journal*, **288**, 751–3.

Logan, R. F. A., Katschinski, B., Somerville, K. W., Pearson, J. C. G., and Langman, M. J. S. (1986). Smoking and inflammatory bowel disease. *Gastroenterology*, **90**, 1525.

Motley, R. J., *et al.* (1987). Time relationships between cessation of smoking and onset of ulcerative colitis. *Digestion*, **37**, 125–7.

Penny, W. J., *et al.* (1983). Mormons, smoking and ulcerative colitis. *Lancet*, **ii**, 1315.

Persson, P. G., Ahlbom, A., and Hellers, G. (1987). Crohn's disease and ulcerative colitis—a review of dietary studies with emphasis on methodologic aspects. *Scandinavian Journal of Gastroenterology*, **22**, 385–9.

Samuelsson, S. V. (1976). Ulcerative colitis in the county of Uppsala 1945–1964. MD Thesis. University of Uppsala.

Sandler, R. and Holland, K. (1988). Smoking and inflammatory bowel disease. *Gastroenterology*, **94**, A398.

Somerville, K. W., Logan, R. F. A., Edmond, M., and Langman, M. J. S. (1984). Smoking and Crohn's disease. *British Medical Journal*, **289**, 954–6.

Thornton, J. R., Emmett, P. M., and Heaton, K. W. (1985). Smoking, sugar, and inflammatory bowel disease. *British Medical Journal*, **290**, 1786–7.

Tobin, M. V., Logan, R. F. A., Langman, M. J. S., McConnell, R. B., and Gilmore, I. T. (1987). Cigarette smoking and inflammatory bowel disease. *Gastroenterology*, **93**, 316–21.

Vessey, M., Jewell, D., Smith, A., Yeates, D., and McPherson, K. (1986). Chronic inflammatory bowel disease, cigarette smoking, and use of oral contraceptives: findings in a large cohort study of women of childbearing age. *British Medical Journal*, **292**, 1101–3.

13. Smoking and Parkinson's disease

Michael Marmot

Abstract

Parkinson's disease is a degenerative disorder of the substantia nigra characterized by a dramatic improvement after treatment with the dopamine precursor L*-dopa. Cigarette smoking is inversely related to the risk of Parkinson's disease, and this appears to be a genuine protective effect. If smoking is, in fact, protective of Parkinson's disease then one would expect not only that patients with Parkinson's disease would be less likely to be smokers but also that they would have a lower risk of smoking-related cancers, which indeed they do.*

13.1. Introduction

In the context of this symposium, the two questions to ask about Parkinson's disease are: to what extent is it a hormone-related disorder? and what role does smoking play in this?

The clinical response to L-dopa provides clues to the first question. The dramatic symptomatic response of Parkinson's disease to L-dopa therapy suggests a role for dopa or a derivative of it. In fact the response is so striking that in the eyes of at least some neurologists, the response to L-dopa is part of the diagnosis. This alone does not of course guarantee a central hormonal role in the disorder; such logic would describe headache as an aspirin-deficiency disorder. However, together with the observation that it is dopaminergic neurons that degenerate in Parkinson's disease it does at least indicate that this disorder is clearly hormone-related, though not oestrogen-related. Smoking could then exert its effect on Parkinson's disease: a therapeutic effect influencing dopaminergic pathways. Another possibility is an effect on the underlying process that is responsible for the dopamine deficiency in Parkinson's disease.

13.2. Association between smoking and Parkinson's disease

This has been well reviewed by Baron (1986) and the present summary draws heavily on his review. Three types of epidemiological study have produced evidence that smoking is inversely related to the occurrence of

Parkinson's disease: longitudinal, case-control, and mortality follow-up studies of Parkinson's disease patients.

Longitudinal studies

Longitudinal studies in USA (Kahn 1966; Hammond 1966), UK (Doll and Peto 1976), and Japan (Hirayama 1985) of cohorts of apparently healthy people showed smokers to have a lower mortality rate from Parkinson's disease than people who never smoked (Table 13.1). In the British doctors' study (Doll and Peto 1976) and the Japanese cohort study (Hirayama 1985), there was an inverse dose–response relationship: the greater the amount smoked, the less the risk of dying of Parkinson's disease. The number of ex-smokers was small, but in general, their risk was intermediate between that for smokers and never smokers.

Table 13.1. Longitudinal studies of cigarette smoking and parkinsonism

	Rate ratio	Statistical significance
Kahn	0.3	Smokers vs. non-smokers
Hammond	0.8*	Not addressed
Doll and Peto	0.4	Trend
Hirayama	0.6	Smokers vs. non-smokers trend

* Subjects 65 to 79 years old.
From Baron (1986).

A potential drawback of these longitudinal studies is their reliance on death certificates. From other data, we know that in England and Wales only about a third of death certificates that list Parkinson's disease as a cause of death have it as an underlying cause (Marmot 1981). Bias would occur if a tendency to list Parkinson's disease as the underlying cause was less in smokers than in non-smokers.

Even accepting these mortality rates as giving an accurate picture, a lower mortality rate from Parkinson's disease in smokers could be the result of decreased incidence, decreased case-fatality ratio, or a combination. Smoking could reduce the chance of getting the disease, or prolong survival among sufferers of it. To distinguish, morbidity studies are needed in addition to studies of mortality.

Case-control studies

A partial clarification is given by case-control studies (Table 13.2). Each of these studies showed a relative risk estimate of less than one, i.e. an apparent protective effect of smoking. However the studies were not limited to newly

Table 13.2. Case-control studies of cigarette smoking and parkinsonism

	Odds ratio*	Statistical significance †
Nefzger *et al.*		
Males	0.4	+
Kessler and Diamond		
Males	0.6	+
Females	0.7	−
Kessler		
Males	0.4	+
Females	0.6	−
Ansari and Johnson		
Males	0.2	+
Marttila and Rinne		
Both sexes	0.7	+
Haack *et al.*		
Males	0.7	−
Females	0.2	+
Ward *et al.*		
Both sexes	‡	?
Godwin-Austen *et al.*		
Males	0.5	+
Females	0.6	+
Barbeau and Pourcher		
Both sexes	0.4§	+
Kondo		
Males	0.4	+
Females	0.6	+
Cazzato *et al.*		
Both sexes	0.4	+
Rajput *et al.*		
Both sexes	0.7	−

* History of ever smoking cigarettes vs. never smoking.
† +, statistically significant results, $0<P<0.05$; −, results not statistically significant, $P<0.05$.
‡ Cases smoked less than twin controls.
§ Parkinson's disease (postencephalitic parkinsonism excluded).
From Baron (1986).

diagnosed (incident) cases. A reasonable speculation would be that the longer the duration of the disease, the greater the chance of being included in a case-control study. If smoking were to increase the case-fatality ratio of Parkinson's disease cases, i.e. shorten the survival, the survivors would have a lower prevalence of smoking for that reason alone. Against this, if case-fatality were higher, one would expect smokers to have a higher, not lower, overall mortality from Parkinson's disease. This would be at variance with the results of the longitudinal studies.

It is potentially difficult to interpret an association detected in a case-control study if both the disease and the 'exposure' can vary over time: smoking could protect against Parkinson's disease or Parkinson's disease could lead to giving up smoking. To eliminate this possibility, it is necessary to look at lifetime non-smokers and at people who gave up smoking before onset of the disease. Godwin-Austen *et al.* (1982) based a case-control study in general practice (Table 13.3). Although a proportion of Parkinson's disease patients did give up smoking after developing symptoms, this was fewer than the proportion of control patients who gave up smoking during the same time period; the relative risk for this group was 0.58. Even for people who gave up smoking before the time when the symptoms of the case began, those who had been smokers had a relative risk less than one. Overall, ex-smokers had a risk intermediate between the low risk of current smokers and the higher risk of never smokers.

Baron (1986) considers a number of possible interpretations of these data other than that of a protective role of smoking. *Chance* is unlikely, as judged by tests of statistical significance. Although there are several possibilities for *artefact* in the case-control studies, the arguments against this accounting for the results include:

(1) the remarkable consistency of the findings in both hospital-based and community-based studies; and
(2) the lack of association with alcohol and coffee make it unlikely that impaired memory of cases made them less likely to recall the use of tobacco.

These results could also be due to *confounding*. Smokers may differ from non-smokers in other respects that make them less likely to develop Parkinson's disease. The strongest argument against confounding is the size of the 'protective' effect of smoking—a relative risk of about 0.5. Nevertheless it remains a possibility.

Causes of death in Parkinson's disease patients

If patients with Parkinson's disease are indeed less likely to be smokers, one might expect that when they die it would be less likely to be from a cause related to smoking. We examined multiple cause coded death certificates and found that certificates that mentioned Parkinson's disease as a contributory cause of death were very much less likely to have recorded a diagnosis of lung cancer, or other smoking-related cancers (Marmot 1981). This is consistent with a lower than average smoking rate in Parkinson's disease patients. There was also a deficit of all cancers regardless of their relationship to smoking.

This has been confirmed recently in a 15-year follow-up study of patients diagnosed as having Parkinson's disease in general practices taking part in

Table 13.3. Distribution of smoking habits in Parkinson's disease cases and controls and relative risk estimates

Smoking habits	Men (179 pairs)			Women (171 pairs)			Combined
	Cases (%)	Controls (%)	Relative risk	Cases (%)	Controls (%)	Relative risk	Relative risk
Never smoked	22.9	12.3	1.00	69.0	58.5	1.00	1.00
Given up smoking:							
more than 10 years before onset of Parkinson's disease	19.6	13.4	0.78	7.6	7.0	0.92	0.84
1–10 years before onset of Parkinson's disease	14.0	12.9	0.58	4.7	5.9	0.68	0.62
after onset of Parkinson's disease	15.1	19.6	0.41	7.6	7.0	0.92	0.58
total	48.6	45.8	0.57	19.9	19.9	0.85	0.71
Still smoking at time of interview	28.5	41.9	0.36	11.1	21.6	0.44	0.40

From Godwin-Austen *et al.* (1982).

the National Morbidity study. Among 220 such patients, the standardized mortality ratio (SMR) from all causes was 165 compared to the England and Wales average. In this cohort, 5.77 smoking-related cancers were expected, none was observed—SMR 0 (confidence interval 0–76.4). For all cancers 18.56 deaths were expected and 8 were observed—SMR 43 (confidence intervals 18.6–84.9). There were several potential methodological problems with this study, but it tends to confirm the suggestion of others (Barbeau and Joly 1963) that Parkinson's disease patients are at lower risk of cancer in general, not only of cancers related to smoking.

13.3. Potential mechanisms

Two types of mechanism have been postulated to mediate the possible effect of smoking in reducing the risk of Parkinson's disease: an effect on dopaminergic pathways, and a possible antioxidant effect of carbon monoxide.

Nicotine appears to stimulate dopaminergic pathways in the central nervous system and there is some evidence that nicotine may have beneficial effects on symptoms in Parkinson's disease. If damage to the substantia nigra with consequent decrease in dopamine release is the primary underlying problem in Parkinson's disease, then perhaps the nicotine in tobacco smoke is to some extent mitigating these effects.

The other type of hypothesis, for which there is somewhat less support, is that carbon monoxide in tobacco smoke, by creating a reducing environment, might protect the substantia nigra from oxidative damage (Calne and Langston 1983). In this context, it is interesting to note that there is speculation that one of the mechanisms by which smoking might *increase* the risk of atherosclerosis is by aiding the formation of free radicals and hence contributing to oxidative damage rather than the reverse as suggested here.

13.4. Conclusion

The data are consistent with a true protective effect of smoking on Parkinson's disease. What is lacking is extensive study of incident cases. Even if the possibility of a causal relationship was accepted, one would of course not recommend smoking to prevent Parkinson's disease. The recognized hazards of smoking far outweigh any potential benefits. The main interest here is in what it may tell us of aetiological pathways. The apparent inverse relation between Parkinson's disease and cancer may similarly hold aetiological clues.

There may also be clues to further therapeutic benefit. If smoking relieves symptoms because of its effect on dopamine, might there be the possibility of therapeutic development?

References

Barbeau, A. and Joly, J. G. (1963). Parkinson et cancer. *Union Medicale du Canada*, 92, 169–74.

Baron, J. A. (1986). Cigarette smoking and Parkinson's disease. *Neurology*, 36, 1490–6.

Calne, D. B. and Langston, J. W. (1983). Aetiology of Parkinson's disease. *Lancet*, ii, 1457–9.

Doll, R. and Peto, R. (1976). Mortality in relation to smoking: 20 years' observations on male British doctors. *British Medical Journal*, 25, 1525–36.

Godwin-Austen, R. B., Lee, P. N., Marmot, M. G., and Stern, G. M. (1982). Smoking and Parkinson's disease. *Journal of Neurology, Neurosurgery and Psychiatry*, 45, 577–81.

Hammond, E. C. (1966). Smoking in relation to the death rates of one million men and women. In *Epidemiological approaches to the study of cancer and other chronic diseases* (ed. W. Haenszel), National Cancer Institute Monograph 19. US Department of Health, Education, and Welfare.

Hirayama, T. (1985). Epidemiological patterns of Parkinson's disease based on a cohort study. Epidemiology of Intractable Diseases Research Committee 1985. Japan Ministry of Health and Welfare, Tokyo.

Kahn, H. A. (1966). The Dorn study of smoking and mortality among US veterans: report on eight and one-half years of observation. In *Epidemiological approaches to the study of cancer and other chronic diseases* (ed. W. Haenszel), National Cancer Institute Monograph 19. US Department of Health, Education, and Welfare.

Marmot, M. G. (1981). Mortality and Parkinson's disease. In *Research progress in Parkinson's disease* (ed. F. C. Rose and R. Capildeo), pp. 9–16. Pitman, London.

V

Smoking and Hormone-Related Cancers

14. Cigarette smoking and the incidence of endometrial cancer

Noel S. Weiss

Abstract

A lower risk of endometrial cancer among cigarette smokers than among non-smokers has been noted in 10 of 11 studies. The negative association has been particularly strong in recent smokers, which would be predicted if smoking were to exert an effect by interfering in some way with the action of oestrogens in endometrial carcinogenesis. The observed difference between smokers and non-smokers has generally been somewhat greater in post-menopausal than in pre-menopausal women, and greater in users than in non-users of post-menopausal oestrogens. Thus, if cigarette smoking does prevent some women from developing endometrial cancer, it is likely to do so in ways other than by reducing ovarian production of oestrogens.

14.1. Introduction

The results of eight case-control studies of cigarette smoking in relation to the incidence of endometrial cancer have now been published (Williams and Horm 1977; Weiss *et al.* 1980; Lesko *et al.* 1985; Baron *et al.* 1986; Stockwell and Lyman 1987; Tyler *et al.* 1985; Franks *et al.* 1987; Lawrence *et al.* 1987; Levi *et al.* 1987). All but one were conducted in the United States. All found a history of smoking to be less common among women with endometrial cancer than among controls, and estimated the incidence of this neoplasm in cigarette smokers to be but 50–70 per cent that of non-smokers. Two cohort studies (Garfinkel and Boffetta, Chapter 1; Ross *et al.*, Chapter 3) obtained similar results. A third (Stampfer *et al.*, Chapter 2), however, found the incidence of endometrial cancer to be similar among smokers and non-smokers though this was mainly among pre-menopausal women.

The occurrence of endometrial cancer is known to be strongly influenced by ovarian sex hormones, whether endogenously produced or exogenously administered (Weiss 1983). Since cigarette smoking is related both to age at menopause and the incidence of post-menopausal fractures (McKinlay *et al.*

Table 14.1. Case-control studies of cigarette smoking in relation to the incidence of endometrial cancer

Author	Location	Cases			Source of controls	Ascertainment of exposures
		Dates of diagnosis	Number	Source		
Williams and Horm (1977)	US	1969–71	358	Population-based registries	Patients with smoking-unrelated cancers	Interview
Weiss *et al.* (1980)	Western Washington	1975–6	322	Population-based registry	Population sample	Interview
Lesko *et al.* (1985)	Eight North American cities	1976–83	510	Hospitals	Patients with smoking-unrelated cancers	Interview
Baron *et al.* (1986)	Buffalo, NY	1957–65	476	Roswell Park Memorial Institute	Patients without cancer or smoking-related primary diagnosis	Interview
Stockwell and Lyman (1987)	Florida	1981	1374	Population-based registry	Patients with smoking-unrelated cancers	Hospital records
Tyler *et al.* (1985)	US	1980–2	437	Population-based registries	Population sample	Interview
Franks *et al.* (1987)	US	1980–2	79	Population-based registries	Population sample	Interview
Lawrence *et al.* (1987)	Upper NY state	1979–81	200	Sample of NY hospitals	Population sample	Interview
Levi *et al.* (1987)	Milan	1983–5	357	Hospitals	Patients without smoking-related primary diagnosis	Interview

1985; Williams *et al.* 1982), two other sex hormone-related phenomena, it seems plausible that if smoking does have an effect on the incidence of endometrial cancer, it would be mediated via sex hormone production and/or metabolism. The past several years have brought discoveries of mechanisms through which cigarette smoking is indeed related to production and metabolism of sex hormones, but it is unclear as yet which if any of these mechanisms might be relevant to the genesis of endometrial cancer.

The goal of the present analysis is to determine if the size of the association between smoking and endometrial cancer varies among certain subgroups of women. The presence of this variation can be useful in guiding our inference as to whether smoking *causes* a decreased risk (Weiss 1981). In addition, it may shed some light on the means by which smoking exerts its influence in discouraging the development of this tumour.

14.2. Summary of results

Table 14.1 provides selected characteristics of the case-control studies. [Though reported in two separate publications, the results of Tyler *et al.* (1985) and Franks *et al.* (1987) emanate from the same investigation, the Cancer and Steroid Hormone Study. The analysis of Franks *et al.* gives particular emphasis to recent smoking and to post-menopausal women.] Given that all were case-control in design and were conducted primarily in the US, the studies nonetheless are fairly heterogeneous:

(1) the study populations arose from a variety of regions; and
(2) while most studies used patients who were diagnosed during the mid-1970s to the early 1980s, two were based on data from women diagnosed 10–20 years earlier than that.

Table 14.2. Cohort studies of cigarette smoking in relation to the occurrence of endometrial cancer

First author	Location	Period of follow-up	Incidence vs. mortality	Number of cases among smokers
Garfinkel (Chapter 1)				
(1)	USA	1959–72	Mortality	68
(2)	USA	1982–6	Mortality	44
Stampfer (Chapter 2)	USA	1976–82	Incidence	150
Ross (Chapter 3)	California	1981–8	Incidence	55

Table 14.3. Relation of intensity/duration of cigarette smoking to risk of endometrial cancer

Author	Cigarette smoking categories	Relative risk
Williams and Horm (1977)	Non-smokers vs. 1–20, 21–39, ≥40 pack years	1, 0.9, 0.8, 0.7
Weiss *et al*. (1980)	Non-smokers vs. maximum consumption of <10, 10–19, 20, ≥21 cigarettes/day	1, 0.4, 0.5, 0.6, 0.4
Lesko *et al*. (1985)	Non-smokers vs. current smokers of 1–14, 15–24, ≥25 cigarettes/day	1, 0.8, 1.0, 0.5
Baron *et al*. (1986)	Non-smokers vs. 1–14, ≥15 pack-years	1, 0.8, 0.6
Stockwell and Lyman (1987)	Non-smokers vs. current smokers of <20, 20–40, >40 cigarettes/day	1, 1.1, 0.8, 0.6
Franks *et al*. (1987)	Average number of cigarettes/day	(Among smokers, 'no consistent trend in risk' with increasing number per day)
Lawrence *et al*. (1987)	Non-smokers vs. current smokers of ≤20, >20 cigarettes/day	1, 0.7, 0.5
Levi *et al*. (1987)	Non-smokers vs. current smokers of <15, ≥15 cigarettes/day	1, 0.5, 0.4
Garfinkel (Chapter 1)		
(1)	Non-smokers vs. current smokers of <20, ≥20 cigarettes/day	1, 0.9, 0.8
(2)	Non-smokers vs. current smokers of <20, ≥20 cigarettes/day	1, 0.6, 0.6
Stampfer (Chapter 2)	Non-smokers vs. current smokers of 1–14, 15–24, ≥25 cigarettes/day	1, 0.5, 1.1, 1.1
Ross (Chapter 3)	Non-smokers vs. ever-smokers of 1–10, 11–20, ≥21 cigarettes/day	1, 0.8, 0.9, 0.2

Seven of the eight case-control studies obtained cigarette smoking histories from interviews with cases and controls.

Table 14.2 indicates some features of the three cohort studies. The age distribution of the subjects in two of them was quite different. In the study by Stampfer *et al.* (Chapter 2)—the Nurse's Health Study—the large majority of the cohort was pre-menopausal at entry. In contrast, the study of Ross *et al.* (Chapter 3) enrolled residents of a retirement community.

With one exception, only the published results from these studies are presented here, and as a consequence not every study has contributed data to every subgroup analysis. That exception is the study conducted by Weiss *et al.* (1980), from which unpublished results relating to subgroups defined by intensity of smoking, menopausal status, and body weight have been included.

Table 14.3 examines the influence of daily smoking consumption (nine studies) or cumulative lifetime cigarette consumption (two studies) on the size of the smoking-cancer association. Weiss *et al.* (1980), Franks *et al.* (1987), and Garfinkel and Boffetta (Chapter 1) found a similar negative association at every level of consumption, while Lesko *et al.* (1985) and Ross *et al.* (Chapter 3) found the negative association largely restricted to the highest category. However, the remaining studies in which there was an association observed a steady decline in risk with increasing level of smoking. It would seem that the latter pattern is a reasonable average across all the studies.

The influence of recency of cigarette smoking was analysed in nine studies

Table 14.4. Relation of recency of cigarette smoking to risk of endometrial cancer

Author	Relative risk* in	
	Current smoker	Ex-smoker
Lesko *et al.* (1985)	0.7	0.9
Stockwell and Lyman (1987)	0.8	0.6
Franks *et al.* (1987)	0.5	0.7
Lawrence *et al.* (1987)	0.6	0.9
Tyler *et al.* (1985)	0.8	1.0
Levi *et al.* (1987)	0.5	0.9
Garfinkel (Chapter 1)		
(1)	0.9	1.1
(2)	0.6	0.7
Stampfer (Chapter 2)	1.0	1.0
Ross (Chapter 3)	0.7	0.7

* Risk relative to that of women who never smoked cigarettes.

(Table 14.4). In all but the ones reported by Stockwell and Lyman (1987) and Ross *et al.* (Chapter 3), the negative association with endometrial cancer was greater for current than for past smokers. Probably more credence can be given to the pattern observed by the majority, since:

(1) Stockwell and Lyman ascertained smoking histories of subjects through medical records, rather than through interviews; and
(2) the analysis by Ross *et al.* was based on a relatively small number of smokers with endometrial cancer (21).

While cigarette smoking is associated with a reduced risk of endometrial cancer in both pre- and post-menopausal women (Table 14.5), it appears that the association is more pronounced in the latter group. Among post-menopausal women the reduced risk is present both in users and non-users of oestrogens (Table 14.6), though the size of the reduction is perhaps greatest in oestrogen users.

Though one case-control study found the negative association between smoking and endometrial cancer to be largely restricted to heavy women (Table 14.7), the three others to examine the issue have found no such pattern. One cohort study (Ross *et al.* Chapter 3) similarly detected no

Table 14.5. Influence of menopausal status on the association between cigarette smoking and endometrial cancer

Author	Comparison	Relative risk in	
		Pre-menopausal women	Post-menopausal women
Weiss *et al.* (1980)	Ever-smoker vs. non-smoker	0.5	0.4
Lesko *et al.* (1985)	≥25 cigarettes/day vs. non-smoker	0.9	0.5
Stockwell and Lyman (1987)	Current smoker vs. non-smoker	1.0*	0.8†
Franks *et al.* (1987)	Current smoker vs. non-smoker	0.7	0.5
Lawrence *et al.* (1987)	Current smoker vs. non-smoker	0.6	0.6
Levi *et al.* (1987)	Current smoker vs. non-smoker	0.5	0.4
Stampfer (Chapter 2)	Current smoker vs. non-smoker	1.0*	1.0†

* Women <50 years of age.
† Women ≥50 years of age.

Table 14.6. Influence of post-menopausal oestrogen use on the association between cigarette smoking and endometrial cancer

Author	Comparison	Relative risk in	
		Oestrogen non-users	Oestrogen users
Weiss *et al.* (1980)	Ever vs. never smokers, age-adjusted	0.4	0.3
Franks *et al.* (1987)	Current smoker vs. non-smoker, post-menopausal women only	0.5	0.3
Levi *et al.* (1987)	Current smoker vs. non-smoker, age-adjusted	0.5	0.2

Table 14.7. Influence of body weight on the association between cigarette smoking and endometrial cancer

Author	Comparison	Relative risk in women who weigh (lbs)			
		<140	140–159	160–189	≥190
Weiss *et al.* (1980)	Ever vs. never smoker	0.5	0.5	0.4	0.6
Lawrence *et al.* (1987)	Current vs. non-smoker	1.1	0.9	0.6	0.3
Franks *et al.* (1987)	Current vs. non-smoker	('No appreciable stratum-specific differences')			
Levi *et al.* (1987)*	Current vs. non-smoker	0.3	0.8	0.7	0.1

* Relative risk in four categories of body mass index (kg/m^2): <20, 20–24.9, 25–29.9, ≥30.

systematic variation in the size of the association across categories of weight (data not shown).

14.3. Why do cigarette smokers have a decreased incidence of endometrial cancer?

A causal interpretation of the negative association between cigarette smoking and endometrial cancer is supported by the presence of the association in nearly all studies, and by the tendency for the reduced risk to be particularly great among the heaviest smokers. The observation of a stronger influence of recent than past smoking on endometrial cancer risk also suggests a causal relationship, since:

(1) the effect of smoking is likely to be mediated via its impact on production/metabolism of oestrogens (see below); and
(2) oestrogens appear to act at a relatively late stage in the pathogenesis of endometrial cancer (Weiss 1983).

Other chapters in this volume document the ways in which cigarette smoking might interfere with oestrogen production and might alter oestrogen metabolism. Theoretically, smoking could also directly antagonize the effect of oestrogens on the endometrium, e.g. by interfering with the binding of oestrogens to their receptors on endometrial cells. While results of epidemiologic studies are crude instruments with which to make mechanistic distinctions, they do tend to argue against an important role for smoking's effect on oestrogen production. The considerable reduction in risk among postmenopausal women who smoke, particularly among those who have been receiving oestrogen hormones, argues that mechanisms other than those involving the production of oestrogens are likely to be the principal ways by which cigarette smoking exerts its beneficial influence.

References

Baron, J. A., Greenberg, E. R., Cummings, K. M., and Swanson, M. (1986). Cigarette smoking in women with cancers of the breast and reproductive organs. *Journal of the National Cancer Institute*, 77, 677–801.

Franks, A. L., Kendrick, J. S., Tyler, C. W., and The Cancer and Steroid Hormone Study Group (1987). Postmenopausal smoking, estrogen replacement therapy, and the risk of endometrial cancer. *American Journal of Obstetrics and Gynecology*, 156, 20–3.

Lawrence, C., *et al.* (1987). Smoking, body weight, and early-stage endometrial cancer. *Cancer*, 59, 1665–9.

Lesko, S. M., *et al.* (1985). Cigarette smoking and the risk of endometrial cancer. *New England Journal of Medicine*, 313, 593–6.

Levi, F., La Vecchia, C., and Decarli, A. (1987). Cigarette smoking and the risk of endometrial cancer. *European Journal of Cancer and Clinical Oncology*, 23, 1025–9.

McKinlay, S. M., Bifano, N. L., and McKinlay, J. B. (1985). Smoking and age at menopause in women. *Annals of Internal Medicine*, 103, 350–6.

Stockwell, H. G. and Lyman, G. H. (1987). Cigarette smoking and the risk of female reproductive cancer. *American Journal of Obstetrics and Gynecology*, 157, 35–40.

Tyler, C. W., Webster, L. A., Ory, H. W., and Rubin, G. L. (1985). Endometrial cancer: How does cigarette smoking influence the risk of women under age 55 years having this tumor? *American Journal of Obstetrics and Gynecology*, 151, 899–905.

Weiss, N. S. (1981). Inferring causal relationships: Elaboration of the criterion of 'dose-response'. *American Journal of Epidemiology*, **113**, 487–90.

Weiss, N. S. (1983). Epidemiology of endometrial cancer: A review of hormonal and non-hormonal risk factors. In *Reviews in cancer epidemiology*, No. 11 (ed. A. M. Lilienfeld). Elsevier.

Weiss, N. S., Farewell, V. T., Szekely, D. R., English, D. R., and Kiviat, N. (1980). Oestrogens and endometrial cancer: Effect of other risk factors on the association. *Maturitas*, **2**, 185–190.

Williams, A. R., Weiss, N. S., Ure, C. L., Ballard, J., and Daling, J. R. (1982). Effect of weight, smoking, and estrogen use on the risk of hip and forearm fractures in postmenopausal women. *Obstetrics and Gynecology*, **60**, 695–9.

Williams, R. R. and Horm, J. W. (1977). Association of cancer sites with tobacco and alcohol consumption and socioeconomic status of patients: Interview study from the Third National Cancer Survey. *Journal of the National Cancer Institute*, **58**, 525–47.

15. Cigarette smoking and cancer of the breast

Brian MacMahon

Abstract

All known published data on the possibility of an association between cigarette smoking and risk of breast cancer have been reviewed. Summary odds ratios and confidence intervals have been calculated for various types of study. The summary odds ratio was significantly below 1.0 only for the category of case-control studies in which controls were hospital patients including patients with diseases related to smoking. This finding is predictable on a priori *grounds. Excluding this category other case-control studies gave an odds ratio of 1.12 with confidence limits 1.06 to 1.19. Cohort studies also gave an odds ratio slightly, though significantly, higher than 1.0–1.14 with confidence interval 1.02–1.27. There was no indication of effect modification by menopausal status. It is concluded that breast cancer risk is not reduced among cigarette smokers. The very small, though significant,* elevation *of risk in smokers is unexplained.*

15.1. Introduction

Interest in the question of whether a relationship exists between a woman's use of cigarettes and her risk of breast cancer originated with the suggestion based on a modicum of data in the literature that breast cancer risk may be slightly lower in smokers than non-smokers and the observation that in pre-menopausal women urine oestrogen levels in the luteal cycle were lower in smokers than in non-smokers (MacMahon *et al.* 1982). If these two observations were related it would have provided additional evidence for the role of oestrogen stimulus in breast cancer aetiology. The question was thoroughly reviewed by Baron (1984) and up until that time the evidence relating cigarette smoking to breast cancer risk showed no clear pattern. However, large studies published subsequent to Baron's paper indicate that there is no important association between cigarette smoking and breast cancer risk.

15.2. Methods

The first question to be addressed is whether there is a difference in breast cancer risk between 'genuine' smokers and 'genuine' non-smokers. Neither of these categories is easy to define but if there was an association between smoking and breast cancer risk it might emerge more clearly in such a comparison than in the more all-inclusive comparison of all smokers and non-smokers. A genuine non-smoker in the terminology used here is a person who has never been a smoker, according to whatever criteria the individual investigator has used to define a smoker. Occasionally, as noted in footnotes to the tables, data for this category have not been provided and those for persons who were not currently smokers have had to be substituted. A genuine smoker is, in this presentation, someone who takes more than the occasional social puff. A variety of category boundaries have been used by different investigators, but generally it has been possible to obtain data for persons who currently smoke either more than 15 cigarettes or more than one pack a day. From here on the category will be referred to simply as 'smokers'. The categories of smokers of lesser amounts and the issue of past smoking are excluded.

Some summary estimates of odds ratios (OR), risk ratios (RR), and confidence limits (CL) are presented for groups of studies having similar methodology. These summary estimates are approximate. They are based on the proposal of Woolf (1955) to weight the natural logarithms of the odds ratios in case-control studies by the inverse of each one's variance, the variance of the weighted estimate being the inverse of the sum of the weights. The approximate nature of the estimates given here stems in part from the fact that some authors have given estimates of OR adjusted for age (AOR), and sometimes other risk factors, but no estimate of the variance around the adjusted point estimate. However, data have been available in some papers to estimate the variance around the unadjusted OR. In these situations the adjusted OR is shown but using the unadjusted variance for weighting purposes and for estimation of CL. While this clearly leads to some inaccuracy the greater inaccuracy was to exclude the series from the pooled estimate altogether. In general, differences between adjusted and unadjusted OR have been small.

In such pooled estimates, case-control studies, because of their greater statistical precision, carry greater weight than cohort studies. On the other hand, cohort studies have virtues that one may not like to see overshadowed to this extent. No pooled estimates have therefore been made combining case-control and cohort studies. All CL presented are approximate 95 per cent limits.

Table 15.1. Odds ratios for smokers in case-control studies in which controls are hospital patients including patients with diseases related to smoking

Authors	Year	Smoking level selected (cigarettes +/day)	Percentage controls at this level	Odds ratio*	Confidence interval †
MacMahon and Feinleib ‡	1960	10	14	1.0	0.6–1.5
Salber *et al.* ‡	1969	16	25	0.7	0.6–0.9
Valaoras *et al.* ‡	1969	16	2	1.2	0.7–2.0
Lowe and MacMahon ‡	1970	16	8	1.0	0.7–1.4
Yuasa and MacMahon ‡	1970	16	6	0.8	0.6–1.1
Ravnihar *et al.* ‡	1971	16	3	0.7	0.4–1.1
Lin *et al.* ‡	1971	16	2	1.3	0.5–3.2
Vessey *et al.*	1983	15	28	0.7	0.6–0.8
Le *et al.*	1984	15	2	1.9	0.8–4.2
Weighted average	—	—	—	0.82	0.73–0.92

* Referent group is never-smokers except in MacMahon and Feinleib and Le *et al.* where it is current non-smokers. All OR are age-adjusted. Estimates of MacMahon and Feinleib and of Vessey *et al.* adjusted for other risk factors.

† Approximate 95 per cent intervals derived by applying the variances derived from unadjusted data to the adjusted point estimates.

‡ These studies were part of a co-ordinated international study. Smoking data were not given in the original publications but have been extracted from the original data for the present paper.

15.3. Results

Case-control studies, hospital controls (A)

One fairly large category of studies is comprised of those case-control studies in which the controls are hospital patients with other diseases when no attempt was made to exclude patients with diseases which themselves are associated with smoking. Such studies are listed in Table 15.1. This type of control group has generally been used when the hypothesis under investigation had to do with something other than smoking. In the first seven studies listed in this table the investigators were investigating the relationship between lactation and breast cancer risk. In the study of Vessey *et al.* (1983) the concern was with contraception. In these studies there was no reason to exclude patients with cigarette-related diseases from the controls; indeed one can imagine circumstances in which it would have been incorrect to do so. However, when attention does turn to smoking in such studies it must be considered that the controls are likely to contain an undue proportion of smokers and that false negative associations with smoking may be seen. In fact, there is an example of this in the study of Salber *et al.* (1969). The AOR of 0.71 was derived from the hospital-based control group used in the published paper. In that study, however, a second control group drawn at random from the general population had also been assembled and analysed but was not included in the final publication, at the request of the editor of the journal in which the paper was published. Use of this population control gave an AOR of 0.81 instead of 0.71 for the same level of cigarette smoking.

The size of this effect will of course vary with time and place and the nature of the particular hospital clientele. The direction of the bias of the OR due to this particular problem is likely to be downwards, but it is not possible to judge whether it has been sufficient to explain the whole difference between 1.0 and the overall weighted average of 0.82. That it was insufficient to do so in one study (Salber *et al.* 1969) does not address the different circumstances of the other studies. However, one can with some confidence believe that the true OR is likely to be higher than that estimated from these studies.

Case-control studies, hospital controls (B)

Some case-control studies have utilized as controls hospital patients from whom patients with smoking-related diseases have been excluded. They are listed in Table 15.2. The results are reasonably homogeneous and centre around an AOR of 1.1. The CL include 1.0 in all studies; in one study the value 1.0 forms the upper bound of the CL and in one it marks the lower bound. The CL of the weighted AOR include 1.0.

Case-control studies in screened populations

Schecter *et al.* (1985) in particular have expressed concern about the

Table 15.2. Odds ratios for smokers in case-control studies in which controls are hospital patients with diseases not known to be related to smoking

Authors	Year	Smoking level selected (cigarettes + /day)	Percentage controls at this level	Odds ratio*	Confidence interval †
Porter and Jick	1983	20	22	1.3	0.6–4.2
Porter and Jick	1983	20	8	0.9	0.4–2.0
Rosenberg *et al.*	1984	15	24	1.0	0.8–1.3
Baron *et al.*	1986	15 ‡	16	0.9	0.8–1.1
Stockwell and Lyman	1987	20	9	1.2	1.0–1.4
Levi	1987	15	9	0.8	0.6–1.0
Weighted average	—	—	—	1.05	0.95–1.16

* Referent group is never-smokers except in Porter and Jick in which it is current non-smokers. All OR are age-adjusted. Data of Porter and Jick and Rosenberg *et al.* adjusted for other risk factors.

† Approximate 95 per cent intervals. Variances based on age-adjusted values as given by the authors.

‡ Refers to 15 or more pack-years.

Table 15.3. Odds ratios for smokers in case-control studies in which cases and controls are derived from screening programmes

Authors	Year	Smoking level selected (cigarettes +/day) ‡	Percentage controls at this level	Odds ratio*	Confidence interval †
Schecter *et al.*	1985	—	12	1.9	1.1–3.4
Brinton *et al.*	1986	20	21	1.2	1.0–1.4
Brownson *et al.*	1988	20	15	1.0	0.7–1.4
Weighted average	—	—	—	1.17	1.02–1.35

* In all studies the referent is never-smokers. All OR are adjusted for age. Data of Schecter *et al.* and Brownson *et al.* are adjusted for other risk factors.

† Approximate 95 per cent intervals. Intervals are age-adjusted CI given by authors, except for Schecter *et al.* for which unadjusted variances have been used.

‡ For Schecter *et al.* smoking is defined as more than 500 pack-years. For Brownson *et al.* the amount includes amounts smoked in the past.

possibility of interaction between smoking habits and participation in screening programmes, wondering whether this may distort the results of case-control studies undertaken in such programmes. Results of three such studies are shown in Table 15.3. The weighted AOR of 1.17 is formally significantly greater than 1.0.

Case-control studies using community controls

Only three case-control studies of breast cancer have been found in which the general community was used as the source of controls. These are shown in Table 15.4. Again, the weighted average OR is above 1.0, but only marginally so.

A summary for all case-control studies, except those listed in Table 15.1, is given in Table 15.5. The weighted average OR is 1.15 and the confidence interval is narrow.

Cohort studies

Risk ratios from nine cohort studies are given in Table 15.6. Data that would permit the first three of these to be included in the overall average are not available. The weighted average AOR is almost identical to that derived from the case-control studies in Table 15.5, and is again marginally significantly higher than 1.0.

Potential effect modifiers

It has been suggested, particularly by Brownson *et al.* (1988), that a direct

Table 15.4. Odds ratios for smokers in case-control studies in which controls are drawn from the general population

Authors	Year	Smoking level selected (cigarettes +/day)	Percentage controls at this level	Odds ratio*	Confidence interval †
Salber *et al.* ‡	1969	16	25	0.8	0.6–1.1
Stroup *et al.*	1987	15	NA	1.2	1.1–1.3
O'Connell *et al.*	1987	20	7	0.6	0.3–1.1
Weighted average	—	—	—	1.15	1.07–1.25

* Referent is never-smokers. All OR are age-adjusted and, except for Salber *et al.*, adjusted for other variables.

† Approximate 95 per cent intervals. Unadjusted variance used for Salber *et al.*

‡ Using not the control group published in the 1969 paper but a matched random community sample drawn and interviewed at the time.

NA, not available.

Table 15.5. Summary odds ratio for the case-control studies reported in Tables 15.2, 15.3 and 15.4

Type of control	Odds ratio	Confidence interval*
Hospital patients (Table 15.2)	1.05	0.95–1.16
Screenees (Table 15.3)	1.17	1.02–1.35
General population (Table 15.4)	1.15	1.07–1.25
Weighted average	1.12	1.06–1.19

* Approximate 95 per cent intervals.

relationship exists between cigarette smoking and breast cancer risk in pre-menopausal women. The relevant data are shown in Table 15.7. Only one study (Stockwell and Lyman 1987) shows an OR significantly above 1.0 and the overall AOR is unimpressive and not significantly different from 1.0. O'Connell *et al.* (1987) also considered menopausal status in multivariate models. No data are given, but this variable was discarded as either a confounder or effect modifier.

Since events in the early years of reproductive life appear to be significant determinants of breast cancer risk, it would be of interest to know the effect,

Table 15.6. Risk ratios for smokers in cohort studies of cigarette smoking and breast cancer

Authors	Year	Smoking level selected (cigarettes + /day)	Percentage controls at this level	Risk ratio (RR)*	Confidence interval †
Hammond	1966	20	NA	0.8	NA
Cederloff *et al.* ‡	1975	1	NA	0.9	NA
Hirayama	1975	1	NA	1.4	NA
Doll *et al.*§	1980	15	15	0.9	0.4–1.6
Ramcharan *et al.*	1981	20	21	1.0	0.7–1.3
Vessey and Yeates‖	1982	15	14	0.8	0.4–1.5
Lund	1985	10	6	1.3	0.8–2.0
Hiatt and Fireman	1986	20	NA	1.1	0.7–1.5
Hiatt *et al.*	1988	20	NA	1.1	0.7–1.5
Weighted average**	—	—	—	1.14	1.02–1.27

* All RR are age-adjusted except in Ramcharan *et al.* Data of Hiatt and Fireman and Hiatt *et al.* are adjusted for numerous other risk factors.

† Variance computed from unadjusted data for Ramcharan *et al.* and Lund. Others confidence intervals are age-adjusted.

‡ Data from Baron (1984).

§ Doll *et al.* (1980), plus personal communication from R. Gray (1988).

‖ M. Vessey and D. Yeates. Personal communication to J. A. Baron (1982).

** Not including the data of Hammond, Cederloff *et al.*, or Hirayama.

NA, not available.

Table 15.7. Odds ratios in studies reporting association of cigarette smoking with breast cancer in women who were pre-menopausal or less than 50 years of age

Author	Year	Odds ratio*	Confidence interval*
Rosenberg *et al.* †	1984	0.9	0.6–1.3
Brinton *et al.* ‡	1986	1.1	0.8–1.5
Stockwell and Lyman§	1987	1.4	1.0–2.1
Brownson *et al.* ‖	1988	1.8	0.9–3.2
Weighted average	—	1.14	0.88–1.48

* See footnotes to previous tables.
† Pre-menopausal; smoking defined as 15 cigarettes or more/day.
‡ Pre-menopausal; all current smokers compared to never-smokers.
§ Age less than 50; smoking defined as 20 cigarettes or more/day.
‖ Pre-menopausal; smoking defined as 20 cigarettes or more/day.

if any, of smoking during those years. Only one relevant set of data has been found. Brinton *et al.* (1986) report AOR for women who started smoking before age 17 and at 17–19 years of age of 1.30 (CL 1.0–1.6) and 1.29 (CL 1.0–1.6), respectively. AOR for women who started at age 20 or older were lower and not significantly higher than 1.0.

On the basis of clinical impression and a very small published series, Daniell (1980) suggested that breast cancers in cigarette smokers were more likely to be receptor-negative for both oestrogen and progesterone and to have unfavourable prognoses. Larger studies have not indicated any significant difference between smokers and non-smokers in proportion of oestrogen-receptor positive tumours (McTiernan *et al.* 1986; Stanford *et al.* 1987). The question of whether cigarette smoking is associated with survival of breast cancer patients, as distinct from incidence of the disease, has not been reviewed for this presentation.

15.4. Discussion

It appears that the conclusion that breast cancer risk is lower in smokers than non-smokers was premature. There now seems little evidence overall that cigarette smoking decreases a woman's risk of cancer of the breast. One might ask why it does not do so, since the evidence is convincing that (1) oestrogen stimulus is a powerful determinant of breast cancer risk (MacMahon and Cole 1972, MacMahon *et al.* 1983) and (2) cigarette smoking reduces oestrogen excretion (and presumably oestrogen stimulus) in pre-menopausal women (MacMahon *et al.* 1982).

Michnovicz *et al.* (1986) showed that increased 2-hydroxylation of oestradiol in pre-menopausal cigarette smokers may be the mechanism of the anti-oestrogenic effect of smoking. Metabolism of oestradiol by the 2-hydroxylation pathway, diminishing the competing pathway of 16-hydroxylation, leads to decreased bioavailability at oestrogen target tissues. However, there are some inconsistencies between our own data and those of Michnovicz *et al.* Michnovicz and his colleagues studied predominantly women in the follicular cycle phase. In a substantially larger series (MacMahon *et al.* 1982) no difference in urinary oestrogen levels between smokers and non-smokers was found in the follicular phase of the cycle—the major difference occurred in luteal phase specimens and there was an indication that it was confined to cycles in which ovulation had occurred. In the five women studied by Michnovicz in both cycle-phases the phenomenon was seen in both phases. Moreover, MacMahon *et al.* (1982) did not see the shift in the urinary oestriol/oestrone ratio which occurred in the data of Michnovicz *et al.* and which, according to them, would be indicative of the implementation of the 2-hydroxylation pathway. Even if the conclusions of Michnovicz *et al.* are correct, however, the mechanism still results in decreased oestrogen stimulus in the peripheral tissues of smokers.

One is also reminded of the 'unopposed oestrogen' theory, under which oestrogens are particularly effective in elevating breast cancer risk when unopposed by progesterone—as in the follicular phase of the menstrual cycle or in cycles which are anovular or have a deficient luteal phase (Sherman and Korenman 1974). While inconsistent with the data of Michnovicz *et al.* (1986), our observations on urine oestrogens suggest that cigarette smoking may be influencing oestrogen stimulus only during periods of progesterone opposition—not during the follicular phase of the cycle or in anovular cycles. It is possible that determinants of the *follicular* oestrogen stimulus—of which cigarettes appear from our data not to be one—are the major determinants of the oestrogen component of breast cancer aetiology. In addition, at least as judged by urinary oestrogen excretion, cigarette smoking does not appear to affect oestrogen stimulus in post-menopausal women (Trichopoulos *et al.* 1987)—a component of total oestrogen stimulus which is not negligible.

Another issue left unresolved by the present review is whether or not the small but statistically significant excess of breast cancer risk among smokers —seen both in case-control and cohort studies—represents a meaningful (causal) excess or is the result of uncontrolled confounding or methodologic bias. While the excess appears very small—point estimates of 12 per cent in case-control and 14 per cent in cohort studies—it would, if real, represent a substantial number of cases in a disease as common as breast cancer—about 15 000 cases per year in the US alone. Alcohol consumption is the most obvious suspect as an uncontrolled confounder. However, the association of breast cancer risk with alcohol consumption as assessed by history is quite weak, and in those studies which have included alcohol consumption among the confounders included in multivariate estimates, the OR or RR associated with cigarette smoking are not consistently elevated. Thus, OR or RR in the studies of Rosenberg *et al.* (1984), Hiatt and Fireman (1986), O'Connell *et al.* (1987) and Hiatt *et al.* (1988) were 1.0, 1.1, 0.6, and 1.1, respectively. Nevertheless, when dealing with OR in the range of 1.1 to 1.2 it is very difficult to rule out the influence of unmeasured confounding by known confounders or the effect of unidentified confounders. It is not clear how this question can be resolved.

References

Baron, J. A. (1984). Smoking and estrogen-related disease. *American Journal of Epidemiology*, **119**, 9-22.

Baron, J. A., Byers, T., Greenberg, E. R., Cummings, K. M., and Swanson, M. (1986). Cigarette smoking in women with cancers of the breast and reproductive organs. *Journal of the National Cancer Institute*, 77, 677-80.

Brinton, L. A., Schairer, C., Stanford, J. L., and Hoover, R. N. (1986). Cigarette smoking and breast cancer. *American Journal of Epidemiology*, **123**, 614-22.

Brownson, R. C., Blackwell, C. W., Pearson, D. K., Reynolds, R. D., Richens, J. W. Jr., and Papermaster, B. W. (1988). Risk of breast cancer in relation to smoking. *Archives of Internal Medicine*, **148**, 140-4.

Cederlof, R., *et al.* (1975). *The relationship of smoking and some social covariables to mortality and cancer morbidity*. Department of Environmental Hygiene, Karolinska Institute, Stockholm. (Quoted by Baron, 1984.)

Daniell, H. W. (1980). Estrogen receptors, breast cancer, and smoking. (Letter to the Editor.) *New England Journal of Medicine*, **302**, 1478.

Doll, R., Gray, R., Hafner, B., and Peto, R. (1980). Mortality in relation to smoking: 22 years' observations on female British doctors. *British Medical Journal*, **280**, 967-71.

Hammond, E. C. (1966). Smoking in relation to the death rates of one million men and women. In *Epidemiological approaches to the study of cancer and other chronic diseases*. National Cancer Institute Monograph No. 19 (ed. E. Haenszel). Superintendent of Documents, US Government Printing Office, Washington.

Hiatt, R. A. and Fireman, B. H. (1986). Smoking, menopause, and breast cancer. *Journal of the National Cancer Institute*, 76, 833-8.

Hiatt, R. A., Klatsky, A. L., and Armstrong, M. A. (1988). Alcohol consumption and the risk of breast cancer in a prepaid health plan. *Cancer Research*, **48**, 2284-7.

Hirayama, T. (1975). Smoking and cancer: a prospective study on cancer epidemiology based on a census population in Japan. In *Proceedings 3rd World Conference Smoking and Health*, Vol. 2 (ed. J. Steinfeld, W. Griffiths, *et al.*), pp. 65-72. US Department of Health, Education, and Welfare, Washington.

Le, M. G., Clavel, F., Hill, C., Kramar, A., and Flamant, R. (1984). Breast cancer and cigarette smoking. (Letter to the Editor.) *New England Journal of Medicine*, **310**, 1532.

Levi, F. (1987). Cigarette smoking and the risk of breast and endometrial cancer. Unpublished M.Sc. thesis. McGill University.

Lin, T. M., Chen, K. P., and MacMahon, B. (1971). Epidemiologic characteristics of cancer of the breast in Taiwan. *Cancer*, 27, 1497–504.
Lowe, C. R. and MacMahon, B. (1970). Breast cancer and reproductive history of women in South Wales. *Lancet*, **i**, 153–7.
Lund, E. (1985). Re 'Smoking and estrogen-related disease'. (Letter to the Editor.) *American Journal of Epidemiology*, **121**, 324–5.
MacMahon, B. and Cole, P. (1972). The ovarian etiology of human breast cancer. *Recent Results in Cancer Research*, **39**, 185–92.
MacMahon, B. and Feinleib, M. (1960). Breast cancer in relation to nursing and menopausal history. *Journal of the National Cancer Institute*, **24**, 733–53.
MacMahon, B., Trichopoulos, D., Cole, P., and Brown, J. (1982). Cigarette smoking and urine estrogens. *New England Journal of Medicine*, **307**, 1062–5.
MacMahon, B., Cole, P., Brown, J. B., Paffenbarger, R., Trichopoulos, D., and Yen, S. (1983). Urine estrogens, frequency of ovulation and breast cancer risk: a case-control study in premenopausal women. *Journal of the National Cancer Institute*, **70**, 247–50.
McTiernan, A., Thomas, D. B., Johnson, L. K., and Roseman, D. (1986). Risk factors for estrogen receptor-rich and estrogen receptor-poor breast cancers. *Journal of the National Cancer Institute*, 77, 849–54.
Michnovicz, J. J., Hershcopf, R. J., Naganuma, H., Bradlow, H. L., and Fishman, J. (1986). Increased 2-hydroxylation of estradiol as a possible mechanism for the anti-estrogenic effect of cigarette smoking. *New England Journal of Medicine*, **315**, 1305–9.
O'Connell, D. L., Hulka, B. S., Chambless, L. E., Wilkinson, W. E., and Deubner, D. C. (1987). Cigarette smoking, alcohol consumption, and breast cancer risk. *Journal of the National Cancer Institute*, **78**, 229–34.
Porter, J. B., and Jick, H. (1983). Breast cancer and cigarette smoking. (Letter to the Editor.) *New England Journal of Medicine*, **309**, 186.
Ramcharan, S., Pellegrin, F. A., Ray, R., and Hsu, J-P. (1981). *The Walnut Creek Contraceptive Drug Study*, Vol. 3, NIH Publication No. 81-564. US Government Printing Office, Washington.
Ravnihar, B., MacMahon, B., and Lindtner, J. (1971). Epidemiologic features of breast cancer in Slovenia, 1965–1967. *European Journal of Cancer*, 7, 295–306.
Rosenberg, L., *et al.* (1984). Breast cancer and cigarette smoking. *New England Journal of Medicine*, **310**, 92–4.
Salber, E. J., Trichopoulos, D., and MacMahon, B. (1969). Lactation and reproductive histories of breast cancer patients in Boston, 1965–66. *Journal of the National Cancer Institute*, **43**, 1013–24.
Schechter, M. T., Miller, A. B., and Howe, G. R. (1985). Cigarette smoking and breast cancer: a case-control study of screening program participants. *American Journal of Epidemiology*, **121**, 479–87.
Sherman, B. M. and Korenman, S. G. (1974). Inadequate corpus luteum function: a pathophysiological interpretation of human breast cancer epidemiology. *Cancer*, **33**, 1306–11.
Stanford, J. L., *et al.* (1987). A case-control study of breast cancer stratified by estrogen receptor status. *American Journal of Epidemiology*, **125**, 184–94.
Stockwell, H. G. and Lyman, G. H. (1987). Cigarette smoking and the risk of female reproductive cancer. *American Journal of Obstetrics and Gynecology*, **157**, 35–40.

Stroup, N. E., Layde, P. M., Webster, L. A., Wingo, P. A., Rubin, G. L., and Ory, H. W. (1987). Cigarette smoking and breast cancer. In *Smoking and reproductive health* (ed. M. J. Rosenberg). PSG Publishing, Littleton, MA.

Trichopoulos, D., Brown, J., and MacMahon, B. (1987). Urine estrogens and breast cancer risk factors among post-menopausal women. *International Journal of Cancer*, **40**, 721–5.

Valaoras, V. G., MacMahon, B., Trichopoulos, D., and Polychronopoulou, A. (1969). Lactation and reproductive histories of breast cancer patients in greater Athens, 1965–67. *International Journal of Cancer*, **4**, 350–63.

Vessey, M., Baron, J., Doll, R., McPherson, K., and Yeates, D. (1983). Oral contraceptives and breast cancer: final report of an epidemiological study. *British Journal of Cancer*, **47**, 455–62.

Woolf, B. (1955). On estimating the relation between blood groups and disease. *Annals of Human Genetics*, **19**, 251–3.

Yuasa, S. and MacMahon, B. (1970). Lactation and reproductive histories of breast cancer patients in Tokyo, Japan. *Bulletin of the World Health Organization*, **42**, 195–204.

16. Cigarette smoking and cancer of the large bowel

John A. Baron and Robert S. Sandler

Abstract

Several aspects of the epidemiology of large bowel cancer suggest that the risks of this malignancy may be affected by oestrogenic stimuli and may therefore also be modified by cigarette smoking. Available data regarding this relationship, however, are contradictory: while several studies suggest a lowered risk of cancer of the colon among smokers, most do not. Further clarification may require consideration of cancer risks at various subsites in the colon.

16.1. Introduction

Several aspects of the epidemiology of large bowel cancer suggest that the risks of this malignancy may be affected by oestrogenic influences (McMichael and Potter 1983). In Western societies, the rates of colon cancer among pre-menopausal women exceed those for men of a similar age, in contrast to the usual male predominance for cancer of non-reproductive organs (Fraumeni *et al.* 1969). After the menopause, women have slightly lower rates. The distribution of cancers within the colon also differs between the sexes: women are more likely to have right-sided cancers than men, especially at older ages (Stewart *et al.* 1983; Vobecky *et al.* 1984; Jensen 1984).

Among women, there may be associations between reproductive history and the risk of colorectal cancer. Several investigators have found that nulliparous women have an increased risk (Dales *et al.* 1979; Fraumeni *et al.* 1969; Potter and McMichael 1983), and others have noted a decreasing risk with increasing parity (Weiss *et al.* 1981), although not all studies have demonstrated this effect (Wu *et al.* 1987; Byers *et al.* 1982). Howe *et al.* (1985) found a strong protective effect of early age at first pregnancy, especially for cancers of the right colon.

Finally, the reports of oestrogen receptor protein in colon cancer specimens are also consistent with a role for oestrogenic influences on the behaviour of these neoplasms (Alford *et al.* 1979; Stedman *et al.* 1980; Bojar *et al.* 1980; Sica *et al.* 1984). To the extent that cancer of the large bowel (especially colon) is an oestrogen-related disease, then one might expect that cigarette smoking would decrease risk through its 'anti-oestrogenic' effect.

An influence of cigarette smoking on large bowel pathology is also suggested by the repeatedly demonstrated inverse association between ulcerative colitis and cigarette smoking, as discussed by Logan (Chapter 12). Little is known about the factors that cause this disorder, and there are few established oestrogenic connections for it. However, the relationship between cigarette smoking and ulcerative colitis indicates that smoking can have important effects on the large bowel, or at least is associated with something that has important effects.

16.2. Epidemiological summary

There are abundant epidemiological data regarding cigarette smoking and colorectal cancer (Tables 16.1–16.3). However, most of the published studies have not focused on that particular relationship, and details such as dose–response trends are not well described. Most studies reported relative risk estimates for ever smoking or current smoking vs. never smoking, controlling only for age (and for sex, in estimates pertaining to both sexes). A variety of relative risk measures are used and reported here, including odds ratios in case-control studies, and odds ratios and risk ratios in cohort studies. Several case-control studies employed a matched design and presented either an unmatched odds ratio, or only smoking percentages from which an unmatched odds ratio could be computed. The use of these statistics will tend to result in underestimation of the magnitude of any associations present.

For cancer of the colon, the data are mixed (Fig. 16.1 and Table 16.1). The reported relative risks associated with smoking varied in the range 0.5

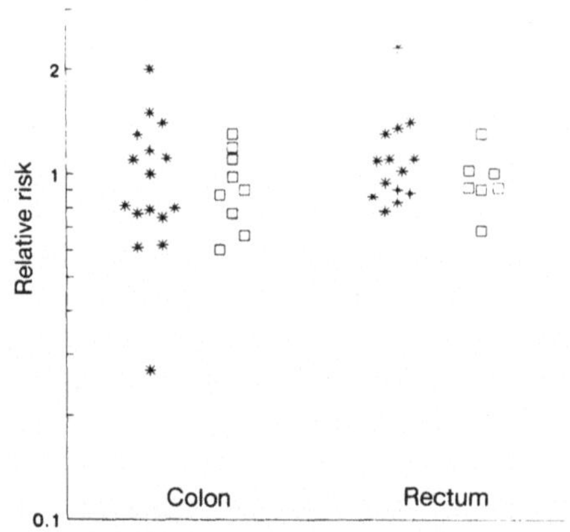

Fig. 16.1. Smoking and large bowel cancer. * , males; □ , females.

to 2.0, with a tendency toward estimates less than one. Only two studies reported statistically significant results, both in a 'protective' direction. Risk estimates for women were similar to those for men. The studies that used colon cancer mortality as an endpoint, in general reported higher relative risks than those that investigated incident cases, although case-control and cohort studies reported estimates in roughly the same range.

For cancer of the rectum, the data also varied, with little suggestion of decreased risks associated with smoking (Fig. 16.1 and Table 16.2). None of the estimates was statistically different from one. As for colon cancer, the results were similar for males and females.

Studies of colorectal cancer in aggregate resembled those for colon cancer: there was a range of relative risk estimates, with more studies showing lower risks than increased, especially among women (Fig. 16.2 and Table 16.3). Two of the individual estimates were statistically lower than one, however, but the control for confounding by age in the studies by Higginson (1966) and Staszewski (1969) appears inadequate. Two studies that did not report relative risks indicated lower risks in smokers (Nakamura *et al.* 1984; Garland *et al.* 1985), while another found, if anything, increased risks (Martinez *et al.* 1979).

Sandler *et al.* (1988) reported a pattern of relative risks decreasing with age among women. Similar patterns for age-related changes in the risks associated with smoking have been found in some studies of endometrial cancer and benign breast disease.

Data regarding pipe or cigar smoking are essentially limited to men (Table 16.4). Relative risk estimates tended to be modestly greater than one, and a few were statistically different from one, though still less than 2.0.

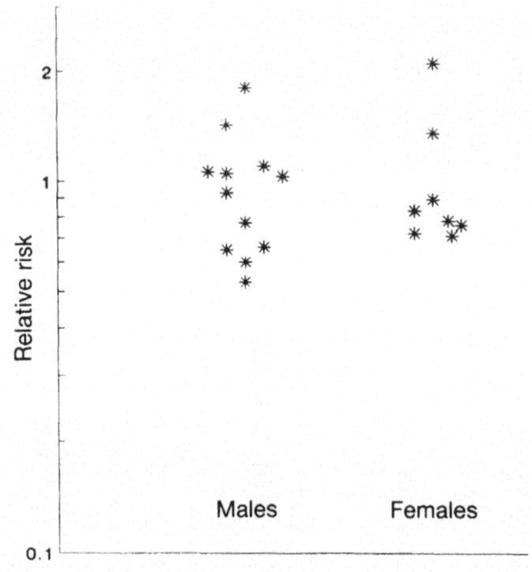

Fig. 16.2. Smoking and colorectal cancer.

Table 16.1. Smoking and cancer of the colon

Study	Study design and source of subjects	Contrast	Relative risk	
			Male	Female
Williams *et al.* (1981)	Cohort incidence (58 cases)	One pack per day of cigarettes vs. non-smoker	0.27 †	less than 1†
Cederlof *et al.* (1975)	Cohort incidence (88 cases) (cancer of the intestine)	Current cigarette smoker vs. not current smoker	0.81	1.19
Carstensen *et al.* (1987)	Cohort mortality (117 deaths)	Current smoker (8–15 g tobacco/day) vs. never smoker	1.5	
Lund and Zeiner-Henriksen (1981)	Cohort (incidence)	Current smoker vs. never smoker	0.8	0.9
Hammond and Horn (1958)	Cohort mortality (193 deaths)	Ever regular cigarette smoker vs. never smoker	0.77	—
Doll and Peto (1976)	Cohort mortality (195 deaths)	Current smoker (any tobacco) vs. never smoker	1.3	—
Rogot and Murray (1980)	Cohort mortality (662 deaths) (cancer of the intestine)	Current cigarette smoker vs. never smoker	1.11	—
Kahn (1966)	Cohort mortality (697 deaths) (cancer of the intestine)	Current cigarette smoker vs. never smoker	1.17	—
Garfinkel (1980)	Cohort mortality (2382 deaths among never smokers)	Ever regular smoker vs. never regular smoker	1.10 ‡	0.98 ‡

Table 16.1. (*cont.*)

Study	Study design and source of subjects	Contrast	Relative risk	
			Male	Female
Tajima and Tominaga (1985)	Hospital case-control (27 cases)	Current smoker vs. never smoker	0.61	—
Schober *et al.* (1987)	Population case-control (72 cases)	Ever cigarette smoker vs. never smoker	(1.13)*	
Enstrom and Godley (1980)	Two national samples (105 cases among never smokers)	Ever cigarette smoker vs. never smoker	0.75 ‡	1.1 ‡
Vobecky *et al.* (1983)	'Community' case-control (207 large bowel cases)	Current cigarette smoker vs. never smoker	2.0	1.3
Wynder and Shigematsu (1967)	Hospital case-control (468 cases)	Cigarette smoker vs. non-smoker	0.62*	0.87*
Byers *et al.* (1986) (unpublished data)	Hospital case-control (481 cases)	39 + pack years (males) or 15 + pack years (females) vs. never smoker	1.0	0.6 †
Pernu (1960)	Hospital case-control (666 cases) (cancer of the intestines)	Ever smoker vs. never smoker	1.4	0.77
Williams and Horm (1977)	Cancer survey case-control (722 cases)	40 + pack years vs. never smoker	0.79	0.66

* Matched design, analysed unmatched; derived from data presented.
† Statistically different from 1, $P<0.05$.
‡ Reciprocal of relative risk for non-smokers vs. entire study population.

Table 16.2. Smoking and cancer of the rectum

Study	Study design and source of subjects	Contrast	Relative risk	
			Male	Female
Cederlof *et al.* (1975)	Cohort incidence (52 cases)	Current cigarette smoker vs. not current smoker	0.88	0.68
Carstensen *et al.* (1987)	Cohort mortality (69 deaths)	Current smoker (8–15 g tobacco/day) vs. never smoker	1.3	—
Doll and Peto (1976)	Cohort mortality (78 deaths)	Current smoker (any tobacco) vs. never smoker	2.3	—
Lund and Zeiner-Henriksen (1981)	Cohort incidence (91 cases)	Current smoker vs. never smoker	1.09	0.4
Hammond and Horn (1958)	Cohort mortality (104 deaths)	Ever regular cigarette smoker vs. never smoker	0.94	—
Rogot and Murray (1980)	Cohort mortality (239 deaths)	Current cigarette smoker vs. never smoker	1.11	—
Kahn (1966)	Cohort mortality (338 deaths)	Current cigarette smoker vs. never smoker	0.90	—
Garfinkel (1980)	Cohort mortality (554 deaths among never smokers)	Ever regular smoker vs. never regular smoker	1.35†	1.02†

Table 16.2. (*contd.*)

Study	Study design and source of subjects	Contrast	Relative risk	
			Male	Female
Tajima and Tominaga (1985)	Hospital case-control (25 cases)	Current cigarette smoker vs. never smoker	1.02	—
Enstrom and Godley (1980)	Two national samples (36 cases among never smokers)	Ever cigarette smoker vs. never smoker	0.86†	1.30†
Vobecky *et al.* (1983)	'Community' case-control (207 colorectal cases)	Current cigarette smoker vs. non-smoker	1.4	1.0
Wynder and Shigematsu (1967)	Hospital case-control (323 cases)	Cigarette smoker vs. non-smoker	0.83*	0.91*
Williams and Horm (1977)	Cancer survey case-control (339 cases)	40+ pack years vs. never smoker	0.78	0.91
Byers *et al.* (1986) (unpublished data)	Hospital case-control (653 cases)	39+ pack years (males) or 15+ pack years (females) vs. never smoker	1.1	0.9

* Matched design, analysed unmatched; derived from data presented.
† Reciprocal of relative risk for non-smokers vs. entire study population.

Table 16.3. Cigarette smoking and colorectal cancer

Study	Study design and source of subjects	Contrast	Relative risk	
			Male	Female
Kono *et al.* (1987)	Cohort mortality (39 deaths)	Current smoker 20+ cigarettes per day vs. non-current	0.93	—
Wu *et al.* (1987)	Cohort incidence (126 cases)	Current cigarette smoker vs. never smoker	1.80	1.35
Sidney *et al.* (1986)	Cohort incidence (245 cases)	Current smoker vs. not current smoker	(1.04)*	
Sandler *et al.* (1988)	Cohort mortality (480 cases)	Ever cigarette smoker vs. never smoker not passively exposed	1.42	0.76
Hammond (1966)	Cohort mortality (695 deaths)	Ever regular cigarette smoker vs. never regular smoker (age 45–64)	1.01	0.78
Hirayama (1981)	Cohort mortality (726 deaths)	Daily cigarette smoker vs. none	(1.26)	
Dales *et al.* (1979)	Hospital case-control (99 cases)	Ever regular cigarette smoker vs. never smoker	(1.0)	
Papadimitriou *et al.* (1984)	Hospital case-control (100 cases)	Current cigarette smoker vs. not current smoker	0.66	2.1

Table 16.3. (*cont.*)

Study	Study design and source of subjects	Contrast	Relative risk	
			Male	Female
Haenszel *et al.* (1973)	Hospital case-control (178 cases)	Any tobacco use vs. no tobacco	1.05	0.71
		20 cigarettes daily vs. <20	0.65	—
Haenszel *et al.* (1980)	Hospital case-control (284 cases)	Ever tobacco use vs. never use	0.77	—
Higginson (1966)	Hospital case-control (340 cases)	Ever cigarette smoker vs. never smoker	0.53* †	0.72*
Schwartz *et al.* (1961)	Hospital case-control (355 cases)	Recent cigarette smoking vs. not	1.06*	—
Staszewski (1969)	Hospital case-control (438 cases)	Ever cigarette smoker vs. never smoker	0.60 † ‡	0.83‡
Jain *et al.* (1980)	Population case-control (542 cases)	Ever cigarette smoker vs. never smoker	1.03*	0.89*

* Matched design, analysed unmatched; derived from data presented.
† Significantly different from 1, $P<0.05$.
‡ No age adjustment (?).

Table 16.4. Pipe and cigar smoking and cancer of the large bowel

Study	Exposure	Relative risk: Cancer of the colon	Relative risk: Cancer of the rectum
Vobecky *et al.* (1983)	Pipe	0.29	1.6
Higginson (1966)	Pipe (ever)	(1.03)	
	Cigars (ever)	(1.17)	
Staszewski (1969)	Pipe or cigar only (ever)	(1.32)	
Pernu (1960)	Pipe	1.76*†	—
Wynder and Shigematsu (1967)	Pipe (ever)	1.23*	0.77*
	Cigar (ever)	1.84*†	1.65*†
Williams and Horm (1977)	Pipe (high use)	1.12	0.70
	Cigar (high use)	1.44	1.06
Kahn (1966)	Pipe and/or cigar only—current	1.20	1.07
Hammond (1966)	Pipe and/or cigar (ever)	(1.31)	
Dales *et al.* (1979)	Pipe—ever	(1.54)*	
	Cigar—ever	(1.37)*	

* Matched design, analysed unmatched; derived from data presented.
† Statistically different from 1, $P<0.05$.

There were no noticeable differences between the patterns for cancer of the colon and cancer of the rectum.

16.3. Discussion

The data regarding the relationship between cancer of the large bowel and cigarette smoking are contradictory. Cancer of the rectum appears unrelated to cigarette smoking, though cancer of the colon (and colorectal cancer) show hints of an inverse association. Many of the studies reported a reduction in risk, although only a few of these estimates were statistically different from one. Other investigations have not found this inverse association.

There are several possible explanations for these varying results regarding colon and colorectal cancer. Most importantly, any association between smoking and the risk of large bowel cancer may vary depending on the site within the large bowel. The proximal colon has been most associated with oestrogenic influences, presumably through an effect on bile acid metabolism

(McMichael and Potter 1983). Therefore the risk of cancers at proximal sites might be more likely to be affected by smoking, and the varying proportion of tumours derived from the right colon could underlie the variable effects. Similarly, an effect may be confined to older women, resulting in mixed results depending on the sex and ages of the subjects in a study.

Several technical considerations may also play a role. In particular, some of the case-control studies using hospitalized controls may have been biased toward an inverse relationship because cigarette smoking may be associated with high smoking rates among controls. Second, unrecognized confounding may have affected the results. For example, smoking may be associated with reproductive history in women, or with alcohol intake, which may be related to the risk of large bowel cancer. Hirayama (1981), in fact, found an interaction between cigarette smoking and alcohol intake: smoking was associated with an increased risk of large bowel cancer only among daily alcohol drinkers. Finally, contamination of the case series with other malignancies could have altered the results. For example, some cases of cancer of the rectum could easily be diagnosed as cancer of the colon and vice versa. Also, a series of colorectal cancer cases may be contaminated with a few malignancies originating in the ovaries, uterus, or other organs.

In summary, there are hints of a negative association between cigarette smoking and cancer of the colon, though most studies have not shown this. Further clarification will require consideration of subsite-specific cancer risks.

References

Alford, T. C., *et al.* (1979). Steroid hormone receptors in human colon cancers. *Cancer*, **43**, 980–4.

Bojar, H., Heim, M. E., Petzinna, D., and Staib, W. (1984). Steroid receptor pattern of human colorectal neoplasms. *Anticancer Research*, **4**, 129–32.

Byers, T., Graham, S., and Swanson, M. (1982). Parity and colorectal cancer risk in women. *Journal of the National Cancer Institute*, **69**, 1059–62.

Carstensen, J. M., Pershagen, G., and Eklund, G. (1987). Mortality in relation to cigarette and pipe smoking: 16 years' observation of 25,000 Swedish men. *Journal of Epidemiology and Community Health*, **41**, 166–72.

Cederlof, R., *et al.* (1975). *The relationship of smoking and some social covariables to mortality and cancer morbidity*. Department of Environmental Hygiene, Karolinska Institute, Stockholm.

Dales, L. G., *et al.* (1979). A case-control study of relationships of diet and other traits to colorectal cancer in American blacks. *American Journal of Epidemiology*, **109**, 132–44.

Doll, R. and Peto, R. (1976). Mortality in relation to smoking: 20 years' observations on male British doctors. *British Medical Journal*, **2**, 1525–36.

Enstrom, J. E. and Godley, F. H. (1980). Cancer mortality among a representative sample of nonsmokers in the United States during 1966–68. *Journal of the National Cancer Institute*, **65**, 1175–83.

Fraumeni, J. F., Lloyd, J. W., Smith, E. M., and Wagoner, J. K. (1969). Cancer mortality among nuns: role of marital status in etiology of neoplastic disease in women. *Journal of the National Cancer Institute*, **42**, 455–68.

Garfinkel, L. (1980). Cancer mortality in nonsmokers: prospective study by the American Cancer Society. *Journal of the National Cancer Institute*, **65**, 1169–73.

Garland, C., Barrett-Connor, E., and Rossof, A. H. (1985). Dietary vitamin D and calcium and risk of colorectal cancer: a 19-year prospective study in men. *Lancet*, **i**, 307–9.

Haenszel, W., *et al.* (1973). Large-bowel cancer in Hawaiian Japanese. *Journal of the National Cancer Institute*, **51**, 1765–79.

Haenszel, W., Locke, F. B., and Segi, M. (1980). A case-control study of large bowel cancer in Japan. *Journal of the National Cancer Institute*, **64**, 17–22.

Hammond, E. C. (1966). Smoking in relation to the death rates of one million men and women. *National Cancer Institute Monograph*, **19**, 127–204.

Hammond, E. C. and Horn, D. (1958). Smoking and death rates—report on forty-four months of follow-up of 187,783 men. II. Death rates by cause. *Journal of the American Medical Association*, **166**, 1294–1308.

Higginson, J. (1966). Etiological factors in gastrointestinal cancer in man. *Journal of the National Cancer Institute*, **37**, 527–45.

Hirayama, T. (1981). A large-scale cohort study on the relationship between diet and selected cancers of digestive organs. In *Gastrointestinal cancer: endogenous factors*, Banbury Report 7 (ed. W. R. Bruce, R. Correa, M. Lipkin *et al.*). Cold Spring Harbor Laboratory, New York.

Howe, G. R., Craib, K. J. P., and Miller, A. B. (1985). Age at first pregnancy and risk of colorectal cancer: a case-control study. *Journal of the National Cancer Institute*, **74**, 1155–9.

Jain, M., *et al.* (1980). A case-control study of diet and colo-rectal cancer. *Journal of the National Cancer Institute*, **26**, 757–68.

Jensen, O. M. (1984). Different age and sex relationship for cancer of subsites of the large bowel. *British Journal of Cancer*, **50**, 825–9.

Kahn, H. A. (1966). The Dorn Study of smoking and mortality among U.S. Veterans: Report on eight and one-half years of observation. *National Cancer Institute Monograph*, **19**, 1–126.

Kono, S., *et al.* (1987). Cigarette smoking, alcohol and cancer mortality: a cohort study of male Japanese physicians. *Japanese Journal of Cancer Research (Gann)*, **78**, 1323–8.

Lund, E. and Zeiner-Henriksen, T. (1981). Roking som risikofaktor for ulike dreftformer blant 26000 norske menn og kvinner. *Tidsskrift for den Norske Laegeforening*, **101**, 1937–40.

McMichael, A. J. and Potter, J. D. (1983). Do intrinsic sex differences in lower alimentary tract physiology influence the sex-specific risks of bowel cancer and other biliary and intestinal disease? *American Journal of Epidemiology*, **118**, 620–7.

Martinez, I., *et al.* (1979). Factors associated with adenocarcinomas of the large bowel in Puerto Rico. In *Advances in medical oncology, research, and education*. Vol. 3, *Epidemiology* (ed. J. H. Birch), pp. 45–52. Pergamon Press, Oxford.

Nakamura, G. J., Schneiderman, L. J., and Klauber, M. R. (1984). Colorectal cancer and bowel habits. *Cancer*, **54**, 1475–7.

Papadimitriou, C., *et al.* (1984). Biosocial correlates of colorectal cancer in Greece. *International Journal of Epidemiology*, **13**, 155–9.

Pernu, J. (1960). An epidemiological study on cancer of the digestive organs and respiratory system. *Annales Medicinae Internae Fenniae*, **49**(suppl. 33), 25–117.

Potter, J. D. and McMichael, A. J. (1983). Large bowel cancer in women in relation to reproductive and hormonal factors: a case-control study. *Journal of the National Cancer Institute*, **71**, 703–9.

Rogot, E. and Murray, J. L. (1980). Smoking and causes of death among U.S. veterans: 16 years of observation. *Public Health Reports*, **95**, 213–22.

Sandler, R. S., Sandler, D. P., Comstock, G. W., Helsing, K. J., and Shore, D. L. (1988). Cigarette smoking and the risk of colorectal cancer in women. *Journal of the National Cancer Institute*, **80**, 1329–33.

Schober, S. E., *et al.* (1987). Serologic precursors of cancer. I. Prediagnostic serum nutrients and colon cancer risk. *American Journal of Epidemiology*, **126**, 1033–41.

Schwartz, D., Flamant, R., Lellouch, J., and Denoix, P. F. (1961). Results of a French survey on the role of tobacco, particularly inhalation, in different cancer sites. *Journal of the National Cancer Institute*, **26**, 1085–108.

Sica, V., *et al.* (1984). Estradiol and progesterone receptors in malignant gastrointestinal tumors. *Cancer Research*, **44**, 4670–4.

Sidney, S., Friedman, G. D., and Hiatt, R. A. (1986). Serum cholesterol and large bowel cancer. A case-control study. *American Journal of Epidemiology*, **124**, 33–8.

Staszewski, J. (1969) Smoking and cancer of the alimentary tract in Poland. *British Journal of Cancer*, **23**, 247–53.

Stedman, K. E., Moore, G. E., and Morgan, R. T. (1980). Estrogen receptor proteins in diverse human tumors. *Archives of Surgery*, **115**, 244–8.

Stewart, R. J., Stewart, A. W., Turnbull, P. R. G., and Isbister, W. H. (1983). Sex differences in subsite incidence of large-bowel cancer. *Diseases of the colon and rectum*, **26**, 658–60.

Tajima, K. and Tominaga, S. (1985). Dietary habits and gastro-intestinal cancers: a comparative case-control study of stomach and large intestinal cancers in Nagoya, Japan. *Japanese Journal of Cancer Research (Gann)*, **76**, 705–16.

Vobecky, J., Caro, J., and DeVroede, G. (1983). A case-control study of risk factors for large bowel carcinoma. *Cancer*, **51**, 1958–63.

Vobecky, J., Leduc, C., and DeVroede, G. (1984). Sex differences in the changing anatomic distribution of colorectal carcinoma. *Cancer*, **54**, 3065–9.

Weiss, N. S., Daling, J. R., and Chow, W. H. (1981). Incidence of cancer of the large bowel in women in relation to reproductive and hormonal factors. *Journal of the National Cancer Institute*, **67**, 57–60.

Williams, R. R. and Horm, J. W. (1977). Association of cancer sites with tobacco and alcohol consumption and socioeconomic status of patients: interview study from the Third National Cancer Survey. *Journal of the National Cancer Institute*, **58**, 525–47.

Williams, R. R., *et al.* (1981). Cancer incidence by levels of cholesterol. *Journal of the American Medical Association*, **245**, 247–52.

Wu, A. H., Paganini-Hill, A., Ross, R. K., and Henderson, B. E. (1987). Alcohol, physical activity and other risk factors for colorectal cancer: a prospective study. *British Journal of Cancer*, **55**, 687–94.

Wynder, E. L. and Shigematsu, T. (1967). Environmental factors of cancer of the colon and rectum. *Cancer*, **20**, 1520–61.

VI

Mechanisms: Hormonal Differences in Smokers and Non-smokers

17. Smoking and endogenous sex hormones in men and women

Elizabeth Barrett-Connor

Abstract

Studies of endogenous hormone levels have confirmed that cigarette smoking can have important hormonal effects. Circulating levels of the adrenal hormones androstenedione and dehydroepiandrosterone sulphate have repeatedly been found to be elevated in smokers. Oestradiol and oestrone levels do not appear to be related to smoking in women, but may be increased in men who smoke. The data regarding testosterone are variable. The net effect of these changes may be that smoking has an androgenic influence in women and an oestrogenic influence in men.

17.1. Introduction

Cigarette smoking is associated with an increased risk of ischaemic heart disease and osteoporosis in both men and women. In women, cigarette smoking is also associated with earlier menopause, and, in some studies, decreased fertility and a reduced risk of breast and endometrial cancer. These observations have suggested an anti-oestrogenic effect of cigarette smoking (see review by Baron 1984). Endogenous sex hormone levels in smokers vs. non-smokers and possible mechanisms for the differences have been described in various reports since 1973. This chapter reviews the published literature in men and women and updates previously reported work in Rancho Bernardo (Barrett-Connor and Khaw 1987; Khaw *et al.* 1988).

17.2. Studies in women

Targett *et al.* (1973) studied urinary oestriol excretion in 1000 consecutive pregnant women; although the number with categorically defined subnormal secretion did not differ significantly when smokers were compared to non-smokers, there was a step-wise increase in those with subnormal oestriol excretion with increasing number of cigarettes smoked. MacMahon *et al.* (1982) studied urinary oestrogen levels in 106 pre-menopausal women aged

25–49 who had provided timed overnight specimens on each of two days of a single menstrual cycle. In the follicular specimens (days 10 and 11) oestrogen levels were similar in smokers and non-smokers, but in luteal specimens (days 21 and 22) current smokers had levels of oestrone, oestradiol, and oestriol that were about one third below those of non-smokers. Mochizuki *et al.* (1984) studied 124 pregnant women and also found urine oestriol levels to be significantly lower in heavy smokers. In contrast, Trichopoulos *et al.* (1987) reported that urine oestrone, oestradiol, and oestriol levels in 220 post-menopausal women from Boston and Greece did not differ by cigarette smoking status; the number of cigarettes smoked was not given. Urine oestrogen studies are summarized in Table 17.1.

Blood levels of oestrogen by smoking status were first investigated by Crawford *et al.* (1981). They found plasma ethinyloestradiol and norgestrel levels in 311 women using oral contraceptives were similar in smokers and non-smokers, although they did not report the day of the menstrual cycle when blood was obtained. Jensen *et al.* (1985) reported serum oestrone and oestradiol levels in 136 post-menopausal women who were treated with one of three different doses of oestrogen and progestin. Baseline oestrogen levels were said to be the same in women who smoked or did not smoke, but the data were not shown. Among non-smoking women receiving low, medium, or high dose replacement oestrogen, there was a clear gradient of serum oestrone and oestradiol with dose. There was no obvious gradient and a significantly smaller increment in serum oestrogen in the hormone-treated smokers. The difference between this effect for oestradiol and the lack of one for ethinyloestradiol is compatible with the studies of Kanarkowski *et al.* (1988), who reported that smoking had no effect on ethinyloestradiol levels.

Table 17.1. Urinary oestrogens in women by cigarette smoking status

Study	Characteristics of women	Oestrogen in smokers vs. non-smokers			
		Number (% smokers)	E_1	E_2	E_3
Targett *et al.* (1973)	Pregnant	1000 (39)	—	—	NS*
MacMahon *et al.* (1982)	Pre-menopausal (luteal phase)	106 (37)	↓	↓	↓
Mochizuki *et al.* (1984)	Pregnant	124 (48)	—	—	↓
Trichopoulos *et al.* (1987)	Post-menopausal	220 (44)	NS	NS	NS

* See text.
NS, not significant; E_1, oestrone; E_2, oestradiol; E_3, oestriol.

Table 17.2. Plasma sex hormones in women by cigarette smoking status

Study	Source of subjects (age)	Number	Hormones in smokers vs. non-smokers					Adjusted/ matched for obesity
			A	DHEAS	T	E_1	E_2	
Jensen *et al.* (1985)	Volunteers (44–56)	136	—	—	—	NS*	NS*	No
Friedman *et al.* (1987)	Volunteers (49.2±6.3–54.2±3.9)	25	↑	NS	↑	NS	NS	No
Longcope and Johnston (1988)	Volunteers (49.4±0.8–52.9±0.5)	88	↑	—	NS	NS	NS	No
Khaw *et al.* (1988)	Rancho Bernardo (60–79)	233	↑	↑	NS	NS	NS	Yes

* See text.

NS, not significant; A, androstenedione; DHEAS, dihydroepiandrosterone sulphate; T, testosterone; E_1, oestrone; E_2, oestradiol.

Blood levels of sex hormones in untreated women are shown in Table 17.2. Friedman *et al.* (1987) studied 25 post-menopausal women volunteers, nine of whom were cigarette smokers. No significant differences were found for oestrone, oestradiol, or dihydrotestosterone between smokers and non-smokers. Cigarette smokers had significantly higher plasma levels of testosterone, androstenedione, and progesterone and 17-hydroxyprogesterone than non-smokers. Dehydroepiandrosterone sulphate (DHEAS) levels were twice as high in smokers as in non-smokers but this difference was not statistically significant. The non-smoking women were significantly older and tended to be heavier than smoking women; however, hormone levels were not adjusted for age or obesity.

Khaw *et al.* (1988) reported sex hormone levels in 233 Rancho Bernardo white women, aged 60–79 years. Oestrone, oestradiol, testosterone, and sex hormone binding globulin levels did not differ by smoking status, but current cigarette smokers had significantly higher mean plasma levels of both adrenal androgens measured, DHEAS, and androstenedione. These differences persisted after adjusting for age and obesity. As shown in Figure 17.1, a dose–response relationship was apparent with levels of androstenedione increasing with increasing numbers of cigarettes smoked per day.

Longcope and Johnson (1988) reported endogenous sex steroid levels in 88 pre- and post-menopausal women, 23 of whom were smokers. They also found that smokers had significantly higher levels of androstenedione than non-smokers. No significant differences were seen in oestrone, oestradiol, or testosterone levels by cigarette smoking status. DHEAS was not measured.

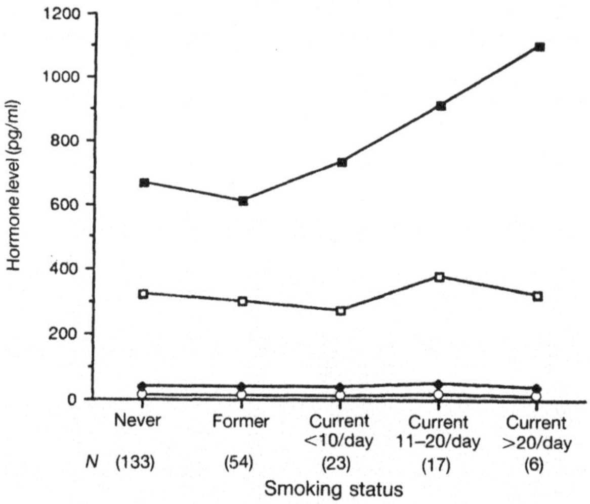

Fig. 17.1. Age- and BMI-adjusted sex hormone levels by cigarette smoking status in Rancho Bernardo women aged 60–79. ■, androstenedione*; □, testosterone; •, oestrone; ○, oestradiol. * $P<0.002$.

17.3. Studies in men

Many more studies of cigarette smoking and plasma sex hormones have been reported for men than for women (Table 17.3). In a letter to the editor Briggs (1973) reported plasma testosterone levels in two groups of healthy men closely matched for age, height, and weight. The six chronic heavy smokers had significantly lower testosterone levels than six non-smokers. After seven days abstinence from smoking, there was a highly significant rise in testosterone in the cigarette smokers; during the same period there was no change in the testosterone level in the non-smokers. Dotson *et al.* (1975) reported a significant increase in testosterone with drinking and smoking behaviour among 89 young men observed during parties; changes in plasma alcohol and smoking were about equally and additively related to testosterone changes, and together accounted for about 12 per cent of the variance in the testosterone. Results were not consistent, however; men who smoked few cigarettes and had relatively low plasma alcohol concentrations showed a decrease in testosterone. Shaarawy and Mahmoud (1982) studied 45 volunteers and found lower testosterone levels in smokers compared to non-smokers. In the same year Tsitouras *et al.* (1982) reported no difference in serum testosterone levels by smoking status in 183 older men. Handelsman *et al.* (1984) studied 119 consecutive healthy men being considered as potential sperm donors. They reported virtually identical plasma testosterone levels in men who smoked or did not smoke cigarettes. Deslypere and Vermeulen (1984) reported on 302 volunteers and found higher free and total testosterone levels in those who smoked cigarettes. In a later report, Vermeulen and Deslypere (1985) reaffirmed these findings and noted that the differences decreased with age. It is not clear whether these were the same subjects reported previously.

At about the same time, Klaiber *et al.* (1984) reported higher oestradiol levels in smokers vs. non-smokers in each of two groups of men, 41 healthy volunteers and 31 men referred for infertility evaluation. In a large population-based study in Denmark, Lindholm *et al.* (1982) reported significantly higher oestradiol levels in smokers than in non-smokers, a difference which persisted after adjusting for obesity. There was no difference in testosterone levels. In a study of 73 sedentary men aged 30–55, 14 of whom were smokers, Stefanick *et al.* (1987) found a strong positive correlation of oestradiol with the number of cigarettes smoked per day, but no significant correlation for testosterone. No adjustment was made for obesity.

Barrett-Connor and Khaw (1987), reported sex hormones by smoking status in 590 Rancho Bernardo men aged 30–79 years. Men who were current cigarette smokers had significantly higher mean DHEAS, androstenedione, oestrone, and oestradiol levels than non-smoking men from the same community. These differences persisted after adjusting for age and obesity. Age-adjusted testosterone levels were marginally higher in male

Table 17.3. Plasma sex hormones in men by cigarette smoking status

Study	Source of subjects (age)	Number	Hormones in smokers vs. non-smokers					Adjusted/ matched for obesity
			A	DHEAS	T	E_1	E_2	
Briggs (1973)	Volunteers (19–26)	12	—	—	↓	—	—	Yes
Dotson *et al*. (1975)	Volunteers (18–32)	89	—	—	↑	—	—	No
Tsitouras *et al*. (1982)	Volunteers (60–79) (Baltimore Study on Aging)	183	—	—	NS	—	—	No
Lindholm *et al*. (1982)	Glostrup (30–60)	443	—	—	NS	—	↑	Yes
Shaarawy and Mahmoud (1982)	Volunteers (25–35)	45	—	—	↓	—	—	No
Klaiber *et al*. (1984)	Volunteers (18–24)	41	—	—	—	—	↑	No
Handelsman *et al*. (1984)	Sperm donors (31.4)	119	—	—	NS	—	—	No
Andersen *et al*. (1984)	Infertility Clinic (28–30±4.5)	233	—	—	↑	—	—	No
Deslypere and Vermeulen (1984)	Volunteers (20–80)	302	—	—	↑	—	—	No

Table 17.3. (*cont.*)

Study	Source of subjects (age)	Number	Hormones in smokers vs. non-smokers					Adjusted/ matched for obesity
			A	DHEAS	T	E_1	E_2	
Vermeulen and Deslypere (1985)	Volunteers (20–80)	181	—	—	↑	—	—	No
Lichtenstein *et al.* (1987)	Caerphilly (45–59)	2512	—	—	↑	—	NS	No
Stefanick *et al.* (1987)	Sedentary men (33–55) (exercise trial)	73	—	—	NS	—	↑	No
Barrett-Connor *et al.* (1986), Barrett-Connor and Khaw (1987)	Rancho Bernardo (30–79)	590	↑	↑	NS	↑	↑	Yes
Dai *et al.* (1988)	High risk men (35–57) (MRFIT trial)	121	↑	—	↑	—	—	Yes
Dai *et al.* (1988)	High risk men (35–57) (MRFIT trial)	326	↑	—	NS	NS	NS	Yes

NS, not significant; A, androstenedione; DHEAS, dihydroepiandrosterone sulphate; T, testosterone; E_1, oestrone; E_2, oestradiol.

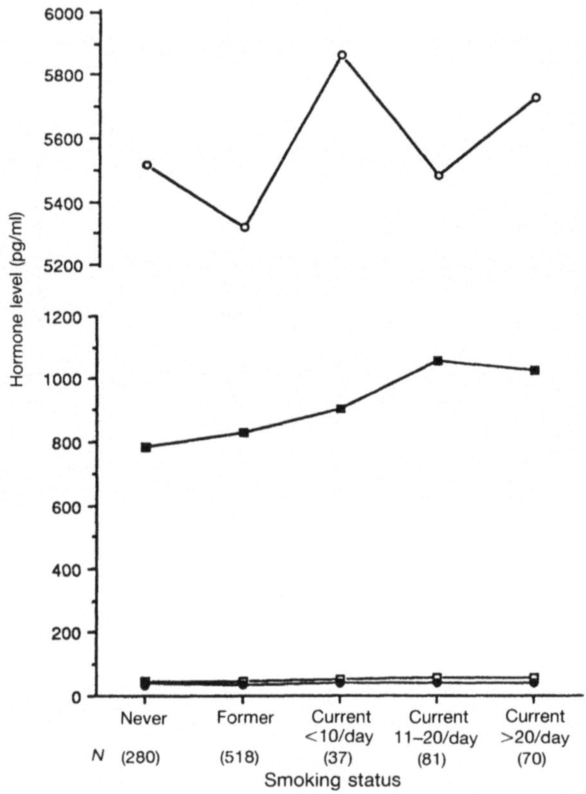

Fig. 17.2. Age- and BMI-adjusted sex hormone levels by cigarette smoking status in Rancho Bernardo men aged 30–79. ■, androstenedione*; ○, testosterone; □, oestrone*; ●, oestradiol. * $P<0.0001$.

smokers ($P=0.08$) but this difference was non-linear and was non-significant after adjusting for obesity ($P=0.14$). Since publication, the sample of men studied has been increased to 986 with similar results, except that oestradiol no longer showed a dose–response relation to the number of cigarettes smoked (Fig. 17.2). However, the overall difference between oestradiol in smokers vs. non-smokers remained highly significant ($P=0.006$).

The Caerphilly Heart Study of 2512 men aged 45–59 years found 15 per cent higher testosterone levels in cigarette smoking men but no dose–response relationship. Oestradiol levels were unrelated to smoking status. Age- and obesity-adjusted comparisons were not reported (Lichtenstein *et al.* 1987).

Dai *et al.* (1988) reported sex hormone levels in two subgroups of men from the MRFIT cohort; these men were aged 35–59 years and had been recruited to a randomized clinical trial on the basis of being at high risk for coronary artery disease. Baseline hormone levels were measured in one group of 121 men who volunteered for a prospective study of sex hormones, and in another group consisting of 163 cases (defined on the basis of an ischaemic heart disease event in the course of the trial) and their age-matched controls. Androstenedione levels were higher at baseline in smokers than in non-smokers in all comparisons—within the prospective study group, the cases, and the controls.

In the case-control group, baseline levels of total and free testosterone, total and free oestradiol, and oestrone were also measured; none differed by smoking status when cases and controls were pooled. When cases and controls were analysed separately, however, testosterone levels were significantly higher in smokers, but only in the control group. In the prospectively studied men, testosterone levels were also higher in smokers at baseline; in these men both androstenedione and testosterone levels were positively and significantly correlated with cigarettes/day and with serum thiocyanate. Four years later the level of testosterone correlated significantly with the change in cigarette smoking. Unfortunately androstenedione was not measured at this visit.

17.4. Discussion

As summarized in Tables 17.2 and 17.3, the most consistent finding in these studies is that both men and women who smoke cigarettes have higher blood levels of androstenedione than those who do not smoke. Although studied less often, DHEAS levels are also higher in smokers of both sexes. Further, whenever a dose–response relationship was sought, there was nearly always a clear gradient of increasing levels of these hormones with increasing number of cigarettes smoked per day. Studies in men and women conducted in the 1960s (Hökfelt and Sjukhuset 1961; Kershbaum *et al.* 1968) showed smoking by habitual smokers caused an acute elevation of cortisol or 11-hydroxycorticosteroids and similar results have been reported more recently (Dotson *et al.* 1975; Winternitz and Quillen 1977; Shaarawy and Mahmoud 1982; Friedman *et al.* 1987). The similar androstenedione and DHEAS increments with smoking in both sexes, coupled with the higher level of cortisol in smokers, point to a direct or indirect adrenal stimulus with cigarette smoking. In animal models, not reviewed here, nicotine increases adrenocorticotropic hormone (ACTH) secretion.

Other results are much less consistent. For testosterone in men, various studies have reported both highly significant differences or no differences. In some studies male smokers also had significantly higher levels of oestrone and/or oestradiol compared to non-smokers. Female smokers, on the other hand, generally had normal endogenous plasma and reduced urinary oestrogen compared to non-smokers. For unknown reasons, observed hormone associations were altered or absent in the presence of known or impending cardiovascular disease in MRFIT and Rancho Bernardo men; for this reason, no studies based on men with known or suspected heart disease were reviewed here. Similar studies have not been done in women.

Some of the conflicting results with regard to testosterone and oestrogen may reflect a failure to control adequately for differences in obesity and body composition between cigarette smokers and non-smokers. Overweight is associated with increased peripheral conversion of testosterone to oestradiol and androstenedione to oestrone (and oestradiol). As a result, oestrogen levels are higher in fatter men and women. The decrease in testosterone and increase in oestrogen observed in older men are often attributed to the ageing process, but this effect is probably due in part to increasing the proportion of body weight that is fat with age (Dai *et al.* 1981). It is also not entirely possible to distinguish the effect of obesity from that of exercise, since physical exercise also causes an increase (Sutton *et al.* 1973; Remes *et al.* 1979) or decrease (Dessypris *et al.* 1976) in plasma androgens. In some of the studies reviewed here, testosterone differences persisted after adjusting for differences in body mass index, suggesting that adiposity is not the sole explanation for the smoking–sex hormone differences. It must be acknowledged, however, that the surrogate measures of obesity (such as body mass index) lack precision, and that a role for differential obesity in determining hormone levels in smokers vs. non-smokers cannot be excluded entirely. Also, if smoking–disease relationships are mediated by weight-induced testosterone or oestrogen differences, correcting for obesity may be inappropriate, obscuring biologically important differences.

With the exception of testosterone, the adrenal gland is the main source of sex hormones in post-menopausal women (Vermeulen 1980). The post-menopausal ovary is predominantly an androgen-secreting endocrine gland; it secretes testosterone and androstenedione, the former in larger and the latter in smaller amounts than in the pre-menopausal woman (Rice 1988). Oestrogen in post-menopausal women is derived from androstenedione, and about a quarter of the latter is derived from DHEA. Any stimulus which increases adrenal androgen production could thereby increase oestrogen levels. In the study by Mochizuki *et al.* (1984), however, pregnant heavy smokers actually showed a reduced conversion of DHEAS to oestrogen compared to non-smokers. Work by Barbieri *et al.* (1986a,b) in two human cell culture models also suggests that nicotine and anabasine from cigarette smoke inhibit the aromatization of androstenedione to oestradiol in a dose-dependent manner. In contrast, Longcope and Johnson (1988) found that the aromatization of androstenedione to oestrone and that of testosterone to oestradiol were similar in women who smoked and those who did not smoke cigarettes.

Over the wide range of plasma concentrations of the principal sex hormones in men and in pre- and post-menopausal women, the average plasma levels generally reflect production rates (Nordin *et al.* 1981). However, any effect of smoking on oestrogens seems unlikely to reflect changed production rates. In a study of 88 pre- and post-menopausal women, Longcope and Johnson (1988) found no evidence of altered production of oestrogen or testosterone in smokers compared to non-smokers. Further, the lower plasma oestrogen levels in cigarette smoking women receiving non-contraceptive oestrogen therapy (Jensen *et al.* 1985) cannot be explained by a production defect.

Longcope and Johnson (1988) also studied metabolic clearance rates in 88 pre- and post-menopausal women grouped by smoking status, using radioactively labelled oestrogens and androgens. Based on the rate of infusion in the peripheral venous blood divided by the mean concentration of radioactivity in the venous blood, metabolic clearance rates for testosterone, androstenedione, and oestrone, but not oestradiol, were significantly decreased in smokers. None of these differences remained significant after adjusting for body weight.

Michnovicz *et al.* (1986) postulate that women who smoked cigarettes had increased 2-hydroxylation of oestradiol. When oestradiol is irreversibly hydroxylated at the C-2 position, the result is a rapidly cleared product with almost no oestrogenic activity. Using radioactively labelled oestradiol in pre-menopausal women, they reported that 14 women smokers had significantly higher oestradiol-2-hydroxylation in plasma than 13 non-smoking women. The smokers also had decreased urinary excretion of oestriol, compatible with the results in pre-menopausal women reported by MacMahon *et al.* (1982) and Mochizuki *et al.* (1984). The predicted biologic consequence of these findings is reduced bioavailability of oestrogen at target tissues. In this scenario, measurement of plasma oestrogen could fail to reflect biologically important changes in oestrogenicity.

Although a number of inconsistencies remain to be resolved, as shown in Table 17.4, overall these results suggest that:

(1) the anti-oestrogenic effect of cigarette smoking may be largely mediated by adrenal hormones; and
(2) when smoking alters the androgen/oestrogen ratio, it makes men more female and women more male in their hormone profiles.

In men, smoking may on balance be oestrogenic because the androgenic effect of any increment in adrenal androgens is obscured by the large amount of endogenous testosterone. In post-menopausal women even a small increase in adrenal androgen (with or without a decrease in biologically available oestrogen) could cause an increased androgen/oestrogen ratio. Overall, these findings are compatible with the hypothesis that the androgen–oestrogen *ratio* is critical in determining the sex-specific risk of some sex hormone-related diseases. This is teleologically attractive, in that these results imply

Table 17.4. Summary of plasma sex hormone differences in studies of smokers vs. non-smokers (proportion of studies reporting elevated levels)

	Men	Women
Androstenedione	3/3	3/3
DHEAS	1/1	1/2
Testosterone	6/14*	1/3
Oestrone (E_1)	1/2	0/4
Oestradiol (E_2)	4/6	0/4

* Vermeulen/Deslypere study counted only once.

that a male hormone pattern is good for men and a female hormone pattern is good for women.

References

Andersen, A. N., Semczuk, M., and Tabor, A. (1984). Prolactin and pituitary-gonadal function in cigarette smoking infertile patients. *Andrologia*, **16**, 391–6.

Barbieri, R. L., McShane, P. M., and Ryan, K. J. (1986a). Constituents of cigarette smoke inhibit human granulosa cell aromatase. *Fertility and Sterility*, **46**, 232–6.

Barbieri, R. L., Gochberg, J., and Ryan, K. J. (1986b). Nicotine, cotinine, and anabasine inhibit aromatase in human trophoblast *in vitro*. *Journal of Clinical Investigation*, 77, 1727–33.

Baron, J. A. (1984). Smoking and estrogen-related disease. *American Journal of Epidemiology*, **119**, 9–22.

Barrett-Connor, E. and Khaw, K.-T. (1987). Cigarette smoking and increased endogenous estrogen levels in men. *American Journal of Epidemiology*, **126**, 187–92.

Barrett-Connor, E., Khaw, K.-T., and Yen, S. C. (1986). A prospective study of dehydroepiandrosterone sulfate, mortality, and cardiovascular disease. *The New England Journal of Medicine*, **315**, 1519–24.

Briggs, M. H. (1973). Cigarette smoking and infertility in men. *The Medical Journal of Australia*, **60-II**, 616–17.

Crawford, F. E., Back, D. J., L'e Orme, M., and Breckenridge, A. M. (1981). Oral contraceptive steroid plasma concentrations in smokers and non-smokers. *British Medical Journal*, **282**, 1829–30.

Dai, W. S., Kuller, L. H., LaPorte, R. E., Gutai, J. P., Falvo-Gerard, L., and Caggiula, A. (1981). The epidemiology of plasma testosterone levels in middle-aged men. *American Journal of Epidemiology*, **114**, 804–16.

Dai, W. S., Gutai, J. P., Kuller, L. H., and Cauley, J. A. (1988). Cigarette smoking and serum sex hormones in men. *American Journal of Epidemiology*, **128**, 796–805.

Deslypere, A. and Vermeulen, A. (1984). Leydig cell function in normal men; effect of age, life-style, residence, diet and activity. *Journal of Clinical Endocrinology and Metabolism*, **59**, 955–62.

Dessypris, A., Kuoppasalmi, K., and Adlercreutz, H. (1976). Plasma cortisol, testosterone, androstenedione and luteinizing hormone (LH) in a non-competitive marathon run. *Journal of Steroid Biochemistry*, 7, 33-7.

Dotson, L. E., Robertson, L. S., and Tuchfield, B. (1975). Plasma alcohol, smoking, hormone concentrations and self-reported aggression; a study in a social-drinking situation. *Journal of Studies on Alcohol*, **36**, 578-86.

Friedman, A. J., Ravnikar, V. A., and Barbieri, R. L. (1987). Serum steroid hormone profiles in postmenopausal smokers and nonsmokers. *Fertility and Sterility*, **47**, 398-401.

Handelsman, D. J., Conway, A. J., Boylan, L. M., and Turtle, J. R. (1984). Testicular function in potential sperm donors: normal ranges and the effects of smoking and varicocele. *International Journal of Andrology*, 7, 369-82.

Hokfelt, B. and Sjukhuset, K. (1961). The effect of smoking on the production of adreno-cortical hormones. *Acta Medicine Scandinavia*, **170**(Suppl.369), 123-4.

Jensen, J., Christiansen, C., and Rodbro, P. (1985). Cigarette smoking, serum estrogens, and bone loss during hormone-replacement therapy early after menopause. *The New England Journal of Medicine*, **313**, 973-5.

Kanarkowski, R., Tornatore, K. M., D'Ambrosio, R., Gardner, M. J., and Jusko, W. J. (1988). Pharmakokinetics of single and multiple doses of ethinylestradiol and levonorgestrel in relation to smoking. *Clinical Pharmacology and Therapeutics*, **43**, 23-31.

Kershbaum, A., Pappajohn, D. J., Bellet, S., Hirabayashi, M., and Shafiiha, H. (1968). Effect of smoking and nicotine on adrenocortical secretion. *Journal of the American Medical Association*, **203**, 275-8.

Khaw, K.-T., Tazuke, S., and Barrett-Connor, E. (1988). Cigarette smoking and levels of adrenal androgens in postmenopausal women. *The New England Journal of Medicine*, **318**, 1705-9.

Klaiber, E. L., Broverman, D. M., and Dalen, J. E. (1984). Serum estradiol levels in male cigarette smokers. *American Journal of Medicine*, 77, 858-62.

Lichtenstein, M. J., *et al.* (1987). Sex hormones, insulin, lipids, and prevalent ischemic heart disease. *American Journal of Epidemiology*, **126**, 647-57.

Lindholm, J., Winkel, P., Brodthagen, U., and Gyntelberg, F. (1982). Coronary risk factors and plasma sex hormones. *American Journal of Medicine*, **73**, 648-51.

Longcope, C. and Johnston, C. C. Jr. (1988). Androgen and estrogen dynamics in pre- and postmenopausal women: a comparison between smokers and nonsmokers. *Journal of Clinical Endocrinology and Metabolism*, **67**, 379-83.

MacMahon, B., Trichopoulos, D., Cole, P., and Brown, J. (1982). Cigarette smoking and urinary estrogens. *The New England Journal of Medicine*, **307**, 1062-5.

Michnovicz, J. J., Hershcopf, R. J., Naganuma, H., Bradlow, H. L., and Fishman, J. (1986). Increased 2-hydroxylation of estradiol as a possible mechanism for the anti-estrogenic effect of cigarette smoking. *The New England Journal of Medicine*, **315**, 1305-9.

Mochizuki, M., Maruo, T., Masulo, K., and Ohtsu, T. (1984). Effects of smoking on fetoplacental-maternal system during pregnancy. *American Journal of Obstetrics and Gynecology*, **149**, 413-20.

Nordin, B. E. C., Crilly, R. G., Marshall, D. H., and Barkworth, S. A. (1981).

Oestrogens, the menopause and the adrenopause. *Journal of Endocrinology*, **89**, 131P–43P.

Remes, K., Kuoppasalmi, K., and Adlercreutz, H. (1979). Effect of long-term physical training on plasma testosterone, androstenedione, luteinizing hormone and sex-hormone-binding globulin capacity. *Scandinavian Journal of Clinical Laboratory Investigation*, **39**, 743–9.

Rice, B. F. (1988). The aging ovary. In *The endocrinology of aging* (ed. J. R. Sowers and J. V. Felicetta), pp. 135–49. Raven Press, New York.

Shaarawy, M. and Mahmoud, K. Z. (1982). Endocrine profile and semen characteristics in male smokers. *Fertility and Sterility*, **38**, 255–7.

Stefanick, M. L., Williams, P. T., Krauss, R. M., Terry, R. B., Vranizan, K. M., and Wood, P. D. (1987). Relationships of plasma estradiol, testosterone, and sex hormone-binding globulin with lipoproteins, apolipoproteins, and high density lipoprotein subfractions in men. *Journal of Clinical Endocrinology and Metabolism*, **64**, 723–9.

Sutton, J. R., Coleman, M. J., Casey, J., and Lazarus, L. (1973). Androgen responses during physical exercise. *British Medical Journal*, **3**, 520–2.

Targett, C. S., Gunesee, H., McBride, F., and Beischer, N. A. (1973). An evaluation of the effects of smoking on maternal estriol excretion during pregnancy and on fetal outcome. *The Journal of Obstetrics and Gynecology*, **80**, 815–21.

Trichopoulos, D., Brown, J., and MacMahon, B. (1987). Urine estrogens and breast cancer risk factors among post-menopausal women. *International Journal of Cancer*, **40**, 721–5.

Tsitouras, P. D., Martin, C. E., and Harman, S. M. (1982). Relationship of serum testosterone to sexual activity in healthy elderly men. *Journal of Gerontology*, **37**, 288–93.

Vermeulen, A. (1980). Sex hormone status of the postmenopausal woman. *Maturitas*, **2**, 81–8.

Vermeulen, A. and Deslypere, J. P. (1985). Testicular endocrine function in the ageing male. *Maturitas*, **7**, 273–9.

Winternitz, W. W. and Quillen, D. (1977). Acute hormonal response to smoking. *Journal of Clinical Pharmacology*, **17**, 389–97.

18. Increased oxidative metabolism of oestrogens in male and female smokers

Jon J. Michnovicz and Jack Fishman

Abstract

The metabolism of oestradiol in humans is principally oxidative, and involves two competing pathways, C-2 and C-16α hydroxylation. Oestradiol 2-hydroxylation generates peripherally inactive catechol oestrogens, and increased activity of this enzyme in smokers could contribute to a hypo-oestrogenic state. Using an in-vivo radiometric technique cigarette smoking in both men and women has been found to be associated with significant induction of 2-hydroxylation, and no change in 16α-hydroxylation. Increased 2-hydroxylation measured radiometrically is accompanied by enhanced urinary excretion of 2-hydroxyoestrone, the end product of the enzyme reaction. The ratio of urinary 2-hydroxyoestrone to oestriol ($[2OHE_1]/[E_3]$) is roughly proportional to the increase in 2-hydroxylation. Furthermore, elevated 2-hydroxylation increases gradually with greater levels of smoke exposure, as judged by serum cotinine levels, suggesting that even breathing other people's smoke may be sufficient, in some individuals, to alter oestrogen metabolism. These studies shed light on the environmental factors capable of modulating hormone metabolism, and may help in developing strategies to reduce the risk for oestrogen-dependent diseases in humans.

18.1. Introduction

An anti-oestrogenic effect of smoking in women has been suggested in epidemiological studies (Baron 1984). The mechanisms which may underlie this biological phenomenon have focused on diminished production as well as enhanced metabolism of circulating oestrogens as a direct consequence of smoking. Work in this laboratory has shown that one of the oxidative pathways of oestrogen metabolism, namely 2-hydroxylation, is greatly enhanced in female and male smokers (Michnovicz *et al*. 1986, 1989). This reaction generates the catechol oestrogens, 2-hydroxyoestrone ($2OHE_1$) and

2-methoxyoestrone ($2MeOE_1$), both of which have low affinity for the oestrogen receptor and therefore little peripheral oestrogenic activity. Increased 2-hydroxylation in men and women, and the resulting diversion of oestrogens into inactive metabolites, may therefore have a significant effect on oestrogen bioavailability and the risk of developing hormone-dependent disease. Furthermore, since the activity of this pathway is readily increased or decreased by a variety of environmental and pharmacologic stimuli, it may serve as a locus for reducing the risk.

18.2. Metabolic pathways of steroids

An outline of sex hormone metabolism is shown in Fig. 18.1, with emphasis on the oxidative transformations of oestradiol. Androgens such as androstenedione and testosterone secreted by the gonads and adrenal glands are converted to oestrone (E_1) and oestradiol (E_2) by the aromatase enzyme (MacDonald *et al.* 1967). Androgens are removed from the aromatizable pool by the enzyme 5α-reductase, yielding dihydrotestosterone.

The metabolism of oestradiol in humans involves two mutually exclusive, irreversible hydroxylations of oestrone at either the C-2 or C-16α positions (Fishman *et al.* 1960). The end products of these two reactions show quite different biological properties. The 2-hydroxyoestrogens are virtually devoid of peripheral oestrogenic activity, and are rapidly cleared from the circulation (Martucci and Fishman 1979). Enhancement of this pathway results in more extensive inactivation of the biologically active oestrogens, thereby leading to an hypooestrogenic environment.

In contrast, the 16α-hydroxylated metabolites, 16α-hydroxyoestrone (16αOHE_1) and oestriol (E_3), retain oestrogen agonist activity (Fishman and

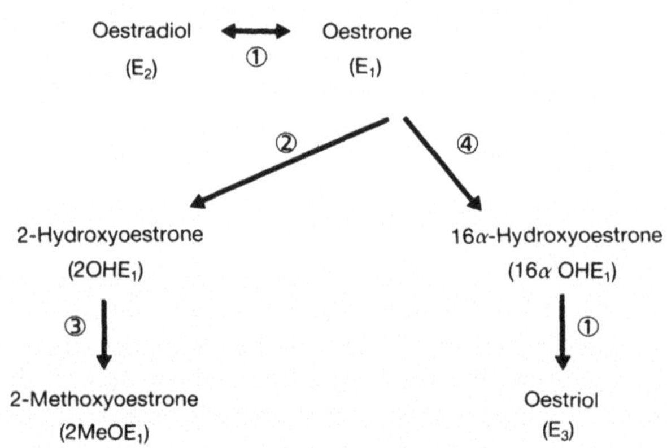

Fig. 18.1. Oxidative metabolism of oestradiol in humans. Pathways include: (1) 17-oxidoreductase; (2) oestradiol 2-hydroxylase; (3) catechol-o-methyltransferase, and (4) 16α-hydroxylase.

Martucci 1980). In particular, 16αOHE$_1$ binds minimally to sex-hormone-binding globulin, thus potentiating its impact on oestrogen-target tissues in humans. Evidence is growing that oestradiol 16α-hydroxylation may be implicated in the genesis of oestrogen-dependent diseases in women. For example, an increase in 16α-hydroxylation was found in peri- and post-menopausal women with breast cancer, and in a separate group with endometrial cancer (Schneider *et al.* 1982; Fishman *et al.* 1984). 16αOHE$_1$ is unique among all of the metabolites in its ability to bind covalently to cellular proteins such as the oestrogen receptor, thereby allowing prolonged oestrogen action by this hormone despite low circulating concentrations (Bucala *et al.* 1984; Swaneck and Fishman 1988).

Cigarette smoking could potentially alter the activity of any of the enzyme reactions shown in Fig. 18.1. There is evidence suggesting that in fact several steps may be affected, including adrenal and gonadal steroid output (Barbieri *et al.* 1987), aromatase activity (Barbieri *et al.* 1986), and 2-hydroxy-oestrogen formation. The possible consequences of these metabolic alterations in pre- and post-menopausal women, as well as men, are only beginning to be understood.

18.3. Elevated 2-hydroxylation in female smokers

The extent of oestradiol 2-hydroxylation in pre-menopausal female smokers and non-smokers has been measured utilizing two separate techniques in order to assess changes in metabolism. The first was an *in vivo* radiometric procedure developed in this laboratory, which yields specific information on the extent of hydroxylation at a given metabolically reactive site (Michnovicz *et al.* 1986). The second involved radioimmunoassay of five important urinary oestrogens (Michnovicz *et al.* 1988). In general, volunteers for these studies were healthy and non-obese, using no prescription or recreational drugs.

The extent of the reaction in smokers and a comparable group of non-smokers is shown in Fig. 18.2. The average for the smokers ($n = 14$) was 53.6 ± 2.2 (SEM) per cent of the administered dose, as compared with 35.1 ± 1.8 per cent for the 13 non-smokers—an increase of about 50 per cent. Despite some overlap between the two groups, smoking had a large effect in nearly every woman. The smokers had cotinine levels between 191 and 345 ng/ml, with a mean of 245 ng/ml. All subjects were tested between days 1–12 of the follicular phase of the menstrual cycle. Further study of five smokers in the luteal phase showed that there was no difference in the extent of this reaction between the two phases: follicular 57.8 per cent vs. luteal 56.8 per cent.

A large cohort of 52 women with widely differing amounts of daily tobacco consumption has been further studied. The subjects (mean age 30.2 ± 2.4 years) smoked between 0 and 60 cigarettes per day. Five of the women were

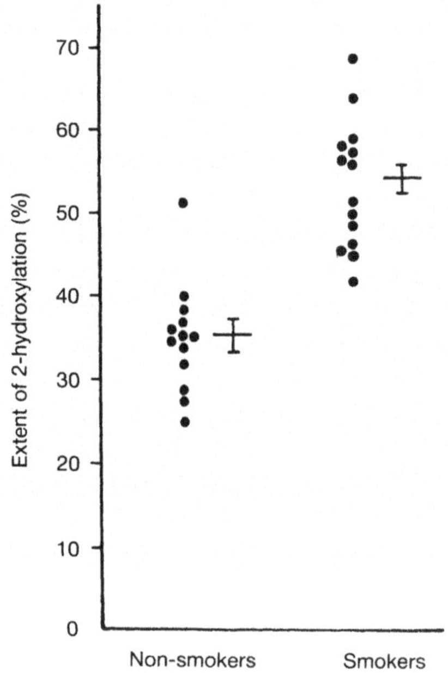

Fig. 18.2. Radiometrically determined extent of 2-hydroxylation in pre-menopausal female smokers ($n = 14$) and non-smokers ($n = 13$). Bars indicate means ± SEM.

post-menopausal; the pre-menopausal women were studied in the follicular phase of the menstrual cycle. Cotinine, a metabolite of nicotine and a biochemical marker of tobacco consumption, was measured in plasma by radioimmunoassay. The average extent of oestradiol 2-hydroxylation (±SD) in the 19 non-smokers was 34.7 ± 5.7 per cent, and varied from 27.3 to 69.6 per cent in the smokers (Fig. 18.3). Light smokers (between 1 and 14 cigarettes daily) had a mean extent of reaction of 41.7 ± 6.7 per cent, while heavier smokers (> 15 daily) averaged 52.7 ± 7.8 per cent. The extent of reaction differed significantly between light and heavy smokers ($P < 0.001$) and between light and non-smokers ($P < 0.005$). Cotinine, which was undetectable in the non-smokers, ranged from 5 to 466 ng/ml among the smokers. The extent of reaction correlated significantly with the cotinine levels ($r = 0.76$, $P < 0.001$).

The data in Fig. 18.3 demonstrate that oestradiol 2-hydroxylation in women is elevated by the active inhalation of smoke from relatively few cigarettes, and that the extent of the reaction is associated with the cotinine level. There is no evidence of a threshold effect. Epidemiological studies have shown that the anti-oestrogenic effects of smoking such as earlier natural menopause can also be detected in women who are passively exposed to sidestream smoke, which in some individuals may reach the equivalent

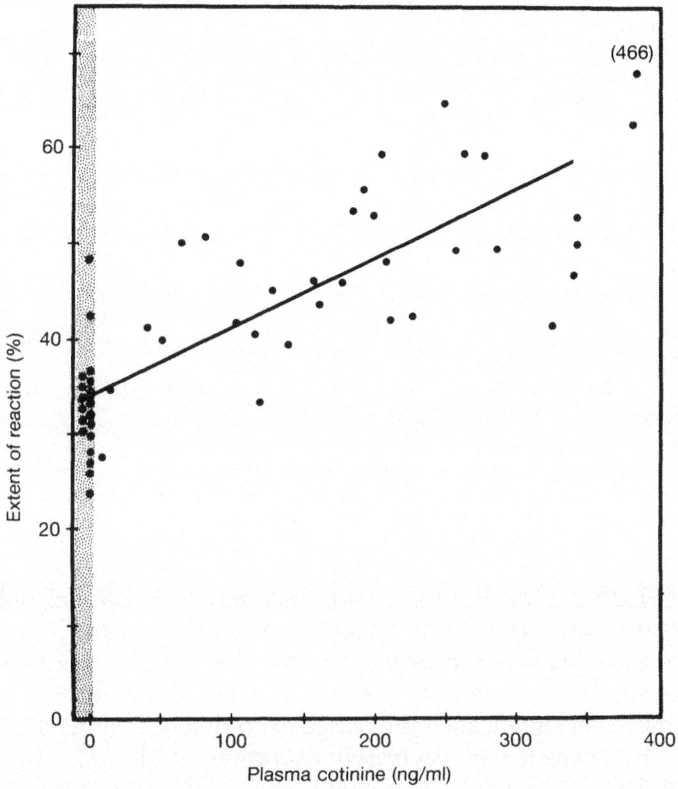

Fig. 18.3. Plot of oestradiol 2-hydroxylation vs. cotinine levels in 52 female smokers and non-smokers. The correlation is significant ($r=0.76$, $P<0.001$).

of actively smoking 1–3 cigarettes daily. The data presented here indicate that increased 2-hydroxylation of oestrogens may play a role in the anti-oestrogenic effects of environmental tobacco smoke as well.

A separate group of female smokers was examined in order to determine whether oestradiol 16α-hydroxylation also changed following use of tobacco. The extent of reaction in the smokers averaged ($\pm$SD) 9.2 ± 1.4 per cent, as compared with 9.3 ± 2.5 per cent in the non-smokers ($n=8$ and 7 respectively). Thus, this pathway is apparently unaffected by smoking.

A detailed analysis of five urinary oestrogen metabolites, including oestradiol, oestrone, oestriol, 2-hydroxyoestrone, and 16α-hydroxyoestrone, was performed in female smokers and non-smokers (Table 18.1). Follicular phase urine samples (days 1–12 following onset of menses) were obtained from subjects in whom radiometric testing had been performed. Significant elevations were found in urinary $2OHE_1$ in the smokers compared with non-

Table 18.1. Summary of urinary oestrogens in smokers (S) and non-smokers (NS)

Metabolite	Women		Men	
	S	NS	S	NS
Oestradiol	5.1±0.6	4.0±1.5	3.9±0.4	3.4±0.3
Oestrone	16.4±1.2	16.5±2.5	9.6±0.8	9.7±1.0
16αOHE$_1$	6.0±0.7	6.1±0.7	3.3±0.5	2.5±0.2
Oestriol	10.6±1.1	15.7±1.8*	7.9±0.8	9.0±0.9
2OHE$_1$	17.2±2.4	9.4±1.2*	10.4±1.3	6.3±0.7*
Total	55.3±4.2	51.7±4.5	35.2±2.7	30.9±1.9
2OHE$_1$/E$_3$	1.67±0.21	0.59±0.08**	1.46±0.19	0.81±0.11**

* $P<0.02$; ** $P<0.01$.

Values are means ± SEM. Oestrogen metabolites are expressed in μg/g creatinine, and all urine samples for women were obtained in the follicular phase. Numbers of smokers and non-smokers for women and men were 15 and 14, and 20 and 16, respectively.

smokers (17.2±2.4 vs. 9.4±1.2 μg/g creatinine). A parallel reduction in urinary E_3 was also observed in female smokers. In contrast, no significant differences were observed in urinary levels of E_2, E_1, or 16αOHE$_1$. Total measured urinary oestrogens were elevated in smokers, although this difference did not reach significance. Increased excretion of 2OHE$_1$ thus occurred largely at the expense of decreased excretion of the 16α-hydroxylated metabolite, E_3.

Various ratios of metabolites were investigated as a means of differentiating the urinary excretion profiles of smokers and non-smokers. A urinary catechol oestrogen index was defined by [2OHE$_1$]/[E_3], using the major end products of the reaction to represent the relative strengths of the two oxidative pathways. While the values for the non-smokers were tightly grouped around the mean value of 0.59±0.08, the average of smokers increased significantly to 1.67±0.21. This urinary catechol oestrogen index correlated well with the extent of 2-hydroxylation ($r=0.84$; see Fig. 18.4). Such results suggest that random urine samples will be sufficient to assess the relative strengths of the two oxidative pathways, particularly following a therapeutic intervention, and therefore eliminate the need for radioisotope infusions.

18.4. Oestradiol metabolism in men

Changes in oestrogen metabolism may play a less significant role in men, given the gender differences in oestrogen physiology and pathophysiology. However, the sex steroids may be a major factor in determining the incidence

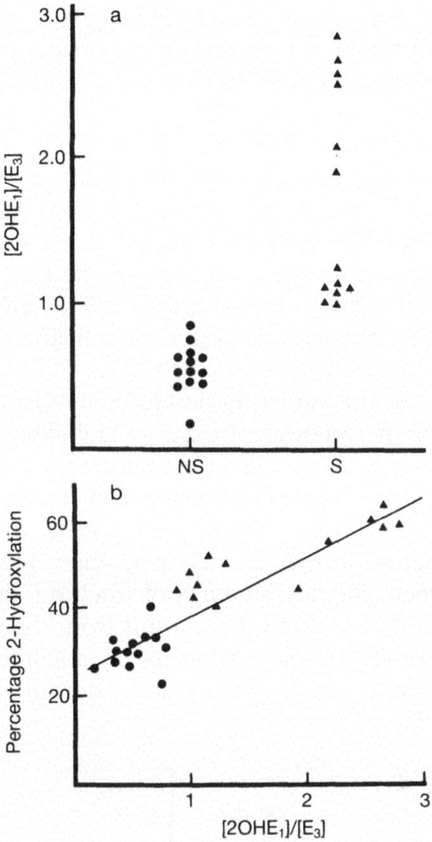

Fig. 18.4. Urinary catechol oestrogens (2OHE$_1$) in female smokers (S) and non-smokers (NS). (a) The urinary catechol oestrogen index ([2OHE$_1$]/[E$_3$]) was significantly greater among the smokers ($P<0.001$). (b) The radiometric measurement correlated strongly with the urinary index ($r=0.84$).

of cardiovascular disease in men. Because cigarette smoking is a strong risk factor for early ischaemic heart disease, and because a role for oestrogens in atherosclerosis is likely, the effect of smoking on oestrogen disposition in men is potentially important.

Epidemiological studies have demonstrated that cigarette smoking in men leads to a modest elevation in circulating oestrogens (Barrett-Connor and Khaw 1987). From this standpoint, smoking could be said to have a pro-oestrogenic effect on men, in contrast to the previous discussion of an anti-oestrogenic effect in women. However, a paradox exists when considering the effect of cigarette smoking on high density lipoprotein cholesterol (HDLC) in men. HDLC is consistently lower in male smokers (Garrison *et al.* 1978), despite numerous investigations demonstrating a positive relationship between oestrogens and HDLC (Bush and Barrett-Connor 1985). The studies outlined below provide a possible explanation for this discrepancy (Michnovicz *et al.* 1989).

Radiometric analysis of oestradiol 2-hydroxylation in men showed that this pathway was significantly induced by smoking, as in women. The average extent of reaction was 43.3 ± 1.9 per cent among the smokers, as compared to 24.6 ± 1.9 per cent among the non-smokers ($P<0.001$) (Fig. 18.5). Urinary oestrogens from male smokers and non-smokers are presented in Table 18.1, and these data are plotted as a urinary catechol oestrogen index ($[2OHE_1]/[E_3]$) alongside the radiometric data for individual subjects in Fig. 18.5. Smokers excreted significantly more 2-hydroxyoestrone than did the non-smokers (10.4 ± 1.3 vs. 6.3 ± 0.7 μg/g creatinine, $P=0.011$). Clearly, in the smoking subjects a significant elevation of 2-hydroxyoestrone relative to oestriol occurs. The elevated ratio of $2OHE_1$ to E_3 correlated strongly with the elevated radiometric extent of 2-hydroxylation ($r=0.71$, $P<0.002$), as was the case in female smokers.

Our results thus indicate that smoking is a potent inducing stimulus for oestradiol 2-hydroxylation in men as well as women. However, in men and post-menopausal women, the overall effect of smoking on oestrogen balance can be affected by changes in androgen output from the adrenals. Increased levels of several adrenal steroids have been documented in smokers, including androstenedione and dehydroepiandrosterone (Khaw *et al.* 1988).

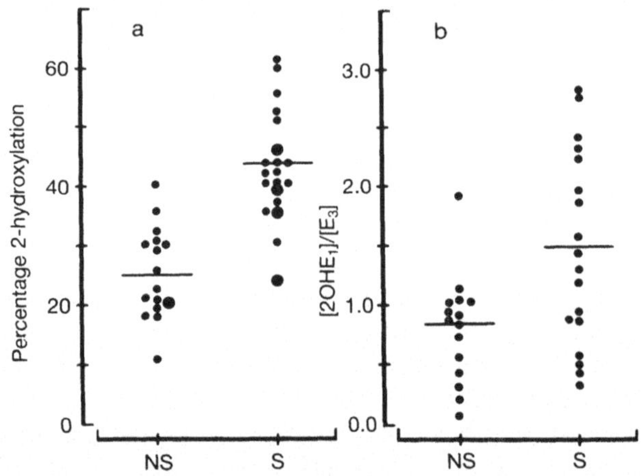

Fig. 18.5. Effects of smoking on 2-hydroxylation among male subjects. (a) The extent of oestradiol 2-hydroxylation was significantly greater among the smokers (S) ($P<0.001$). Subjects reporting a heavy alcohol consumption are indicated by a large circle. (b) The catechol oestrogen index, $[2OHE_1]/[E_3]$, was also elevated among the smokers ($P=0.006$).

Androstenedione is converted to oestrone via peripheral aromatization in adipose and muscle tissue. Furthermore, adipocytes have the enzymatic capacity to interconvert androstenedione and testosterone, as well as oestrone and oestradiol (see Fig. 18.1) (Perel and Killinger 1979). Therefore, increased production of androgen precursors in male smokers could result in greater oestrogen formation, particularly since the overall activity of *in vivo* aromatization is unaltered by smoking (Longcope and Johnston 1988). Taken together, these findings suggest that the increased production of androstenedione serving as a substrate for an unaltered rate of peripheral aromatization provide an explanation for elevated circulating oestrogens in male smokers. The alternative possibility, a decrease in metabolic clearance of oestrogens, is ruled out by the data presented above.

The liver is the principal site of 2-hydroxylation (Barbieri *et al.* 1978). The findings described above suggest that increased hepatic inactivation of circulating oestrogens as a result of greater 2-hydroxylation could directly affect lipoprotein production in male smokers. Production of the major protein of HDLC, apolipoprotein A-I, is highly oestrogen-responsive, and takes place largely in the liver (Tam *et al.* 1985). Our results suggest that smoking shunts hepatic oestrogens into the catechol oestrogen pathway, followed by urinary excretion. By diminishing the relative flux through the 16α-hydroxylative pathway, the total oestrogen stimulation in the hepatocyte is probably diminished. Furthermore, E_3 and 16αOHE_1 are excreted in large amounts in the bile, and thus returned to the liver via the enterohepatic circuit (Adlercreutz *et al.* 1978). Enhanced 2-hydroxylation of oestradiol thus has numerous ways of decreasing the ongoing hepatic oestrogenic stimulation. A mechanism of increased adrenal androgen output and elevated 2-hydroxylation helps to reconcile the disparate observations that smoking in men may both elevate circulating oestrogens while severely reducing oestrogen-sensitive HDLC.

18.5. Summary

A recent detailed study of production rates, metabolic clearance rates, and aromatization of sex hormones in pre- and post-menopausal women showed no significant effect of smoking on these variables (Longcope and Johnston 1988). Thus, the only specific metabolic alteration among smokers uncovered thus far is enhanced oestradiol 2-hydroxylation. A shift in the pattern of oestrogen metabolism as described in this paper could explain some of the results in the study of MacMahon *et al.* (1982), in which luteal phase urinary oestrogens (sum of E_1, E_2, and E_3) were decreased in female smokers. The greatest difference in their study was found in urinary E_3 (14.2 vs. 9.8 μg/g creatinine), and was very similar to our results, although our data were obtained in the follicular phase (15.7 vs. 10.6 μg/g creatinine; Table 18.1). Inclusion of 2OHE_1 in their analysis might have demonstrated greater total urinary oestrogen excretion, rather than less. However, the mechanism discussed here would not directly explain the different findings regarding E_1 and E_2 excretion in the two studies.

The full consequences of altered oxidative metabolism of oestrogens are not yet understood. The relative flux of oestradiol through the C-2 vs. C-16α pathways may play a key role in determining the overall oestrogen stimulation in various tissues. Certainly, the metabolic pattern will influence the excretion of oestrogen metabolites via the urinary and biliary routes, the latter of which returns oestrogens to the circulating pool through the enterohepatic circuit. Recent experiments in male volunteers have demonstrated that pharmacological suppression of 2-hydroxylation by about 40 per cent can elevate circulating oestradiol levels in these individuals (Galbraith and Michnovicz 1989). Thus, increasing or decreasing the C-2 oxidative metabolism of oestradiol may prove to be a useful route for controlling oestrogen balance, and ultimately a method for influencing the risk of developing oestrogen-dependent diseases.

References

Adlercreutz, H., Martin, F., and Lindström, B. (1978). Gas chromatographic and mass spectrometric studies on oestrogens in bile—2. Men and non-pregnant women. *Journal of Steroid Biochemistry*, **9**, 1197–205.

Barbieri, R. L., Canick, J. A., and Ryan, K. J. (1978). Estrogen 2-hydroxylase: Activity in rat tissues. *Steroids*, **32**, 529–38.

Barbieri, R. L., McShane, P. M., and Ryan, K. J. (1986). Constituents of cigarette smoke inhibit human granulosa cell aromatase. *Fertility and Sterility*, **46**, 232–6.

Barbieri, R. L., York, C. M., Cherry, M. L., and Ryan, K. J. (1987). The effects of nicotine, cotinine, and anabasine on rat adrenal 11beta-hydroxylase and 21-hydroxylase. *Journal of Steroid Biochemistry*, **28**, 25–8.

Baron, J. A. (1984). Smoking and estrogen-related disease. *American Journal of Epidemiology*, **119**, 9–22.

Barrett-Connor, E. and Khaw, K.-T. (1987). Cigarette smoking and increased endogenous estrogen levels in men. *American Journal of Epidemiology*, **126**, 187–92.

Bucala, R., Fishman, J., and Cerami, A. (1984). The reaction of 16α-hydroxyestrone with erythrocytes *in vitro* and *in vivo*. *European Journal of Biochemistry*, **140**, 593–8.

Bush, T. L. and Barrett-Connor, E. (1985). Noncontraceptive estrogen use and cardiovascular disease. *Epidemiological Reviews*, **7**, 80–104.

Fishman, J. and Martucci, C. (1980). Biological properties of 16α-hydroxyestrone: implications in estrogen physiology and pathophysiology. *Journal of Clinical Endocrinology and Metabolism*, **51**, 611–15.

Fishman, J., Bradlow, H. L., and Gallagher, T. F. (1960). Oxidative metabolism of estradiol. *Journal of Biological Chemistry*, **235**, 3104–7.

Fishman, J., Schneider, J., Hershcopf, R. J., and Bradlow, H. L. (1984). Increased estrogen-16α-hydroxylase activity in women with breast and endometrial cancer. *Journal of Steroid Biochemistry*, **20**, 1077–81.

Galbraith, R. A. and Michnovicz, J. J. (1989). The effects of cimetidine on the oxidative metabolism of estradiol. *New England Journal of Medicine*, **321**, 269–74.

Garrison, R. J., Kannel, W. B., Feinleib, M., Castelli, W. P., McNamara, P. M., and Padgett, S. J. (1978). Cigarette smoking and HDL cholesterol. *Atherosclerosis*, **30**, 17–25.

Khaw, K.-T., Tazuke, S., and Barrett-Connor, E. (1988). Cigarette smoking and levels of adrenal androgens in postmenopausal women. *New England Journal of Medicine*, **318**, 1705–9.

Longcope, C. and Johnston, C. C. Jr. (1988). Androgen and estrogen dynamics in pre- and postmenopausal women: a comparison between smokers and nonsmokers. *Journal of Clinical Endocrinology and Metabolism*, 67, 379–83.

MacDonald, P. C., Rombaut, R. P., and Siiteri, P. K. (1967). Plasma precursors of estrogen. Extent of conversion of plasma androstenedione to estrone in normal males and non-pregnant normal, castrate, and adrenalectomized females. *Journal of Clinical Endocrinology and Metabolism*, **27**, 1103–11.

MacMahon, B., Trichopoulos, D., Cole, P., and Brown, J. (1982). Cigarette smoking and urinary estrogens. *New England Journal of Medicine*, **307**, 1062–5.

Martucci, C. P. and Fishman, J. (1979). Impact of continuously administered catechol estrogens in uterine growth and luteinizing hormone secretion. *Endocrinology*, **105**, 1288–92.

Michnovicz, J. J., Hershcopf, R. J., Naganuma, H., Bradlow, H. L., and Fishman, J. (1986). Increased 2-hydroxylation of estradiol as a possible mechanism for the anti-estrogenic effect of cigarette smoking. *New England Journal of Medicine*, **315**, 1305–9.

Michnovicz, J. J., Naganuma, H., Hershcopf, R. J., Bradlow, H. L., and Fishman, J. (1988). Increased urinary catechol estrogens in female smokers. *Steroids*, **52**, 69–83.

Michnovicz, J. J., Hershcopf, R. J., Haley, N. J., Bradlow, H. L., and Fishman, J. (1989). Cigarette smoking alters hepatic estrogen metabolism in men: implications for atherosclerosis. *Metabolism*, **38**, 537–41.

Perel, E. and Killinger, D. W. (1979). The interconversion and aromatization of androgens by human adipose tissue. *Journal of Steroid Biochemistry*, **10**, 623–7.

Schneider, J., *et al*. (1982). Abnormal oxidative metabolism of estradiol in women with breast cancer. *Proceeding of the National Academy of Sciences, USA*, **79**, 3047–51.

Swaneck, G. E. and Fishman, J. (1988). Covalent binding of the endogenous estrogen 16α-hydroxyestrone to estradiol receptor in localization. *Proceedings of the National Academy of Sciences, USA*, **85**, 7831–5.

Tam, S.-P., Archer, T. K., and Deeley, R. G. (1985). Effects of estrogen on apolipoprotein secretion by the human hepato-carcinoma cell line, HepG2. *Journal of Biological Chemistry*, **260**, 1670–5.

19. The effect of smoking on hormone levels *in vivo* and steroid hormone biosynthesis *in vitro*

Jacob A. Canick and Robert L. Barbieri

Abstract

The effect of smoking on the levels of oestrogens and other hormones, in vivo, *and on steroidogenic enzymes,* in vitro, *was examined. Maternal serum concentrations of the fetoplacental hormones, human chorionic gonadotropin, unconjugated oestriol, and progesterone, were significantly reduced in second trimester pregnant smokers. In contrast, serum levels of the adrenal steroids, cortisol, 17α-hydroxyprogesterone, progesterone, and androstenedione, were significantly elevated in postmenopausal smokers. The results regarding oestriol and adrenal steroids are consistent with the inhibitory effects of smoke constituents on placental and adrenal steroidogenic enzymes found* in vitro. *In addition to previous data on inhibition of steroidogenic enzymes by constituents of smoke, in the present study, carbon monoxide inhibited the human placental aromatization of 16α-hydroxytestosterone to oestriol, and nicotine inhibited human adrenal 11β- and 21-hydroxylation. Therefore, serum oestriol levels may be reduced because of inhibition of placental aromatase, and adrenal steroid levels may be increased because of compensatory adrenal hyperfunction caused by partial inhibition of adrenal steroidogenic enzymes.*

19.1. Introduction

Cigarette smoking appears to be associated with alterations in oestrogen-related metabolic and disease processes, perhaps through a decrease in the levels of active hormones (Baron 1984). Such a decrease could be accomplished through mechanisms involving diminished rates of oestrogen biosynthesis or increased rates of metabolism, or both. Experiments *in vitro* demonstrate that biosynthesis of oestrogens can be inhibited by constituents of cigarette smoke (Barbieri *et al.* 1986a,b). It is not clear, however, whether oestrogen biosynthesis *in vivo* can also be affected. In two reports, women who smoked were found to have lower urinary oestrogen levels during the third trimester of pregnancy (Mochizuki *et al.* 1984) and in the luteal phase of the menstrual cycle (MacMahon *et al.* 1982), although neither finding could be attributed directly to inhibition of oestrogen production. However, other investigators have not found smoking to alter the levels of circulating oestrogen (see Barrett-Connor, Chapter 17).

This chapter examines the effect of smoking on oestrogens and on other hormones using two distinct models. The first model involves measurement of hormone levels in the maternal serum of smokers and non-smokers during the second trimester of pregnancy and is an outgrowth of ongoing studies on hormonal markers for Down's syndrome screening in pregnancy (Canick *et al.* 1988; Wald *et al.* 1988a,b). This model categorizes smokers and non-smokers objectively by measuring the level of cotinine, a nicotine metabolite, in the patient's serum sample. In addition, data are presented on circulating adrenal steroids in smoking and non-smoking post-menopausal women which indicate that smoking may cause an altered pattern of adrenal steroidogenesis. In neither case, however, are the *in vivo* results sufficient to determine if altered hormone levels in smokers are caused by altered rates of biosynthesis or metabolism.

In contrast, the second model specifically examines the effect of various constituents of cigarette smoke on the biosynthesis of oestrogens and adrenal steroids using a variety of *in vitro* systems (Barbieri *et al.* 1986a, 1987; Canick and Ryan 1976). The results *in vitro* can then be discussed in relation to observations on the circulating levels of these hormones in smokers and non-smokers.

19.2. Methods

In vivo studies on pregnant women

Stored sera from 731 patients in the second trimester of pregnancy who were participating in pre-natal screening at the Women & Infants Hospital during April and May, 1986, were assayed using commercially available radioimmunoassay kits for four analytes, unconjugated oestriol, progesterone, human chorionic gonadotropin, and α-fetoprotein. To assess smoking status, the nicotine metabolite, cotinine, an objective biochemical marker for absorbed tobacco smoke, was measured. Non-smokers were defined as having cotinine levels ≤ 10 ng/ml. For each analyte, weekly median values (completed gestational weeks 14–21) were calculated and results were expressed as the multiple of the median (MoM) for non-smokers of a given gestational age. A two-tailed Student's *t*-test on the transformed MoMs ($\log_{10}$ for human chorionic gonadotropin, progesterone, and α-fetoprotein) and on the untransformed unconjugated oestriol MoMs was used to determine statistical significance between smokers and non-smokers for each analyte.

In vivo studies on adrenal hormones

Serum from 25 post-menopausal women classified as heavy, moderate, or non-smokers was drawn at 8 a.m., extracted, chromatographed, and cortisol, progesterone, 17α-hydroxyprogesterone, and androstenedione measured by radioimmunoassay. For each steroid, the mean ($\pm$SD) was calculated by smoking category and the smokers vs. non-smokers compared by analysis of variance. Individual groups were compared using Tukey's multiple comparison procedure.

In vitro studies

The activities of three enzymes of steroid hormone biosynthesis (aromatase, 11β-hydroxylase, 21-hydroxylase) were measured in cell-free preparations of placenta and adrenal gland as previously described in detail elsewhere (Barbieri *et al.* 1986a, 1987; Canick and Ryan 1976). Four constituents of tobacco smoke, nicotine, cotinine, anabasine, and carbon monoxide were tested for their ability to inhibit these enzymes and to interact with the cytochrome P450 in these preparations as determined spectrally.

19.3. Results

In vivo studies on pregnant women

The effect of smoking on the serum levels of three hormones, unconjugated oestriol, progesterone, and human chorionic gonadotropin, and of α-fetoprotein in second trimester pregnant women is shown in Table 19.1. Smokers had significantly lower concentrations of all three hormones than

Table 19.1. Effect of smoking on second trimester maternal serum levels of unconjugated oestriol, progesterone, human chorionic gonadotropin, and α-fetoprotein

Cotinine level (ng/ml)	*n*	median MoM †			
		uE3	prog	hCG	αFP
≤10	528	1.02*	1.02*	1.06*	1.00
≥11	203	0.87*	0.93*	0.89*	1.01
11-69	61	0.93	0.94	1.02	0.90
70-169	73	0.86	0.91	0.86	1.04
>169	69	0.86	0.95	0.83	1.12
all	731	1.00	1.00	1.00	1.00

* Statistically significant difference between means, $P<0.001$.

† MoM, multiple of median; uE3, unconjugated oestriol; prog., progesterone; hCG, human chorionic gonadotropin; αFP, α-fetoprotein.

did non-smokers. Oestriol was reduced by 15 per cent in smokers, progesterone was reduced by 9 per cent, and human chorionic gonadotropin was reduced by 16 per cent. In contrast, the level of α-fetoprotein was unchanged. When the smokers were divided into three groups (low, moderate, and heavy) based on their cotinine concentrations, it appeared that oestriol and human chorionic gonadotropin reached their lowest levels in both moderate and heavy smokers, whereas the same level of reduction in progesterone was apparent in all three groups. To determine the validity of the patient sample for this study, the effect of maternal weight and age on the concentrations of the four analytes was determined (data not shown). In the case of maternal weight, there was a statistically significant effect on all four analytes; the greater the weight the lower the median concentration, as would be predicted based on dilution by increasing fluid volume. No effect of maternal age was observed.

These results were replicated in a separate study on a smaller number of women in the second trimester of pregnancy. In addition, the adrenal steroid, dehydroepiandrosterone sulphate (DHEAS), was measured and was found to be 15 per cent higher in smokers than in non-smokers, indicating either decreased utilization of DHEAS in oestrogen biosynthesis or inhibition of the enzymes of adrenal corticosteroid biosynthesis.

In vivo studies on adrenal hormones

The effect of smoking on steroid levels in post-menopausal women is shown in Table 19.2. In this study smoking was determined by self-report rather than by measurement of serum cotinine levels. Cortisol, progesterone, 17α-hydroxyprogesterone, and androstenedione were all significantly higher in heavy smokers than in non-smokers, with the latter three steroids markedly elevated. These results are consistent with a partial inhibition of the cortisol biosynthetic pathway resulting in compensatory hyperfunction.

Table 19.2. Serum steroid levels in postmenopausal smokers and non-smokers

Subjects	No.	Cortisol (ng/ml)	Progesterone (pg/ml)	17-OH Progesterone (pg/ml)	Androstenedione (pg/ml)
NS	18	111±28*	62±33*	209±71*	537±254*
MS	7	152±35	68±39	387±211	554±260
HS	9	161±40*	122±51*	747±409*	1149±438*

* $P<0.01$.
NS, non-smokers; MS, moderate smokers; HS, heavy smokers.

In vitro studies on steroid hormone biosynthesis

Barbieri *et al.* (1986a,b) have previously reported that dialysed extracts of tobacco smoke and the tobacco constituents, nicotine, cotinine, and anabasine, inhibited oestrogen biosynthesis (aromatase) in choriocarcinoma cells and in human ovarian granulosa cells in culture.

The same constituents of tobacco competitively inhibited aromatase activity when tested in microsomal preparations from term human placenta (Barbieri *et al.* 1986a). Nicotine was shown to bind to human placental microsomal cytochrome P450, the steroid and oxygen binding component of the aromatase system. Addition of nicotine produced type II difference spectra, suggesting that inhibition was at the level of the cytochrome P450 active site.

Canick and Ryan (1975, 1976) found that carbon monoxide, another constituent of tobacco smoke, had mixed effects on human placental aromatase. Carbon monoxide effectively inhibited the conversion of 16α-hydroxytestosterone to oestriol but had no effect on the conversion of androstenedione to oestrone. The lack of effect of carbon monoxide on the aromatization of

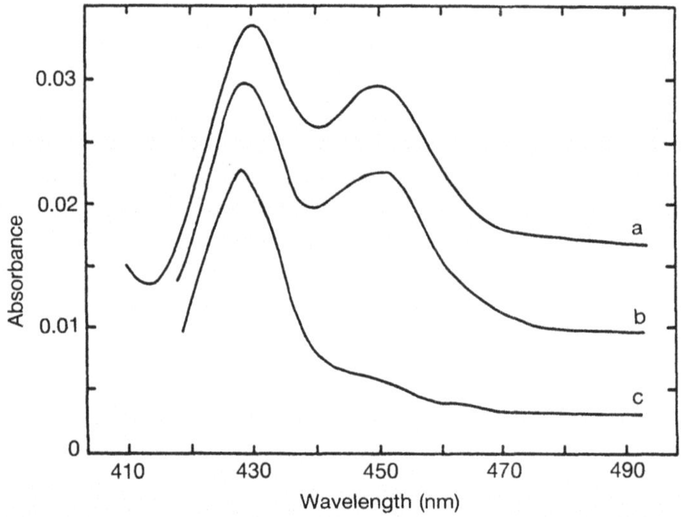

Fig. 19.1. Cytochrome P450 difference spectra in microsomal preparations of human placenta. (a) Carbon monoxide + NADPH in the sample cuvette and carbon monoxide in the reference cuvette. Two peaks are seen. One at 450 nm represents reduced, carbon monoxide-bound cytochrome P450, and the other at 425 nm represents reduced cytochrome b_5. (b) Same as in (a) but with 16α-hydroxytestosterone (50μmol/l) added to both cuvettes. Both peaks are seen. (c) Same as in (a) but with androstenedione (50μmol/l) added to both cuvettes. The 450 nm peak is eliminated, demonstrating that androstenedione prevents the binding of carbon monoxide to cytochrome P450.

androstenedione has historical significance because it delayed for a number of years the classification of aromatase as a cytochrome P450-linked enzyme. The reason for the mixed effect of carbon monoxide is not understood, but is illustrated in the ability of androstenedione to prevent carbon monoxide binding to placental P450. Figure 19.1 shows that addition of androstenedione to an NADPH difference spectrum prevented carbon monoxide from inducing a peak at 450 nm. In contrast, addition of the equally important aromatase substrate, 16α-hydroxytesterone, to another preparation had no effect on the ability of carbon monoxide to induce a peak at 450 nm. Clearly, aromatization of certain substrates is susceptible to carbon monoxide, while aromatization of others is not.

Recently, Barbieri *et al.* (1987) reported that nicotine, cotinine, and anabasine could inhibit the activity of two key adrenocortical enzymes in the rat, the 11β-hydroxylase, which catalyses the conversion of deoxycorticosterone to corticosterone, and the 21-hydroxylase, which catalyses the conversion of progesterone to deoxycorticosterone. Inhibition was competitive with K_i values in the micromolar range. The same type of experiments have now been done using subcellular fractions prepared from human fetal adrenal tissue. Both nicotine ($K_i = 9.8$ μmol/l) and cotinine ($K_i = 9.0$ μmol/l) competitively inhibited the 11β-hydroxylase (conversion of 11-deoxycortisol to cortisol). Nicotine competitively inhibited the 21-hydroxylase (conversion of 17α-hydroxyprogesterone to deoxycortisol) while cotinine did not have an inhibitory effect.

19.4. Discussion

The results presented here clearly demonstrate that the levels of oestrogens and other hormones of fetoplacental origin are reduced in the circulation of pregnant women who smoke. In addition, it appears that post-menopausal women who smoke have a pattern of circulating adrenal steroids consistent with adrenal hyperfunction. In this regard, it is interesting that levels of the major adrenal androgen, DHEAS, appear to be higher in pregnant smokers. Together with the *in vitro* findings that aromatization, 11β-hydroxylation, and 21-hydroxylation are inhibited by various constituents of smoke, these results support the hypothesis that inhibition of steroidogenic enzymes at least in part causes the alterations in circulating steroid hormones.

The levels of the various constituents of smoke needed to inhibit steroidogenic enzymes *in vitro* are in the micromolar range. Presumably, these constituents must be present at similar concentrations *in vivo* if they are to affect steroid hormone biosynthesis. Barbieri *et al.* (1986a,b, 1987) have determined that the range of nicotine and cotinine concentrations found *in vivo* may be sufficient to affect the activity of steroid biosynthetic enzymes. Hypothalamic-pituitary-adrenal compensatory mechanisms appear to have caused the alterations in circulating adrenal steroids which were observed. Other reports have noted similar increases in the levels of circulating adrenal androgens in smokers (Longo 1977; Barrett-Connor *et al.* 1986; Longcope and Johnston 1988). A compensatory system involving the hypothalamic-pituitary-ovarian axis may not function as well, thus leading to the decreased levels of oestrogen seen in the luteal phase (MacMahon *et al.* 1982).

Nicotine, cotinine, and anabasine are most likely not the only constituents of tobacco smoke which inhibit steroid hormone biosynthesis. The inhibitory effect of carbon monoxide on placental oestriol biosynthesis suggests that this constituent of smoke may also affect steroid hormone levels *in vivo*. In this regard, studies by Longo (1977) indicate that various aspects of placental function are altered by carbon monoxide.

One of the hallmarks of the cytochrome P450 family of enzymes, of which aromatase is one, is the ability of carbon monoxide to inhibit their activity. It is reasonable to predict that carbon monoxide may alter the pattern of adrenal steroids in the same way that nicotine does, by inhibiting the 11β- and 21-hydroxylases, both of which are cytochrome P450-linked enzymes and both of which are inhibited by carbon monoxide *in vitro*. We have shown that the aromatization of 16α-hydroxytestosterone to oestriol is inhibited by carbon monoxide but the aromatization of androstenedione to oestrone is not. This finding may explain in part why unconjugated oestriol is lower in pregnant smokers. Investigation of oestrone and oestradiol levels in maternal serum may help to clarify further the *in vitro* results on the effect of carbon monoxide.

The placental steroid, progesterone, is lower in the maternal serum of smokers than of non-smokers. While the effect of the constituents of smoke on the enzymes of progesterone biosynthesis has not yet been studied, it is reasonable to expect that cholesterol side-chain cleavage enzyme, which catalyses the synthesis of the progesterone precursor, pregnenolone, may be sensitive to nicotine, cotinine, or anabasine. It is well known that this enzyme is inhibited by carbon monoxide *in vitro*.

The levels of the placental glycoprotein hormone, human chorionic gonadotropin, are lower in the serum of pregnant smokers than in non-smokers. Other protein products of the placenta, such as human placental lactogen and pregnancy-specific β_1-glycoprotein, have also been reported to be lower in smokers (Moser *et al.* 1974; Lee *et al.* 1981), although another report found human placental lactogen levels to be higher in smokers (Spellacy *et al.* 1977). There are no published studies on inhibition of the biosynthesis or secretion of placental proteins by constituents of smoke. However, major alterations in the microanatomy of term placentas from smokers have been demonstrated which may contribute to decreased placental output (Asmussen 1977; Mochizuki *et al.* 1984).

The link between the findings presented in this paper and the role of smoking in hormone-related processes is clear. If in model systems constituents of smoke can be demonstrated to inhibit hormone biosynthesis, then it is probable that such inhibition can occur at sites of potential clinical significance. For example, if the aromatase enzyme found in an oestrogen-dependent tumour of the breast is inhibited by nicotine, perhaps the tumour's growth will be retarded. Or, if aromatase in the bone marrow of a post-menopausal woman is inhibited by nicotine, perhaps the level of locally produced oestrogen needed for maintenance of the bone will decrease and osteoporosis will result. Other examples are readily apparent. Further studies relating *in vitro* and *in vivo* findings will help clarify the role of smoking in hormone-related processes.

Acknowledgements

We greatly appreciate the collaboration of Nicholas J. Wald, Howard S. Cuckle of The Medical College of St. Bartholomew's Hospital, London, and James E. Haddow, George J. Knight, and Glenn E. Palomaki, of the Foundation for Blood Research, Scarborough, Maine, in the studies described on the levels of hormones in pregnancy.

References

Asmussen, I. (1977). Ultrastructure of the human placenta at term. Observations on placentas from newborn children of smoking and non-smoking mothers. *Acta Obstetrica Gynecologica Scandinavica*, 56, 119–26.

Barbieri, R. L., Gochberg, J., and Ryan, K. J. (1986a). Nicotine, cotinine, and anabasine inhibit aromatase in human trophoblast in vitro. *Journal of Clinical Investigation*, 77, 1727–33.

Barbieri, R. L., McShane, P. M., and Ryan, K. J. (1986b). Constituents of cigarette smoke inhibit human granulosa cell aromatase. *Fertility and Sterility*, 46, 232–6.

Barbieri, R. L., York, C. M., Cherry, M. L., and Ryan, K. J. (1987). The effects of nicotine, cotinine, and anabasine on rat adrenal 11beta-hydroxylase and 21-hydroxylase. *Journal of Steroid Biochemistry*, 28, 25–8.

Baron, J. A. (1984). Smoking and estrogen-related disease. *American Journal of Epidemiology*, 119, 9–22.

Barrett-Connor, E., Khaw, K.-T., and Yen, S.S.C. (1986). A prospective study of dehydroepiandrosterone sulfate, mortality, and cardiovascular disease. *New England Journal of Medicine*, 315, 1519–24.

Canick, J. A. and Ryan, K. J. (1975). The inhibition of 16alpha-hydroxytestosterone aromatization by carbon monoxide. *Biochemical and Biophysical Research Communications*, 63, 496–501.

Canick, J. A. and Ryan, K. J. (1976). Cytochrome P-450 and the aromatization of 16alpha-hydroxytestosterone and androstenedione by human placental microsomes. *Molecular and Cellular Endocrinology*, 6, 105–15.

Canick, J. A., Knight, G. J., Palomaki, G. E., Haddow, J. E., Cuckle, H. S., and Wald, N. J. (1988). Low second trimester maternal serum unconjugated oestriol in pregnancies with Down's syndrome. *British Journal of Obstetrics and Gynaecology*, 95, 330–3.

Lee, J. N., Grudzinskas, J. G., and Chard, T. (1981). Effect of smoking on maternal blood SP_1 levels in late pregnancy. *Obstetrics and Gynecology*, 57, 220–3.

Longcope, C. and Johnston, C. C. Jr. (1988). Androgen and estrogen dynamics in pre- and postmenopausal women: a comparison between smokers and nonsmokers. *Journal of Clinical Endocrinology and Metabolism*, 67, 379–83.

Longo, L. D. (1977). The biological effects of carbon monoxide on the pregnant woman, fetus, and newborn infant. *American Journal of Obstetrics and Gynecology*, 129, 69–103.

MacMahon, B., Trichopoulos, D., Cole, P., and Brown, J. (1982). Cigarette smoking and urinary estrogens. *New England Journal of Medicine*, **307**, 1062–5.

Mochizuki, M., Maruo, T., Masuko, K., and Ohtsu, T. (1984). Effects of smoking on fetoplacental-maternal system during pregnancy. *American Journal of Obstetrics and Gynecology*, 149, 413–20.

Moser, R. J., Hollingsworth, D. R., Carlson, J. W., and Lamotte, L. (1974). Human chorionic somatomammotropin in normal adolescent primiparous pregnancy. I. Effect of smoking. *American Journal of Obstetrics and Gynecology*, **120**, 1080–6.

Spellacy, W.N., Buhi, W. C., and Birk, S. A. (1977). The effect of smoking on serum human placental lactogen levels. *American Journal of Obstetrics and Gynecology*, 127, 232–4.

Wald, N. J., *et al*. (1988a). Maternal serum unconjugated oestriol as an antenatal screening test for Down's syndrome. *British Journal of Obstetrics and Gynaecology*, 95, 334–41.

Wald, N. J., *et al*. (1988b). Maternal serum screening for Down's syndrome in early pregnancy. *British Medical Journal*, 297, 883–7.

VII

Mechanisms: Hormones of Possible Relevance to Smoking-Related Diseases

20. Oestrogens and smoking-related disease: theoretical considerations

Jacob A. Canick

Abstract

Oestrogen action, in vivo, *is dependent on a combination of factors. 1. In cycling and pregnant women, the primary site of oestrogen production is glandular and circulating oestrogen levels are high, whereas after the menopause, oestrogen production takes place in peripheral tissues, circulating oestrogen levels are low, and locally produced oestrogen probably functions at its site of synthesis. 2. The availability of androgen substrates, especially in post-menopausal women, is critical to the amount of oestrogen that is produced. 3. Ultimately, the concentration of oestrogen, or perhaps the ratio of androgen to oestrogen, at the target cell will determine the target cell response. The above factors and the possible effect of smoking on them are discussed.*

20.1. Introduction

Smoking appears to affect a variety of oestrogen-mediated physiologic and disease processes. To better understand the interrelationship between constituents of smoke and oestrogen action, the various elements leading to oestrogen–receptor interaction, *in vivo*, should be considered. First, the site of oestrogen biosynthesis is critical, i.e. is the oestrogen glandular in origin or is it made at the target cell? If oestrogen is primarily glandular in origin, as it is in cycling women, then the concentration of oestrogen attained in the blood must be directly related to its ultimate effect at target sites. If on the other hand the oestrogen is made primarily in peripheral tissues, as is the case after the menopause, then its site of action might logically be at its site of synthesis. In that case, oestrogen is acting as a paracrine or autocrine effector, rather than as a blood-borne agent. In addition, if the oestrogen is produced peripherally, then the serum concentrations of the aromatizable androgens will determine the degree of saturation of the aromatase enzyme and therefore the rate of oestrogen production at extra-glandular sites. The tissue concentration of oestrogen to which the receptor is exposed will then determine the degree of receptor occupancy and the extent of the oestrogenic effect. Finally, the concept that the *ratio* of androgen to oestrogen rather than the absolute level of oestrogen is critical to the ultimate responsiveness of the target tissue should be considered. Experiments of nature have shown that oestrogen action is more fully expressed when unimpeded by the presence of androgen.

20.2 Localization of oestrogen biosynthesis and the levels of circulating oestrogens

In pre-menopausal women, serum levels of oestradiol are relatively high, about 40 to 350 pg/ml. These and other oestrogens in the circulation are derived from both ovarian and extra-glandular sources. As the ovarian follicle ripens and during the luteal phase, the ovary is the dominant source of circulating oestrogen; it is this source of hormone which is associated with oestrogenic stimulation of the genital tract and the breast. There are suggestions, however, that peripheral sources of oestrogen are necessary for acquisition and maintenance of cyclicity. Frisch (1985) believes that a critical percentage of body fat is required for menarche and proper functioning of the menstrual cycle. She argues that the contribution of oestradiol and oestrone derived from aromatization of androgen in adipose tissue is essential for normal regulation of gonadotropin secretion.

After the menopause, oestrogen in the circulation is derived exclusively from peripheral aromatization. The serum level of oestradiol is low (approx. 20–30 pg/ml) and the weaker oestrogen, oestrone, is the predominant type in the blood (serum levels approx. 50–70 pg/ml). Since the levels of circulating oestrogens are so low in the post-menopausal period, it is probable that after the menopause local production of oestrogen is the primary mechanism by which the hormone is placed at or near its site of action. For instance, the maintenance of bone density is to some degree oestrogen-dependent (Law, Chapter 7; Baron 1984) and in fact oestradiol receptors have been described recently in human osteoblast cells (Komm *et al.* 1988; Eriksen *et al.* 1988). While the ability of human osteoblasts to aromatize androgen to oestrogen has not yet been demonstrated, Frisch *et al.* (1980) have reported that preparations of human fatty marrow can aromatize androgen to oestrogen, placing newly synthesized oestrogen in close proximity to the bone cells. Previously, Vittek *et al.* (1974) reported that rat mandibular bone has aromatase activity. Thus, oestrogen may be able to act in a paracrine or autocrine fashion in bone to help maintain bone density.

A now classic example of peripheral aromatization linked to the local action of oestrogen is neonatal defeminization of the male rat hypothalamus (MacLusky and Naftolin 1981). In that model, oestradiol is produced within hypothalamic neurons from testosterone supplied from the circulation. The locally produced oestradiol then acts through its receptor located in the same or neighbouring neurons to cause behavioural and physiologic defeminization (McEwen *et al.* 1977; Canick *et al.* 1986). Oestradiol in the circulation is prevented from acting on target sites because it is sequestered by a serum binding protein, α-fetoprotein. Thus, only male rats, which have sufficient levels of circulating testosterone to serve as the substrate for hypothalamic aromatization, are defeminized.

20.3. Levels of circulating androgens

What, then, are sufficient levels of androgens to maximally stimulate peripheral aromatization? The aromatase enzyme complex exhibits unusually high affinity for its androgen substrates. The Michaelis constant (K_m) for the two most potent substrates, androstenedione and testosterone is in the range of 10–40 nmol/l (Barbieri *et al.* 1981). In pre-menopausal women, the concentration of androstenedione in the circulation is 1–3 ng/ml, while testosterone levels are lower (approximately 0.2–0.8 ng/ml). On a molar basis, therefore, the concentration of aromatizable androgens (androstenedione plus testosterone) in the circulation is 4–10 nmol/l. Presumably, a substantial portion of the testosterone is not available to peripheral tissues because it is bound to sex hormone binding globulin (SHBG). In fact, so-called free testosterone, the fraction of testosterone in the circulation that is not bound to SHBG or albumin, is only about 2 per cent of the total. Androstenedione does not bind with high affinity to SHBG so that presumably most of it is available for entry into peripheral tissues followed by aromatization.

Even if all the testosterone and androstenedione in the circulation were available for aromatization in tissues, the concentration would be barely in the range of the K_m for the enzyme. As a consequence it would be the availability of these two hormones which would limit oestrogen synthesis. In contrast, within the functioning ovary, androgen concentrations are very high. For example, follicular fluid levels of androstenedione and testosterone reach 3500 nmol/l (1000 ng/ml) and 500 nmol/l (140 ng/ml), respectively (McNatty *et al.* 1979). Clearly, the aromatase within granulosa cells of the functioning ovary is constantly saturated and aromatase is the limiting factor.

In the post-menopausal woman, the circulating levels of androstenedione and testosterone are approximately half what they are pre-menopausally (Vermeulen 1976) because the ovary is secreting very little steroid hormone. It is clear, therefore, that unless an active uptake system exists to drive androgens into target cells, the aromatase in peripheral tissues will operate both pre- and post-menopausally at subsaturating concentrations of substrate, making the rate of aromatization sub-optimal.

20.4. Oestrogen concentrations and oestrogen receptor occupancy

The oestrogen receptor binds oestradiol with very high affinity; its dissociation constant (K_d) is in the range of 10^{-11}–10^{-10} mol/l (0.01–0.10 nmol/l). This means that very little oestradiol is needed to cause receptor activation. Not surprisingly, the concentration range of circulating oestradiol in cycling women (0.2–1.3 nmol/l) is appropriate for stimulation of receptor activity. In post-menopausal women, the serum levels of oestradiol are much lower (0.07–0.10 nmol/l) and would appear to be insufficient to stimulate a high level of receptor activity. Oestrone levels, which are about twice as high as oestradiol after the menopause also are probably not sufficient to activate receptors because the affinity of the receptor for oestrone is one-tenth that for oestradiol.

It appears, therefore, that aromatization of androgen to oestrogen at the target site may be necessary, at least in part, to provide target cell oestrogen receptors with enough ligand for activation. However, it is very difficult to estimate the concentration of oestrogen within the target that is provided by local production. Experiments, in which aromatase activity of various human peripheral tissues is determined *in vitro*, show that 0.2–1.0 pmol of oestrogen can be produced in a gram of tissue per hour (Frisch *et al.* 1980; Forney *et al.* 1981). Such levels of aromatase activity indicate that nanomolar amounts of oestrogen could be produced locally, levels which would be sufficient to activate oestrogen receptors.

Table 20.1 summarizes the concentrations of androgen and oestrogen in the circulation of pre- and post-menopausal women as well as the affinity constants of the aromatase and the oestrogen receptor for the hormones. Concentrations are given in the same unit (nanomolar) so that comparisons

Table 20.1. Typical androgen and oestrogen concentrations in serum and the affinity constants for aromatase and the oestrogen receptor. The concentration unit for all values is nanomolar

	A	T	E1	E2
Serum:				
Pre-menopausal women	7	2	0.2	0.5
Post-menopausal women	4	1	0.2	0.07
Men	6	25	0.2	0.07
Affinity constants:				
Aromatase K_m	20	20	—	—
Oestrogen receptor	—	—	1.0	0.08

can be drawn more readily. No attempt is made to consider the role of serum binding proteins in the calculation of hormone levels.

20.5. The role of androgen to oestrogen ratio in modulating oestrogen action

While androgens are unable to bind to the oestrogen receptor with high affinity, it appears that their presence can impede the biological effects of oestrogen. Presumably, androgens attenuate oestrogen action through mechanisms involving androgen receptor interaction. Evidence for this is provided by the experiment of nature known as testicular feminization syndrome or androgen insensitivity, an X-linked disorder in which the androgen receptor is greatly reduced or very poorly functional (Griffin and Wilson 1980). Despite the presence of normal male levels of circulating androgens, a female rather than male phenotype is expressed in such an XY individual. Feminization in this case is caused by levels of oestrone and oestradiol in the range that are normally present in the male (20–50 pg/ml, i.e. 0.07–0.15 nmol/l), however, their action is unimpeded because of the lack of an androgen effect. The same or higher concentrations of oestrogens in a normal male with functional androgen receptors would not cause breast development, for example (MacDonald *et al.* 1979).

There is evidence from experiments using cell-free preparations of neural tissue which contain both androgen and oestrogen receptors that there is cross talk between the two receptor types. Fox (1975) found that testosterone can block binding of oestradiol to the oestrogen receptor and that oestradiol can block testosterone binding to the androgen receptor. It is not known whether these mechanisms are operative physiologically, but they also lend support to the notion that androgens and oestrogens can affect each other's functions.

20.6. Relevance to smoking-related disorders

This discussion of steroid hormone levels in the blood and in oestrogen target tissues is intended to show that ultimate receptor occupation and activation are dependent on many factors. While smoking has an effect on oestrogen-induced processes, this effect is generally not reflected in reduced circulating levels of oestrogen. Only in pregnancy, when oestrogen levels are high, is a reduction in serum oestrogen levels clearly seen (Mochizuki *et al.* 1984; Bernstein *et al.* 1989; Canick and Barbieri, Chapter 19). In the non-pregnant, pre-menopausal woman, a reduction in oestrogen levels, measured in urine, has been seen only during the luteal phase of the cycle (MacMahon *et al.* 1982). Smoking has never been shown to reduce circulating oestrogen levels in post-menopausal women (Barrett-Connor, Chapter 17). These findings indicate that unless circulating oestrogen levels are initially high, it is unlikely that they will reflect the inhibitory effects of the constituents of cigarette smoke.

Thus, the effect of smoking on oestrogen-mediated disease processes such as osteoporosis, which affects post-menopausal women in high numbers, must be localized to events other than modulation of circulating oestrogen levels. Perhaps changes in the androgen/oestrogen ratio are responsible for the negative effect of smoking on osteoporosis. New data indicate that the biosynthesis of adrenal androgens is increased in smoking women (Canick and Barbieri, Chapter 19; Barrett-Connor, Chapter 17) leading to the hypothesis that an effect of smoking on osteoporosis is caused by an increased ratio of androgen to oestrogen which attenuates the action of oestrogens through receptor-mediated mechanisms.

It is also possible that constituents of smoke inhibit the production or the action of oestrogens at selective peripheral targets. Perhaps, for example, local aromatization in cells of the fatty marrow is more sensitive to certain tobacco products than are other sites of aromatization. Perhaps receptor binding or activation is sensitive to constituents of smoke. Experiments are currently underway which test these possibilities. New answers to the puzzling relationship between oestrogen-related processes and smoking will be most welcome.

References

Barbieri, R. L., Canick, J. A., and Ryan, K. J. (1981). High affinity steroid binding to rat testis 17alpha-hydroxylase and human placental aromatase. *Journal of Steroid Biochemistry*, **14**, 387–93.

Baron, J. A. (1984). Smoking and estrogen-related disease. *American Journal of Epidemiology*, **119**, 9–22.

Bernstein, L., Pike, M. C., Lobo, R. A., Depue, R. H., Ross, R. K., and Henderson, B. E. (1989). Cigarette smoking in pregnancy results in marked decrease in maternal hCG and oestradiol levels. *British Journal of Obstetrics and Gynaecology*, 96, 92–6.

Canick, J. A., Vaccaro, D. E., Livingston, E. M., Leeman, S. E., Ryan, K. J., and Fox, T. O. (1986). Localization of aromatase and 5alpha-reductase to neuronal and non-neuronal cells in fetal rat hypothalamus. *Brain Research*, **372**, 277–82.

Eriksen, E. F., *et al.* (1988). Evidence of estrogen receptors in normal human osteoblast-like cells. *Science*, **241**, 84–6.

Forney, J. P., *et al.* (1981). Aromatization of androstenedione to estrone by human adipose tissue *in vitro*. Correlation with adipose tissue mass, age, and endometrial neoplasia. *Journal of Clinical Endocrinology and Metabolism*, **53**, 192–9.

Fox, T. O. (1975). Androgen- and estrogen-binding macromolecules in developing mouse brain: biochemical and genetic evidence. *Proceedings of the National Academy of Science (USA)*, **72**, 4303–7.

Frisch, R. E. (1985). Fatness, menarche, and female fertility. *Perspectives in Biology and Medicine*, **28**, 611–33.

Frisch, R. E., Canick, J. A., and Tulchinsky, D. (1980). Human fatty marrow

aromatizes androgen to estrogen. *Journal of Clinical Endocrinology and Metabolism*, **51**, 394-6.
Griffin, J. E. and Wilson, J. D. (1980). The syndromes of androgen resistance. *New England Journal of Medicine*, **302**, 198-209.
Komm, B. S., *et al.* (1988). Estrogen binding, receptor mRNA, and biologic response in osteoblast-like osteosarcoma cells. *Science*, **241**, 81-4.
MacDonald, P. C., Madden, J. D., Brenner, P. F., Wilson, J. D., and Siiteri, P. K. (1979). Origin of estrogen in normal men and in women with testicular feminization. *Journal of Clinical Endocrinology and Metabolism*, **49**, 905-16.
MacLusky, N. J. and Naftolin, F. (1988). Sexual differentiation of the central nervous system. *Science*, **211**, 1294-303.
MacMahon, B., Trichopoulos, D., Cole, P., and Brown, J. (1982). Cigarette smoking and urinary estrogens. *New England Journal of Medicine*, **307**, 1062-5.
McEwen, B. S., Lieberburg, I., Chaptal, C., and Krey, L. C. (1977). Aromatization: important for sexual differentiation of the neonatal rat brain. *Hormones and Behavior*, **9**, 249-63.
McNatty, K. P., Smith, D. M., Makris, A., Osathanondh, R., and Ryan, K. J. (1979). The microenvironment of the human antral follicle: interrelationships among the steroid levels in antral fluid, the population of granulosa cells, and the status of the oocyte *in vivo* and *in vitro*. *Journal of Clinical Endocrinology and Metabolism*, **49**, 851-60.
Mochizuki, M., Maruo, T., Masuko, K., and Ohtsu, T. (1984). Effects of smoking on fetoplacental-maternal system during pregnancy. *American Journal of Obstetrics and Gynecology*, **149**, 413-20.
Vermeulen, A. (1976). The hormonal activity of the postmenopausal ovary. *Journal of Clinical Endocrinology and Metabolism*, **42**, 247-53.
Vittek, J., Altman, K., Gordon, G. G., and Southren, A. L. (1974). The metabolism of 7alpha-3H-testosterone by rat mandibular bone. *Endocrinology*, **94**, 325-9.

21. Hormonal factors and cancers of the endometrium and breast

Malcolm C. Pike

Abstract

Ovarian hormones play a key role in the aetiology of endometrial cancer and of breast cancer. The manner in which these hormones affect the risk of cancer differs according to site. For the endometrium, the concept that oestrogenic stimulation definitely increases cancer risk, while added progestational exposure protects against this risk, explains much of the available laboratory and epidemiological data. For breast cancer, current data are not consistent with a similar hypothesis, and instead suggest that oestrogens alone increase cancer risk and that progestins either have no effect, or are actually cancer-promoting.

21.1. Introduction

Ovarian hormones play a key role, probably the key role, in the aetiology of endometrial cancer and of breast cancer. A key epidemiological observation leading to this conclusion is the marked protective effect of early menopause (natural or artificial, i.e. bilateral ovariectomy) on both these cancers. For endometrial cancer 'unopposed oestrogen', i.e. oestrogen in the absence of progesterone, provides the stimulus to normal endometrial cell division and to increased risk of endometrial cancer. For breast cancer 'unopposed oestrogen' is not the critical hormonal state. Oestrogen is clearly a normal breast cell mitogen and there is much evidence that increased exposure to oestrogens (at least up to some limit) leads to an increased breast cancer risk. Oestrogen plus progesterone may, however, be considerably more mitogenic than an equal exposure to oestrogen alone, and, if this is so, such exposure is then more likely to increase breast cancer risk than the equivalent exposure to oestrogen alone. Epidemiologic data to resolve this issue may be available soon.

The evidence that ovarian cancer is affected by ovarian hormones is weak. The risk of ovarian cancer is much reduced by early menopause, but the key event does not appear to be the reduction of exposure to ovarian steroids but rather the stopping of the recurrent rupture of the ovarian surface with each ovulation (see Pike 1987). Ovarian cancer will not be discussed further here.

21.2. Endometrial cancer

Epidemiological studies have shown that the risk of developing endometrial cancer is decreased by an early age at menopause and by high parity. Risk increases markedly with increasing weight and with use of oestrogen replacement therapy (ORT), and decreases markedly with combination-type oral contraceptive (COC) use (see Key and Pike 1988a for references). These risk factors can all be explained in terms of the 'unopposed oestrogen hypothesis' for endometrial cancer (Siiteri 1978; Henderson *et al.* 1982). This hypothesis maintains that endometrial cancer risk is increased by exposure to endogenous or exogenous oestrogen which is not opposed by progesterone or a synthetic progestin. One description of the hypothesis suggests that this increased risk is caused by the increased mitotic activity of the endometrium induced by such exposure (Key and Pike 1988a).

Mitotic rate of endometrial cells

Oestrogens stimulate mitosis in endometrial cells. Progestins dramatically reduce mitotic activity, mainly by reducing the concentration of oestrogen receptors. Progestins also increase the metabolism of oestradiol, the predominant intracellular oestrogen in the endometrium (Whitehead *et al.* 1981) to

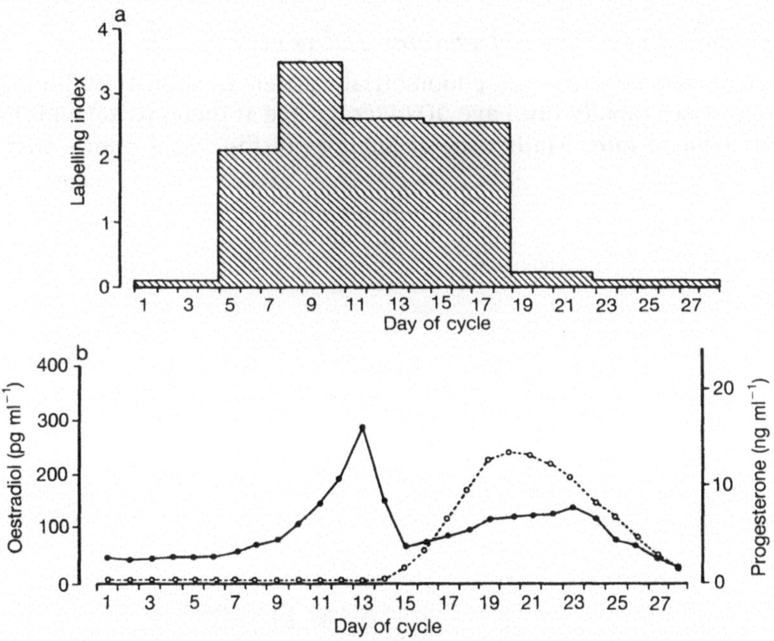

Fig. 21.1. (a) Endometrial mitotic rate by day of cycle (day 1 is first day of menses and 28-day cycle assumed with ovulation on day 14). (b) Serum concentrations of oestradiol (●) and progesterone (○) by day of cycle.

the less active oestrogen oestrone, and stimulate differentiation of endometrial cells to a secretory state. Figure 21.1a shows the mitotic rate of the glandular endometrial cells (Ferenczy *et al.* 1979) and Fig. 21.1b the fluctuating serum concentrations of oestradiol and progesterone during the normal menstrual cycle (Key and Pike 1988a). The two most important points to note from Fig. 21.1 are:

(1) The mitotic rate rises rapidly from a very low level during menses to reach a near maximal level early on in the cycle, probably by day 5, and then stays roughly constant for 14 days until day 19, after which it drops again to a very low level in the face of the post-ovulation increase in progesterone.
(2) The maximal endometrial mitotic rate is induced by the basal early follicular serum oestradiol concentration; later increases in follicular oestradiol levels do not induce any further increase in the mitotic rate.

There thus appears to be an 'effective upper limit' to the serum concentration of unopposed oestradiol: this upper limit is not greater than 50 pg/ml. Very low unopposed oestradiol concentrations (5 pg/ml or less) in slender post-menopausal women are associated with an atrophic endometrium, but there is little information available about the nature of the dose–effect relationship between unopposed oestradiol concentration and mitotic rate between such low concentrations and the 50 pg/ml upper limit.

The age–incidence curve of endometrial cancer

The age–incidence curve of endometrial cancer is shown in Fig. 21.2. Incidence arises rapidly until age 50 (average age at menopause) and then at a much reduced rate. Mathematical analysis of Fig. 21.2 shows that it is

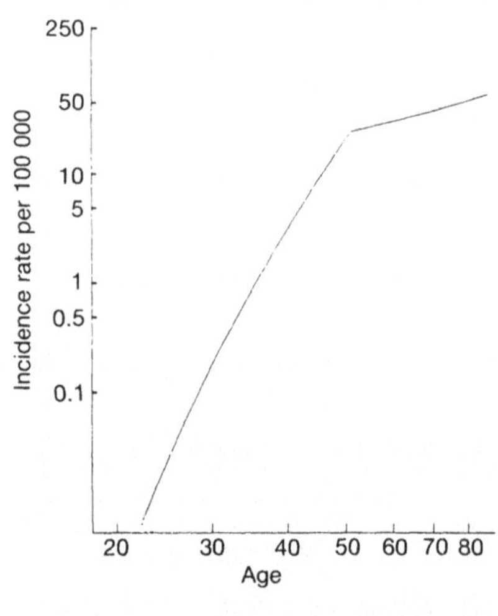

Fig. 21.2. Age-incidence curve of endometrial cancer (from data for West Midlands Region of England, 1968–72 (see Pike 1987)).

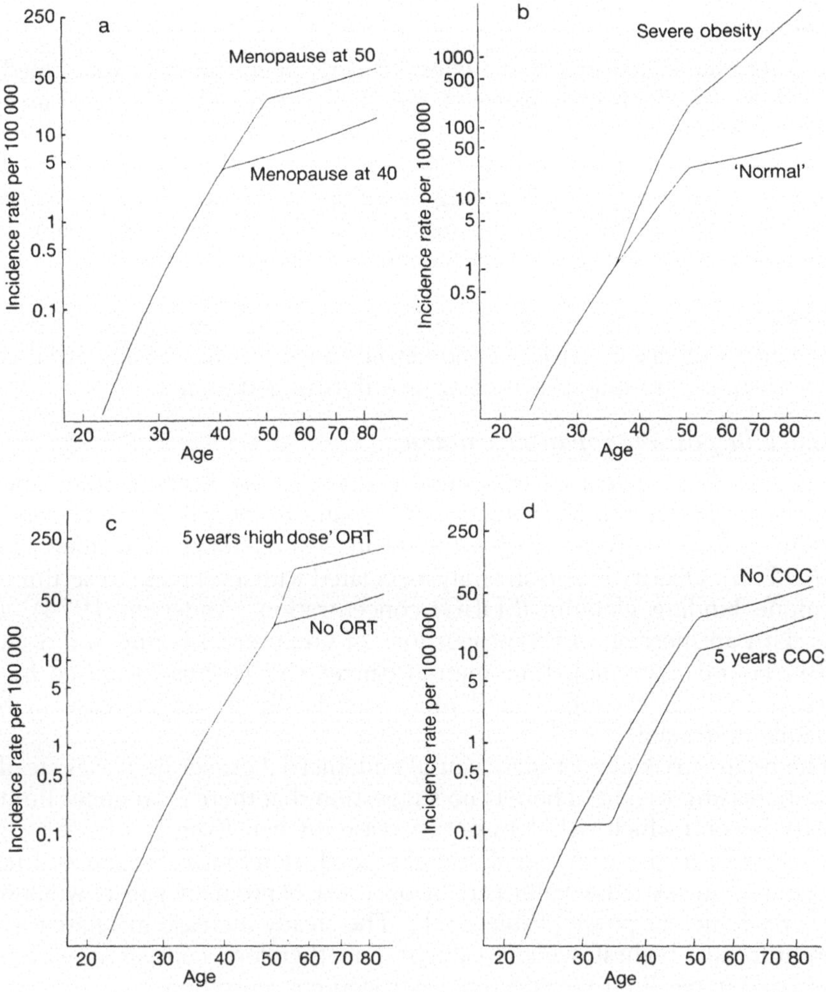

Fig. 21.3. Predicted effects of various 'hormonal' events on the age-incidence curve for endometrial cancer (see text). (a) Menopause; (b) Obesity; (c) ORT; (d) COC.

completely compatible with the mitotic rate ideas intrinsic to the unopposed oestrogen hypothesis (Pike 1987), and the effects of the various risk factors can be most clearly understood by noting their effects on the age-incidence curve. Figure 21.3 shows these effects. It is most important to notice from the figure how long-term (lifelong) the effects are, in particular how the increased risk from ORT use, and the protection from COC use, are predicted to continue almost unabated after the ORT and COC are stopped. The basis of the effects is explained immediately below.

Menopause

The long-established protective effect of early menopause is illustrated in Fig. 21.3a, in which menopause at age 50 is compared with menopause at age 40. The obvious change here is that the curve for early menopause has the reduced slope of the post-menopausal period starting at age 40. Early menopause reduces risk by reducing the unopposed oestradiol concentration from the relatively high level during the follicular phase of every menstrual cycle to the low level of the post-menopausal period.

Parity

Pregnancies reduce the risk of endometrial cancer because endometrial cells are not exposed to unopposed oestrogen during gestation.

Obesity in post-menopausal women

Obesity leads to increased peripheral production of oestrone from androstenedione (Siiteri and MacDonald 1973), and to increased serum concentrations of both oestrone and oestradiol in post-menopausal women (Judd *et al.* 1976). Obesity is also strongly associated with a decrease in serum sex-hormone binding globulin (SHBG) concentration (Anderson 1974), and thus with an increase in the proportions of non-protein bound and of non-SHBG bound oestradiol. Endometrial cancer risk is thus increased by an increase in total oestradiol, and more specifically by an increase in bioavailable oestradiol.

The relative risk of post-menopausal endometrial cancer increases steadily with increasing weight. There is no suggestion that there is an upper limit of obesity beyond which risk does not increase further. Even at a body weight of 110 kg (200 per cent 'ideal' weight) total, non-SHBG bound and non-protein bound oestradiol values are below those of pre-menopausal women in the early follicular phase (Table 21.1). The steady increase in relative risk, even into the highest weight category, is therefore consistent with the postulated upper limit for effective oestrogen concentration.

Obesity in pre-menopausal women

Recent epidemiological studies have consistently found that obesity markedly increases the risk of endometrial cancer in pre-menopausal, as well as in post-menopausal, women. Obesity has not been associated with an increase in serum total oestradiol concentration in pre-menopausal women (Zumoff 1982), but it is certainly associated with a decrease in SHBG and therefore with an increase in bioavailable oestradiol. It is clear, however, that increased bioavailable oestradiol levels cannot be the cause of the increased risk in obese pre-menopausal women, since the serum concentration of oestradiol in pre-menopausal women is always at or above the upper limit for effective oestrogen action. The mechanism by which obesity increases risk in pre-

Table 21.1. Estimates of oestradiol, SHBG, non-protein bound oestradiol, and non-SHBG bound oestradiol*

Menopausal status	Dose of CEO (mg/day)	Weight (kg)	Oestradiol (pg/ml)	SHBG (nmol/l)	Non-protein bound oestradiol (pg/ml)	Non-SHBG bound oestradiol (pg/ml)
Pre			50	60	0.9	34
Post		55	11	50	0.2	8
Post		110	25	27	0.5	19
Post	0.625		50	130	0.7	24
Post	1.25		75	180	0.9	26

* See Key and Pike (1988a) for details.
CEO, conjugated equine oestrogens; SHBG, serum sex-hormone binding globulin.

menopausal women appears rather to involve progesterone deficiency rather than oestradiol excess: obesity is associated with amenorrhoea, with subnormal luteal phase progesterone concentration, and with irregular menstrual periods (see Key and Pike 1988a for references). The endometrium of a woman with normal ovulatory cycles proliferates for 14 days in the cycle, i.e. for only some 50 per cent of the time. Since it is the periods of proliferation that increase endometrial cancer risk under the unopposed oestrogen hypothesis, a pre-menopausal woman with anovulatory cycles will be at an increased risk of endometrial cancer since her endometrium will proliferate for much more than 50 per cent of the time (her serum oestradiol level will be consistently above 50 pg/ml as she will have some follicle development).

Figure 21.3b illustrates the effect of obesity on the age–incidence curve, using as an illustration the predicted curve for a woman whose obesity makes her anovular from age 35. Her endometrial mitotic rate for ages 35 to 50 is twice the normal pre-menopausal rate. After menopause her mitotic rate is equal to the normal pre-menopausal rate [half the follicular rate because bioavailable oestradiol is approximately half the basal follicular level (see Table 21.1), but for double the time (no luteal phase)]. Although the curves continue to separate further after menopause, i.e. the relative risk continues to increase, a large proportion of the increased risk in the post-menopausal period is due to the increased mitotic rate in the pre-menopausal period.

Oestrogen replacement therapy

The endometrial mitotic activity of a post-menopausal woman is greatly increased during ORT. Table 21.1 shows that the serum level of non-SHBG bound oestradiol of a woman using conjugated equine oestrogens ('Premarin') as ORT is approximately two-thirds the early follicular level. Conjugated equine oestrogen contains other potent oestrogens and it therefore seems appropriate to assume that the endometrial mitotic rate of a woman on continuous conjugated equine oestrogen will be between 67 and 100 per cent of that during the follicular phase of the menstrual cycle, and the total mitotic activity over a 28-day period will be thus between 1.33-and 2-times that of a pre-menopausal woman. The twofold figure is illustrated in Fig. 21.3c for 5 years of ORT use starting at menopause (taken as at age 50). Instead of the slope of the incidence curve decreasing at age 50, the slope will actually be steeper for the 5 years of ORT use. The increased risk will be lifelong, and the figure predicts that 5 years of such ORT use will increase lifelong risk by some 280 per cent.

Combination-type oral contraceptives

Since endometrial mitotic activity is near zero in women on COCs, the incidence curve will be very nearly flat during the time COCs are used. When COCs are stopped the curve will increase as before. This is illustrated in Fig. 21.3d for 5 years of COC use starting at age 28. The protection against endometrial cancer is lifelong. The figure shows that 5 years of COC use will decrease risk by some 60 per cent.

The magnitudes of the risks illustrated in Fig. 21.3 and discussed above are close to those observed in epidemiological studies. The long-term effects of menopause are well known. The long-term risks of ORT use have been observed in a number of studies, as have the long-term benefits of COC use (Centers for Disease Control 1983; Shapiro *et al.* 1985).

21.3. Breast cancer

Epidemiologic studies of breast cancer have demonstrated that there are several major risk factors related to hormonal factors (see Key and Pike 1988b for references). For the discussion here the important risk factors are: late menarche and early menopause, both of which decrease risk. The overall effect of obesity is to increase the risk of breast cancer, but this increased risk is restricted to older post-menopausal women. ORT use in post-menopausal women causes a relatively small increase in the risk of breast cancer, while studies of COC use have found either no effect or an increase in risk. Breast cancer cases have been found to have a history of a deficit of long and irregular cycles.

The success of the unopposed oestrogen hypothesis in explaining and predicting the epidemiology of endometrial cancer has stimulated the effort to develop an equivalent hypothesis for breast cancer. This requires an understanding of the hormonal control of breast cell division.

Mitotic rate of breast cells

Biopsy and autopsy studies (Anderson *et al.* 1982; Longacre and Bartow 1986), show clearly that there is some breast epithelial cell division during the follicular phase of the menstrual cycle, but that the mitotic rate of breast cells is approximately fourfold higher during the luteal phase, with a peak at days 23–25. Two interpretations of these data have to be seriously considered. The most straightforward is that oestradiol alone (in the follicular phase) induces some cell division, but that oestradiol and progesterone together (in the luteal phase) induce considerably more cell division . . . the 'oestrogen plus progestin hypothesis'. The failure of *in vitro* studies (see Key and Pike 1988b for references and discussion) to show a significant mitogenic effect of progesterone suggests, however, a need to consider an alternative interpretation, i.e. that breast cell division may only be induced by oestrogens with progesterone having little or no effect. This 'oestrogen alone hypothesis' requires there to be a dose–response relationship between breast cell division and oestradiol serum concentration in the range of oestradiol concentrations occurring during the normal menstrual cycle. As noted above, there is no such relationship with endometrial cell division.

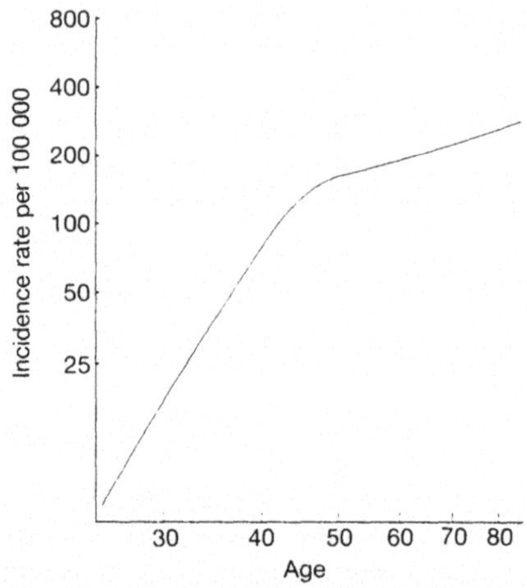

Fig. 21.4. Age–incidence curve of breast cancer (from data for US whites 1969–71).

Many authors have considered an 'unopposed oestrogen hypothesis' for breast cancer, that is, that the effect of oestrogens and progestins on the breast is the same as their effect on the endometrium, with unopposed oestrogen increasing risk and progestins (including progesterone in the physiological range) being protective. The direct observational studies of breast cell mitoses show that, in the physiological range, progesterone cannot be effectively opposing the mitogenic effects of oestrogen on breast cells.

The following sections briefly review the 'important' epidemiological evidence, and then consider the consistency of this evidence with the alternative hypotheses.

The age–incidence curve of breast cancer

The age–incidence curve of breast cancer is shown in Fig. 21.4. When the logarithm of incidence is plotted against the logarithm of age, as in Fig. 21.4, there is a steeply sloping line during the pre-menopausal period, a line with a much shallower slope in the post-menopausal period, and a gradual transition between the two lines during the peri-menopausal period. As with endometrial cancer, the effects of the various risk factors can be most clearly understood by noting their effect on the age–incidence curve. Figure 21.5 shows a number of these effects.

Menarche

Early menarche increases breast cancer risk, and, most importantly, for a given age at menarche (first menstrual period) the sooner regular cycles are established the greater the risk of breast cancer (Henderson *et al.* 1985). Early menarche is itself associated with the rapid onset of regular cycles (Wallace *et al.* 1978; Apter and Vihko 1983).

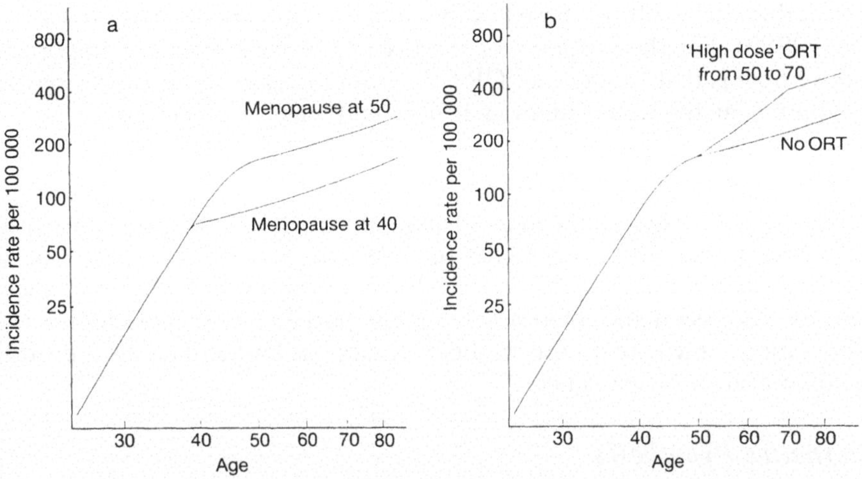

Fig. 21.5. Predicted effects of various 'hormonal' events on the age-incidence curve for breast cancer (see text). (a) Menopause; (b) ORT.

Menopause

The long-established protective effect of early menopause is illustrated in Fig. 21.5a, in which menopause at age 50 is compared with menopause at age 40. The obvious change here is that the curve for early menopause has the reduced slope of the post-menopausal period starting at age 40.

Obesity

The overall effect of obesity is to increase the risk of breast cancer (Lubin *et al.* 1985), but this increased risk is restricted to older post-menopausal women. In pre-menopausal women, recent evidence suggests that obesity is associated with a reduction in risk (Willett *et al.* 1985).

Oestrogen replacement therapy

Epidemiological studies of ORT and breast cancer risk, which have used population controls, have shown that an increase in exposure to exogenous oestrogen (unopposed by a progestin) causes a small increase in breast cancer risk (Key and Pike 1988b). These studies relate essentially to ORT given as conjugated equine oestrogens at daily doses of between 0.625 mg and 1.25 mg (with a mean dose roughly midway between these, i.e. of approximately 0.94 mg) for 21 to 28 days in each 28-day cycle (mean duration of approximately 26 days per cycle). From these studies it appears that 20 years of such ORT use causes an approximately 75 per cent increase in risk of breast cancer (Fig. 21.5b). In contrast, epidemiological studies which have used hospital controls have found little evidence of an increase in risk of breast cancer from even extended use of ORT. For a number of reasons it appears that the results of these hospital-based studies are incorrect (Key and Pike 1988b). For the purposes of the discussion here the most important point to note is that 'high dose' ORT does not increase breast cancer risk to anywhere near the same extent as it does endometrial cancer risk.

Combination-type oral contraceptives

Recent studies which included a substantial number of long-term users of COCs have found either that COCs have no effect on breast cancer risk or that they slightly increase risk (see McPherson and Drife 1986 and Lancet 1986 for discussion and references). For the purposes of this discussion the main point to note is that none of these studies has found that COCs protect a woman against breast cancer.

Alternative hypotheses

The absence of an increased risk of breast cancer in pre-menopausal obese women is strong evidence against the 'unopposed oestrogen hypothesis' for breast cancer. It is also difficult to make this hypothesis compatible with the increased risk associated with the rapid onset of regular cycles and a history of regular cycles in breast cancer cases. The critical evidence against this hypothesis is, however, that COCs have no protective effect against breast cancer, in contrast to their marked protective effect against endometrial cancer. In comparison with hormonal exposure during a normal menstrual cycle, COC use very significantly reduces breast exposure to unopposed oestrogen.

The 'oestrogen alone hypothesis' is consistent with the observed effects of age at menarche, age at menopause, and COCs on breast cancer risk. The consistency of this hypothesis with the observed relatively small effects of ORT and post-menopausal obesity depends on the dose–response relationship between oestrogens and breast cell division. ORT and post-menopausal obesity produce effective oestrogen levels that are sufficient to induce substantial endometrial cell division, but this does not require high oestrogen levels, since, as noted above, an oestrogen level equivalent to the early follicular phase induces maximal stimulation of endometrial cells. The breast cell division rate induced by the early follicular phase oestradiol level is much less than that induced (on this hypothesis) by the late follicular and luteal phase oestrogen levels. The much smaller increase in breast cancer risk, compared to endometrial cancer risk, caused by ORT and post-menopausal obesity is thus compatible with this hypothesis. A slight reduction in risk with pre-menopausal obesity is also compatible with this hypothesis, since there is no luteal phase oestrogen peak in anovular cycles.

The 'oestrogen plus progestin hypothesis' is consistent with the observed small increase in risk associated with the increased level of unopposed oestrogen in ORT and in post-menopausal obesity, with the increase in risk associated with early menarche, with the small protective effect of premenopausal obesity, and with the evidence for regular cycles in breast cancer cases. The hormonal content of COCs suggests that if oestrogens plus progestins increase breast cell proliferation then COCs should cause more mitoses than in a normal cycle and hence should increase breast cancer risk; calculations suggest that 5 years of COC use should give a relative risk for breast cancer of about 1.3 derived using the model in Pike (1987), which is compatible with the risks observed. Against this hypothesis is the evidence for low progesterone found in cases in case-control studies, and for an increased risk of breast cancer in women with 'luteal phase deficiency' (see Key and Pike 1988b); this evidence is contradictory to that obtained in case-control studies of a history of regular cycles in cases. The conflict can only be removed by supposing that low progesterone production is an early consequence of disease, which occurs some time before diagnosis. Current case-control studies (Pike, unpublished data) of this issue in luteal phase serum specimens, have found that when cases and controls who have not ovulated are excluded (more cases than controls), the remaining cases have higher serum levels of both oestradiol and progesterone.

Thus current evidence provides no real support for the unopposed oestrogen hypothesis, but both the oestrogen alone hypothesis and the oestrogen plus progestin hypothesis are tenable. Several areas of research should produce valuable information for choosing between these hypotheses. In particular, the effect of depot medroxyprogesterone acetate (DMPA, Depo Provera) on risk must be established, since this may provide a critical test of the oestrogen alone hypothesis. DMPA use causes complete suppression of ovulation and is associated with low levels of endogenous oestrogen production. The oestrogen alone hypothesis therefore predicts that DMPA use will be associated with a marked decrease in breast cancer risk. Currently available epidemiological studies of DMPA and breast cancer risk suggest the opposite, but they are really inadequate to allow any definite conclusions to be drawn; critical evidence from a New Zealand study should be available soon.

21.4. Conclusion

Our current, rather detailed and quite deep, understanding of the epidemiology (aetiology) of endometrial cancer is based on the knowledge of serum levels of oestrogen (or bioavailable oestrogen) and progesterone. This understanding does not require any particular alterations of metabolic pathways with unobservable effects on serum hormone levels in cancer cases, and before accepting the need for such to explain any effects of cigarette smoking on the risk of this disease, every attempt should be made to explain such effects by alterations of the serum levels of (bioavailable) oestradiol and progesterone or alterations of oestrogen receptor levels.

The success of the 'unopposed oestrogen hypothesis' for endometrial cancer entitles one to be most optimistic that the ideas discussed here in regard to breast cancer are in essence correct. Thus, as for endometrial cancer, any effects of cigarette smoking should be sought *via* effects of cigarette smoking on serum levels of oestradiol and progesterone or alterations of oestrogen receptor status and progesterone receptor status.

References

Anderson, D. C. (1974). Sex-hormone binding globulin. *Clinical Endocrinology*, **3**, 69–96.

Anderson, T. J., Ferguson, D. J. P., and Raab, G. M. (1982). Cell turnover in the 'resting' human breast: influence of parity, contraceptive pill, age and laterality. *British Journal of Cancer*, **46**, 376–82.

Apter, D. and Vihko, R. (1983). Early menarche, a risk factor for breast cancer, indicates early onset of ovulatory cycles. *Journal of Endocrinology and Metabolism*, **57**, 82–6.

Centers for Disease Control (1983). Oral contraceptive use and the risk of endometrial cancer. *Journal of the American Medical Association*, **249**, 1600–4.

Ferenczy, A., Bertrand, G., and Gelfand, M. M. (1979). Proliferation kinetics of human endometrium during the normal menstrual cycle. *American Journal of Obstetrics and Gynecology*, **133**, 859–67.

Henderson, B. E., Ross, R. K., Pike, M. C., and Casagrande, J. T. (1982). Endogenous hormones as a major factor in human cancer. *Cancer Research*, **42**, 3232–9.

Henderson, B. E., Ross, R. K., Judd, H. L., Krailo, M. D., and Pike, M. C. (1985). Do regular ovulatory cycles increase breast cancer risk? *Cancer*, **56**, 1206–8.

Judd, H. L., Lucas, W. E., and Yen, S. S. C. (1976). Serum 17-beta-estradiol and estrone levels in postmenopausal women with and without endometrial cancer. *Journal of Clinical Endocrinology and Metabolism*, **43**, 272–8.

Key, T. J. A. and Pike, M. C. (1988a). The dose-effect relationship between 'unopposed' estrogens and endometrial mitotic rate: its central role in explaining and predicting endometrial cancer risk. *British Journal of Cancer*, **57**, 205–12.

Key, T. J. A. and Pike, M. C. (1988b). The role of oestrogens and progestogens in the epidemiology and prevention of breast cancer. *European Journal of Cancer and Clinical Oncology*, **24**, 29–43.

Lancet (1986). Editorial: oral contraceptives and breast cancer. **ii**, 665–6.

Longacre, T. A. and Bartow, S. A. (1986). A correlative morphologic study of human breast and endometrium in the menstrual cycle. *American Journal of Surgical Pathology*, **10**, 382–93.

Lubin, F., Ruder, A. M., Wax, Y., and Modan, B. (1985). Overweight and changes in weight throughout adult life in breast cancer etiology. *American Journal of Epidemiology*, **122**, 579–88.

McPherson, K. and Drife, J. O. (1986). The pill and breast cancer: why the uncertainty? *British Medical Journal*, **293**, 709–10.

Pike, M. C. (1987). Age-related factors in cancers of the breast, ovary and endometrium. *Journal of Chronic Diseases*, **40**(Suppl.II), 59–69.

Shapiro, S., *et al.* (1985). Risk of localized and widespread endometrial cancer in relation to recent and discontinued estrogens. *New England Journal of Medicine*, **313**, 969–72.
Siiteri, P. K. (1978). Steroid hormones and endometrial cancer. *Cancer Research*, **38**, 4360–6.
Siiteri, P. K. and MacDonald, P. C. (1973). Role of extraglandular estrogen in human endocrinology. In *Handbook of physiology* (ed. Geiger *et al.*), p. 615. American Physiological Society, Washington DC.
Wallace, R. B., Sherman, B. M., Bean, J. A., Leeper, J. P., and Treloar, A. E. (1978). Menstrual cycle patterns and breast cancer risk factors. *Cancer Research*, **38**, 4021–4.
Whitehead, M. I., Townsend, P. T., Pryse-Davies, J., Ryder, T. A., and King, R. J. B. (1981). Effects of estrogens and progestins on the biochemistry and morphology of the postmenopausal endometrium. *New England Journal of Medicine*, **305**, 1599–1605.
Willett, W. C., *et al.* (1985). Relative weight and risk of breast cancer among premenopausal women. *American Journal of Epidemiology*, **122**, 731–40.
Zumoff, B. (1982). Relationship of obesity to blood estrogens. *Cancer Research*, 42(Suppl.), 3289s–94s.

VIII

Mechanisms: The Role of Nicotine and Other Agents in Tobacco Smoke

22. Influence of nicotine and other components of tobacco smoke on oestradiol metabolism

Jon J. Michnovicz, H. Leon Bradlow, and Jack Fishman

Abstract

The oxidative metabolism of oestradiol, particularly C-2 hydroxylation, is significantly enhanced by cigarette smoking in humans. The biochemical mechanism for this metabolic induction may help to explain the anti-oestrogenic effect of smoking on various hormone-dependent diseases in humans. Therefore, it is of considerable interest to know which chemicals in tobacco smoke have the capacity to alter oestrogen metabolism. This paper reviews the various mammalian P450 drug metabolizing isozymes capable of catalysing 2-hydroxylation and the factors influencing their activity. Current research strongly indicates that the polycyclic aromatic hydrocarbons in cigarette smoke are primarily responsible for induction of the cytochrome P450 isozymes (P450I) that perform oestradiol 2-hydroxylation, although other constitutive isozymes may be active in the non-induced individual. While nicotine has the capacity in some experimental systems to induce P450 metabolism, isozymes other than those in the P450I family are more likely to be affected. Further research into the effects of cigarette smoking on oestradiol metabolism should help to develop strategies that reduce the risk of hormone-dependent diseases without the adverse consequences of smoking.

22.1. Introduction

Cigarette smoke is composed of hundreds of different chemical compounds which are routinely inhaled in significant quantities during both voluntary and passive smoking (Stedman 1968). In addition to nicotine, nor-nicotine, and anabasine, cigarette smoke contains a host of pyrolysis products concentrated largely in the tar fraction. These latter compounds include such polycyclic aromatic hydrocarbons (PAH) as benzpyrene (BP), methylcholanthrene, and anthracene, which have been implicated in several studies as the principal agents responsible for the induction of cytochrome P450 drug-metabolizing enzymes (Welch *et al.* 1969).

The aggregate effect of smoking on the hepatic metabolism of endogenous hormones such as oestradiol or testosterone results from the effect of each chemical on a given metabolic pathway, catalysed by a specific isozyme of cytochrome P450. Thus, the effect of smoking on hormone metabolism can be analysed in part by considering the capacity of a particular compound in smoke to influence the enzyme reaction under consideration. This paper will compare the relative capabilities of nicotine and PAH to influence oestrogen metabolism in humans. Although much of the evidence reviewed here is derived from animal or cell culture experiments, strong inferences can be made regarding the effect of smoking on human oestradiol metabolism.

22.2. Modifiability of oestradiol metabolism

The metabolism of oestradiol in humans is principally oxidative in nature (Fishman *et al.* 1960). Oestradiol is reversibly converted to oestrone, which then serves as the proximal substrate for a pair of mutually exclusive irreversible hydroxylations at either the C-16α or C-2 position. The former leads to the formation of 16α-hydroxyoestrone and oestriol, while the latter yields the catechol oestrogens, 2-hydroxyoestrone and 2-methoxyoestrone. The former metabolites retain their oestrogen agonist activity, while the latter do not (Martucci and Fishman 1979; Fishman and Martucci 1980). Increases in the activity of one of these two oxidative pathways will therefore have biological effects opposite to increases in the other. Furthermore, the transformation of the substrate by one pathway might be predicted to influence the total oestrogens available to others. For example, a large increase in hepatic 2-hydroxylation would result in a relative decrease in the production of 16α-hydroxyoestrone and oestriol, without actually changing 16α-hydroxylase activity (Michnovicz *et al.* 1988).

Table 22.1. 2- and 16α-hydroxylation of oestradiol in normal men and women

Subjects	% dose hydroxylated (mean ± SE)	
	C-2	C-16α
Men	29.8 ± 8.8 (38)	10.6 ± 1.6 (20)
Pre-menopausal women	34.3 ± 5.7 (20)	10.7 ± 2.1 (7)
Post-menopausal women	34.1 ± 3.2 (13)	8.5 ± 1.4 (9)

Numbers in parentheses represents the number of subjects.

Table 22.2. Stimuli that affect oestradiol metabolism

Increased	Decreased
2-Hydroxylation	
Cigarette smoking	Obesity
Anorexia nervosa	Very high fat diets (65% fat—chimps)
High protein diets	
Hyperthyroidism	Hypothyroidism
Severe endurance training	Cimetidine
Cruciferous vegetables (indoles)	
Charbroiled meats (polycyclic hydrocarbons)	
16α-Hydroxylation*	
Very high fat diets (65% fat—chimps)	

* Breast cancer and systemic lupus erythematosus have also been associated with increased 16α-hydroxylation, which may be an aetiologic factor in these diseases.

Using an *in vivo* radiometric technique, we have determined the relative activities of the competing 16α- and 2-hydroxylative pathways in men and women, under a wide variety of experimental and pathophysiological conditions. These studies involve the intravenous infusion of a small amount of oestradiol labelled with tritium at a metabolically active site (C-16α, C-2, C-17α, etc.), which generates tritiated water upon hydroxylation at that site. The content of tritium in water from any body fluid sampled 48 h after the dose administration, along with an estimation of the total body water volume, allows the extent of reaction to be calculated. Using this methodology, it has been established that oxidation at C-2 is quantitatively greater than at C-16α (normal in pre- and post-menopausal women 32–39 per cent vs. 8–11 per cent; and in men 20–30 per cent vs. 7–9 per cent, respectively; Table 22.1) (Fishman *et al.* 1980).

A significant finding to emerge in these studies is that the extent of C-2 hydroxylation can be readily modified to higher or lower values by several pharmacological, environmental, and physiological stimuli (Table 22.2). Factors which elevate 2-hydroxylation in humans include cigarette smoking (Michnovicz *et al.* 1986), high protein diets (Anderson *et al.* 1984), hyperthyroidism (Fishman *et al.* 1964), and anorexia (Fishman and Bradlow 1977). Preliminary studies suggest that C-2 hydroxylation is also stimulated by diets containing cruciferous vegetables or charbroiled meats (Anderson 1988). In contrast, variables which are known to lower C-2 hydroxylation are obesity (Schneider *et al.* 1983), hypothyroidism (Fishman *et al.* 1964), use of cimetidine (Galbraith and Michnovicz 1989), and possibly very high fat diets (measured radiometrically in chimpanzees eating a 65 per cent fat diet; Musey *et al.* 1987). Thus, oestradiol 2-hydroxylation has proven to be a highly modifiable enzymatic pathway, responding to a wide variety of stimuli.

By comparison, the extent of C-16α hydroxylation of oestradiol is refractory to most of the stimuli thus far examined. When tested radiometrically, 16α-hydroxylation was unaffected by smoking, cimetidine, dietary composition, or obesity. (The aforementioned 65 per cent fat diet fed to chimpanzees increased the extent of 16α-hydroxylation, although the relevance to human nutrition of such an extreme dietary change is unknown.) Thus, 16α-hydroxylase activity in humans appears to be largely constitutive, i.e. set at a given level.

Two disease states have been reported to be associated with higher average rates of 16α-hydroxylation, namely, systemic lupus erythematosus and breast cancer (Lahita *et al.* 1981; Schneider *et al.* 1982). It is possible that a genetic predisposition toward greater 16α-hydroxylase activity plays an aetiological factor in these diseases. 16α-Hydroxyoestrone is unique as an oestrogen metabolite in its ability to form covalent bonds non-enzymatically with the primary amino acid group of proteins. These adducts occur via Schiff base formation followed by a thermodynamically-favoured Heyn's rearrangement (Bucala *et al.* 1985). Adduct formation to oestrogen receptor proteins might lead to an inappropriately prolonged activation state, with pathophysiological consequences (Swaneck and Fishman 1988). An interesting confirmation of this link between the extent of 16α-hydroxylation and oestrogen-dependent disease has been obtained in studies of mice strains differing in their spontaneous incidence of mammary tumours (Bradlow *et al.* 1985; Table 22.3).

Table 22.3. Comparison of mammary tumour incidence and the extent of 16α-hydroxylation in mice

Strain	Tumour incidence (%)	% 16α-hydroxylation
RIII	100	21.5±0.70
C3H/OuJ	100	18.4±0.86
C3H/HeJ	100	19.1±1.92
CBA/J	40	15.8±0.90
DBA/J	≈30	12.0±1.96
BALB/c/By	10–20	12.1±1.00
C57BL/6J	<1	10.1±1.06
C57L/J	<1	10.3±0.37
C57BR/CdJ	0	3.8±0.14

All studies were carried out in 6- to 8-week-old mice well before the appearance of tumours. Each point is the mean ± SEM of six to eight animals.

The extent of 16α-hydroxylation corresponded well with the overall rates of tumour formation. In these studies, measurements of 16α-hydroxylation were carried out well before the appearance of the tumours, and therefore were not a reflection of tumour presence.

Taken together, these studies suggest that while the extent of 16α-hydroxylation may have a profound impact on incidence of hormone dependent disease in humans, efforts to directly alter it will prove difficult. Since a given manipulation is more likely to affect the extent of 2-hydroxylation, control of the C-2 oxidative pathway offers a more accessible focus for therapeutic hormonal manipulation.

22.3. Effect of tobacco smoke on oestrogen P450 metabolism

Nicotine and the PAHs in smoke are all capable of increasing the activity of cytochrome P450 drug metabolizing enzymes. However, they are likely to differ fundamentally in their effects on various P450s. PAHs induce a specific family of P450s, collectively referred to as P450I (Nebert and Gonzalez 1985; Nebert *et al.* 1987). The P450I genes are defined as those induced by compounds capable of binding with high affinity to a cytosolic aromatic hydrocarbon (Ah receptor. It is particularly noteworthy in this context that PAH induction of a P450I gene product in humans, P_3450, is clearly correlated with increased oestradiol 2-hydroxylase activity (Ryan *et al.* 1982; Tuteja *et al.* 1985). Thus, in assessing the influence of smoking on hormone metabolism, two specific questions must be addressed. First, are nicotine or other components of cigarette smoke capable of inducing the P450I regulatory locus? Second, can these substances induce other P450 enzymes capable of augmenting oestrogen 2-hydroxylation?

The P450I family of monooxygenase enzymes has been well characterized in numerous species, and is believed to give rise upon induction to two distinct forms of P450. The first, cytochrome P_1450, hydroxylates benzpyrene and related polycyclic compounds, while the second, P_3450, hydroxylates such substrates as 2-acetylaminofluorene (AAF) and oestradiol at C-2 (Tuteja *et al.* 1985). Inducers of genes for these enzymes are known to bind with high affinity to a cytosolic Ah receptor. Upon binding, the inducer–receptor complex translocates into the nucleus to generate induction-specific RNA (Nebert 1979). Gene products of the Ah regulatory locus include the cytosolic receptor as well as the two cytochromes. Among the compounds capable of strongly inducing the Ah system are the pyrolysis products of cigarette smoke, β-naphthoflavone, and 2,3,7,8-tetrachlorodibenzo-*p*-dioxin (Tuteja *et al.* 1985). Dioxins in tissue culture have been shown to be potent inducers of oestradiol 2-hydroxylation (Gierthy *et al.* 1988).

Several other families of P450 have been identified that can perform oestradiol 2-hydroxylation, as summarized in Table 22.4 (Waxman 1988).

Table 22.4. P450 isozymes metabolizing oestradiol-17β at C-2

Aromatic hydrocarbon-inducible (P450I family)	
P450IA1	Mouse and human: P_1450 Rabbit: P450 form 6 Rat: $P450_c$ (also: P450 βNF-B, P450 MC-1)
P450IA2	Mouse and human: P_3450; Rabbit: P450 form 4 Rat: $P450_d$ (also: P450 ISF, MC-2, P448 HCB)
Phenobarbital-inducible (P450II)	
P450IIB2	Rat: $P450_e$, P450 PB-5
Testosterone-dependent (P450IIC11)	
$P450_{UT\text{-}A}$ (rat)	Also: P450-2c, $P450_h$, RLM5, P450-male
Steroid-inducible (P450III)	
P450IIIA1	P450 PCN-E, P450 pcn1, PB-2a
Constitutive enzymes	
$P450_{C\text{-}M/F}$ (rat)	

See: Dannan *et al.* 1986; Nebert *et al.* 1987; Ryan *et al.* 1982; and Waxman 1988.

(Note that equivalent names for individual forms of P450 are identified when possible.) Both P450I isozymes may be capable of 2-hydroxylation of oestrogens, although P_3450 is apparently more efficient (Tuteja *et al.* 1985). Also, the relative increase of the two P450I enzymes by different Ah inducers varies considerably. The heterogeneous mixture of inducers such as found in burning tobacco smoke would likely induce all Ah-responsive P450s, with a significant increase in oestrogen 2-hydroxylation as a result.

Other classes of P450 catalysing 2-hydroxylation of oestradiol are either non-inducible, or are instead regulated by compounds that do not act through the Ah receptor. For example, $P450_{UT\text{-}A}$ in rats possesses potent 2-hydroxylase activity, is male-specific and stimulated by testosterone, and is refractory to β-naphthoflavone treatment (Dannan *et al.* 1986). Other P450 enzymes, such as P450IIIA1 and $P450_{C\text{-}M/F}$ (Sugita *et al.* 1987), contribute to 2-hydroxylation of oestrogens in the absence of Ah inducers, and change little when such inducing agents are introduced.

Thus, the overall activity of the 2-hydroxylase pathway in non-smoking humans is likely to involve contributions from such constitutive enzymes as $P450_{C\text{-}M/F}$, gender specific and steroid-inducible isozymes similar to $P450_{UT\text{-}A}$ and P450 PCN-E, and baseline environmental stimulation of the P450I genes. Smoking impacts on 2-hydroxylation largely as a result of P450I activation.

22.4. Inducing effects of nicotine

The effect of nicotine on Ah-inducible P450s has not been well characterized, but most evidence suggests it is at best only a weak inducer. In an early report, it was demonstrated that a single high dose of nicotine (40 mg/kg) in corn oil given intraperitoneally to rats was about half as potent as polycyclic hydrocarbons in increasing hydroxylation of BP or AAF (Yamamoto *et al.* 1966). The pharmacological response to nicotine was quite unusual, however, in that repeating the dose for 2 or 3 days no longer led to increased AAF hydroxylation. The use of 40 mg/kg probably constituted a near-lethal dose (LD_{50} in saline about 25 mg/kg). These researchers reported that administration of a protein synthesis inhibitor 30 min before receiving high-dose nicotine prevented increases in BP and AAF hydroxylation, and interpreted this as evidence that nicotine induced new P450 synthesis. However, in view of the toxic dose of nicotine used (there was evidence of hepatocellular degeneration), the case for Ah induction by nicotine is weak. Nicotine given in convulsive doses acutely to rats was previously shown to produce transient elevations in microsomal drug metabolism, and was postulated to be a stress-related phenomenon (Ruddon and Cohen 1970).

Chronic oral nicotine administered alone to rats in non-toxic doses has been observed to induce other cytochrome P450 reactions, including amidopyrine N-demethylation (Ali *et al.* 1980), ethylmorphine N-dealkylation (Ruddon and Cohen 1970), and increased meprobamate inactivation (Wenzel and Broadie 1966). Again, induction by nicotine was unlike that occurring

Table 22.5. Effect of nicotine on oestradiol 2-hydroxylation in rats. Percent conversion of radiolabelled substrate [2-^{3}H]-oestradiol*

Experiment 1	
Control female	12.0
Control male	55.7
Nicotine-treated (♀) (2.4 mg/kg/d)	13.6 (↑ 13%)
Benzpyrene-treated (♀)	25.7 (↑ 114%)
Experiment 2	
Control female	11.6
Nicotine 4 mg/kg/d	13.3 (↑ 15%)
8 mg/kg/d	13.7 (↑ 18%)
12 mg/kg/d	12.2 (↑ 5%)

* Mean of two animals run in duplicate.

with aromatic hydrocarbons, in that prolonged stimulation by nicotine (>7 days) was often required in order to produce measurable changes in enzyme activity (Kaur and Ali 1982).

Preliminary experiments have been performed in female rats in order to determine whether oestradiol 2-hydroxylation can be specifically stimulated by nicotine alone (Michnovicz *et al.* unpublished data). Because the oral route of nicotine administration differs greatly from that of mainstream cigarette smoking, nicotine has been infused continuously into the circulation via a subcutaneously implanted osmotic pump. Animals received from 2.5 to 12 mg/kg/day for 8 days, after which hepatic microsomes were prepared and assayed. The results are summarized in Table 22.5. Note that female rats perform oestradiol 2-hydroxylation to a lesser extent than male rats, due to the absence of testosterone-dependent isozymes such as $P450_{UT\text{-}A}$. It is evident that while PAHs like BP readily induce 2-hydroxylation, nicotine had only a slight effect. These data further suggest that nicotine is not a potent inducer of P450I enzymes.

22.5. Summary

As pointed out here and elsewhere in these proceedings oestradiol 2-hydroxylation is the pathway that changes most readily in response to the inducing components of tobacco smoke. Enhancement of 2-hydroxylation probably contributes to the hypo-oestrogenic effects of cigarette smoking (Michnovicz *et al.* 1986). Several P450 isozymes may participate in the 2-hydroxylation of oestrogens in a non-smoker, yet in response to nicotine and the combustion products of smoke, Ah-responsive P450I genes are most likely to provide the added capacity for the C-2 oxidation. While definitive studies of the effects of nicotine on oestrogen 2-hydroxylation in human subjects have not been performed, the bulk of studies suggests that nicotine is not likely to have a strong inducing effect. Future clinical studies involving prolonged nicotine administration (>2 weeks) to naive subjects will be required to settle this question.

References

Ali, B., Kaur, S., Kumar, A., and Bhargava, K. P. (1980). Comparative evaluation of stimulatory effects of oral tobacco and nicotine consumption on hepatic microsomal N-demethylations. *Biochemical Pharmacology*, 29, 3087–92.

Anderson, K. E. (1988). Influences of diet and nutrition on clinical pharmacokinetics. *Clinical Pharmacokinetics*, 14, 325–46.

Anderson, K. E., Kappas, A., Conney, A. H., Bradlow, H. L., and Fishman, J. (1984). The influence of dietary protein and carbohydrates on the principal oxidative biotransformations of estradiol in normal subjects. *Journal of Clinical Endocrinology and Metabolism*, 59, 103–7.

Bradlow, H. L., Hershcopf, R. J., Martucci, C. P., and Fishman, J. (1985). Estradiol

16α-hydroxylation in the mouse correlates with mammary tumor incidence and presence of murine mammary tumor virus: a possible model for the hormonal etiology of breast cancer in humans. *Proceedings of the National Academy of Sciences, USA*, **82**, 6295–9.

Bucala, R., Lahita, R. G., Fishman, J., and Cerami, A. (1985). Increased levels of 16α-hydroxyestrone-modified proteins in pregnancy and in systemic lupus erythematosus. *Journal of Clinical Endocrinology and Metabolism*, **60**, 841–7.

Dannan, G. A., Porubek, D. J., Nelson, S. D., Waxman, D. J., and Guengerich, F. P. (1986). 17β-Estradiol 2- and 4-hydroxylation catalyzed by rat hepatic cytochrome P-450: roles of individual forms, inductive effects, developmental patterns, and alterations by gonadectomy and hormone replacement. *Endocrinology*, **118**, 1952–60.

Fishman, J. and Bradlow, H. L. (1977). Effect of malnutrition on the metabolism of sex hormones in man. *Clinical Pharmacology and Therapeutics*, **22**, 721–8.

Fishman, J. and Martucci, C. (1980). Biological properties of 16α-hydroxyestrone: implications in estrogen physiology and pathophysiology. *Journal of Clinical Endocrinology and Metabolism*, **51**, 611–15.

Fishman, J., Bradlow, H. L., and Gallagher, T. F. (1960). Oxidative metabolism of estradiol. *Journal of Biological Chemistry*, **235**, 3104–7.

Fishman, J., Hellman, L., Zumoff, B., and Gallagher, T. F. (1964). Effect of thyroid on hydroxylation of estrogen in man. *Journal of Clinical Endocrinology and Metabolism*, **25**, 365–8.

Fishman, J., Bradlow, H. L., Schneider, J., and Kappas, A. (1980). Radiometric analysis of biological oxidations in man: sex differences in estradiol metabolism. *Proceedings of the National Academy of Sciences, USA*, **77**, 4957–60.

Galbraith, R. A. and Michnovicz, J. J. (1989). The effects of cimetidine on the oxidative metabolism of estradiol. *New England Journal of Medicine*, **321**, 269–74.

Gierthy, J. F., *et al.* (1988). Enhancement of 2- and 16α-estradiol hydroxylation in MCF-7 human breast cancer cells by 2,3,7,8-tetrachlorodibenzo-*p*-dioxin. *Biochemical and Biophysical Research Communications*, **157**, 515–20.

Kaur, S. and Ali, B. (1982). Stimulation of drug and carcinogen metabolism by prolonged oral tobacco consumption. *Biochemical Pharmacology*, **31**, 1595–7.

Lahita, R. G., Bradlow, H. L., Kunkel, H. G., and Fishman, J. (1981). Increased 16α-hydroxylation of estradiol in systemic lupus erythematosus. *Journal of Clinical Endocrinology and Metabolism*, **53**, 174–8.

Martucci, C. P. and Fishman, J. (1979). Impact of continuously administered catechol estrogens in uterine growth and luteinizing hormone secretion. *Endocrinology*, **105**, 1288–92.

Michnovicz, J. J., Hershcopf, R. J., Naganuma, H., Bradlow, H. L., and Fishman, J. (1986). Increased 2-hydroxylation of estradiol as a possible mechanism for the anti-estrogenic effect of cigarette smoking. *New England Journal of Medicine*, **315**, 1305–9.

Michnovicz, J. J., Naganuma, H., Hershcopf, R. J., Bradlow, H. L., and Fishman, J. (1988). Increased urinary catechol estrogens in female smokers. *Steroids*, **52**, 69–83.

Musey, P. I., Collins, D. C., Bradlow, H. L., Gould, K. G., and Preedy, J. R. K. (1987). Effect of diet on oxidation of 17β-estradiol *in vivo*. *Journal of Clinical Endocrinology and Metabolism*, **65**, 792–5.

Nebert, D. W. (1979). Multiple forms of inducible drug-metabolizing enzymes: a reasonable mechanism by which any organism can cope with adversity. *Molecular and Cellular Biochemistry*, 27, 27–46.

Nebert, D. W. and Gonzalez, F. J. (1985). Cytochrome P450 gene expression and regulation. *Trends in Pharmacological Sciences*, 6, 160–4.

Nebert, D. W., *et al.* (1987). The P450 gene superfamily: recommended nomenclature. *DNA*, 6, 1-11.

Ruddon, R. W. and Cohen, A. M. (1970). Alteration of enzyme activity in rat liver following the acute and chronic administration of nicotine. *Toxicology and Applied Pharmacology*, 16, 613–25.

Ryan, D. E., Thomas, P. E., and Levin, W. (1982). Purification and characterization of a minor form of hepatic microsomal cytochrome P-450 from rats treated with polychlorinated biphenyls. *Archives of Biochemistry and Biophysics*, 216, 272–88.

Schneider, J., *et al.* (1982). Abnormal oxidative metabolism of estradiol in women with breast cancer. *Proceedings of the National Academy of Sciences, USA*, 79, 3047–51.

Schneider, J., Bradlow, H. L., Strain, G., Levin, J., Anderson, K., and Fishman, J. (1983). Effects of obesity on estradiol metabolism: decreased formation of non-uterotropic metabolites. *Journal of Clinical Endocrinology and Metabolism*, 56, 973–8.

Stedman, R. L. (1968). The chemical composition of tobacco and tobacco smoke. *Chemical Reviews*, 68, 153–207.

Sugita, O., *et al.* (1987). Cytochrome P-$450_{C\text{-}M/F}$, a new constitutive form of microsomal cytochrome P-450 in male and female rat liver with estrogen 2- and 16α-hydroxylase activity. *Biochemistry*, 27, 678–86.

Swaneck, G. E. and Fishman, J. (1988). Covalent binding of the endogenous estrogen 16α-hydroxyestrone to estradiol receptor in human breast cancer cells: characterization and intranuclear localization. *Proceedings of the National Academy of Sciences, USA*, 85, 7831–5.

Tuteja, N., Gonzalez, F. J., and Nebert, D. W. (1985). Developmental and tissue-specific differential regulation of the mouse dioxin-inducible P_1-450 and P_3-450 genes. *Developmental Biology*, 112, 177–84.

Waxman, D. J. (1988). Interactions of hepatic cytochromes P-450 with steroid hormones. *Biochemical Pharmacology*, 37, 71–84.

Welch, R. M., Harrison, Y. E., Gommi, B. W., Poppers, P. J., Finster, M., and Conney, A. H. (1969). Stimulatory effect of cigarette smoking on the hydroxylation of 3,4-benzpyrene and the N-demethylation of 3-methyl-4-monoethylaminoazobenzene by enzymes in human placenta. *Clinical Pharmacology and Therapeutics*, 10, 100–9.

Wenzel, D. G. and Broadie, L. L. (1966). Stimulatory effect of nicotine on the metabolism of meprobamate. *Toxicology and Applied Pharmacology*, 8, 455–9.

Yamamoto, I., Nagai, K., Kimura, H., and Iwatsubo, K. (1966). Nicotine and some carcinogens in special reference to the hepatic drug-metabolizing enzymes. *Japanese Journal of Pharmacology*, 16, 183–90.

23. Oestrogen 2-hydroxylation in rat and human liver

David Back, Simon Ball, Lesley Forrester, and Roland Wolf

Abstract

Hydroxylation at C-2 effectively terminates the peripheral activity of oestradiol. There is evidence that cigarette smoking increases the rate of 2-hydroxylation of oestradiol by induction of cytochrome P450. However in recent years it has become evident that there are multiple forms (isozymes) of the P450 haemoprotein. This reviews attempts to define more closely the enzymatic catalysts of oestradiol 2-hydroxylation. Data from studies using purified rat liver isozymes show that oestradiol is metabolized by both forms of cytochrome P450 that are phenobarbitone and 3-methylcholanthrene inducible; in contrast the related contraceptive steroid ethinyloestradiol is metabolized only by phenobarbitone inducible isozymes. In human liver there is a weak correlation between oestradiol and ethinyloestradiol 2-hydroxylase activity and differential immunoinhibition is seen with antibodies raised against specific isozymes. Oestradiol appears to be metabolized by a protein within the P450IA family. As proteins within the family are induced by cigarette smoke this may explain changes in 2-hydroxylation rates in smokers.

23.1. Introduction

Endoplasmic reticulum-bound cytochromes P450 play a central role in the oxidative metabolism of lipophilic compounds in mammalian cells. The microsomal P450s are particularly important in hepatic tissue where they catalyse NADPH-dependent monooxygenation of structurally diverse agents, including many drugs, carcinogens, and other foreign chemicals, as well as endogenous compounds such as steroid hormones (Waxman *et al.* 1987). The products of metabolism are polar and often hydroxylated derivatives. In the case of steroid hormones, hydroxylation can lead to products with reduced or altered hormonal properties. Thus hydroxylation at C-2 effectively terminates the peripheral activity of oestradiol (Michnovicz *et al.*

Table 23.1. Nomenclature for rat hepatic P450 enzymes*

Wolf[1]	Waxman[2]	Levin[3]	Guengerich[4]	Schenkman[5]	Steroid hydroxylation †	Human protein from the gene family
PB1a	—	—	—	—		
PB1b	PB-1	k	PB-C	RLM5a		$P450_{MP}$
PB2c	PB-2a	p	PCN-E	—	6β	$P450_{NF}$
PB2a	PB-2c	h	UT-A	RLM5	16α; 2α	
PB2b	2d	i	UT-I	fRLM4		
UT1	PB-3	a	UT-F	—	7α	
PB3a	PB-4	b	PB-B	PBRLM5	16β	
PB3b	PB-5	e	PB-D	PBRLM6		
	PB-6	—	—	—		
MC1a	ISF-G	d	ISF-G	—		$P450_{PA}$
MC1b	BNF-B	c	BNF-B	—		
—	—	f	—			
—	—	g	—	RLM3		
—	—	j	—	RLM6		
—	—	—	UT-H	—		$P450_{DB}$

* The designations of the major rat hepatic P450s characterized in the laboratories of the workers listed. 1. Wolf (1986); 2. Waxman (1986); 3. Ryan *et al.* (1984); 4. Guengerich *et al.* (1982); 5. Jansson *et al.* (1985).

† Regioselectivity of androstenedione and testosterone metabolism (Waxman 1988).

1986). Considerable interest has focused on this particular P450 catalysed reaction because of the evidence that cigarette smoking increases 2-hydroxylation of oestradiol, and this is consequently likely to lead to decreased availability of active hormone at oestrogen target tissues (Michnovicz *et al.* 1986).

In order to assess better the biochemical and clinical data on smoking and oestrogen metabolism it is important to define more closely the enzymatic catalysts of oestradiol 2-hydroxylation. In recent years it has become evident that there are multiple forms (isozymes) of the P450 haemoprotein. At least twenty distinct forms have been isolated from rat liver and characterized biochemically (Waxman 1988). The criteria for distinction of different P450s include the response to inducers, sex specificity, characteristic catalytic activity, spectral properties, immunoinhibition, and amino acid analysis (N-terminal and C-terminal sequencing). Table 23.1 summarizes rat P450 nomenclatures currently in use and indicates proteins identified in humans belonging to the same gene families. As knowledge of the system increases so it becomes essential to have generally accepted names for the isozymes. This chapter will be using the nomenclature of Wolf (1986) or referring other designations to that of Wolf.

23.2. The role of individual isozymes in the 2-hydroxylation of 17β-oestradiol

Ryan *et al.* (1982) examined the oestradiol 2-hydroxylase activity of five purified forms of cytochrome P450 (forms a, b, e, d and c of Levin; equivalent to forms UT1, PB3a, PB3b, MC1a and MC1b) and found the highest catalytic activity present in forms d (MC1a), c (MC1b) and e (PB3b). Later the same group (Ryan *et al.* 1984) extended their observations to three additional purified isozymes, forms f, g and h (PB2a), and found high catalytic activity towards oestradiol in P450h.

These observations are in agreement with the findings of Ball *et al.* (1988b). In the latter study, incubations contained cytochrome P450 isolated enzyme, cytochrome P450 reductase, substrate (either oestradiol or the contraceptive steroid ethinyloestradiol, ascorbic acid (necessary to protect the labile catecholoestrogen), NADPH, and Tris buffer. The incubations were terminated by ether extraction after 30 min. 2-Hydroxyoestradiol and 2-hydroxyethinyloestradiol were quantified by high performance liquid chromatography (hplc). Table 23.2 shows oestradiol 2-hydroxylase and ethinyloestradiol 2-hydroxylase activity of the purified forms. Oestradiol 2-hydroxylation was catalysed by P450 from a variety of families and subfamilies including forms inducible by both phenobarbitone (PB) and 3-methylcholanthrene (3-MC) (principally PB2a and PB3b from family P450II and MC1a and MC1b from family P450I—designation into families and subfamilies from Nebert *et al.* 1987). Ethinyloestradiol, however, appeared to be

Table 23.2. Oestradiol and ethinyloestradiol 2-hydroxylase activity of purified forms of cytochrome P450

Purified enzyme	Oestradiol 2-hydroxylase (nmol min^{-1} nmol $P450^{-1}$)	Ethinyloestradiol 2-hydroxylase (nmol min^{-1} nmol $P450^{-1}$)
PB1a	0.00	0.51
PB1b	0.12	0.20
PB2a	0.46	0.18
PB2c	0.30	0.06
PB3a	0.04	0.01
PB3b	0.65	0.05
MC1a	0.49	0.00
MC1b	0.47	0.02

metabolized only by the P450 isozymes from family P450IIc (principally PB1a, PB1b, PB2a). The implications of the different catalytic activity towards the two steroids will be discussed later.

Dannan *et al.* (1986) have examined oestradiol 2-hydroxylase activity of 10 forms of cytochrome P450 purified from rats pretreated with a variety of inducing agents. Forms UT-A and ISF-G (equivalent to PB2a and MC1a) had high catalytic activity. However, in contrast to the findings of Ryan *et al.* (1982) and Ball *et al.* (1988b), PB-D (PB3b) had relatively low enzyme activity. An additional isozyme catalysing the 2-hydroxylation reaction was PCN-E.

Cheng and Schenkman (1984) have also reported oestradiol 2-hydroxylase activity for form PB2a which they refer to as isozyme RLM5. This isozyme also catalysed the 2-hydroxylation of progesterone. Waxman (1988) has reported that PB2a (RLM5) in the rat is male specific, developmentally induced, and catalyses 2α- and 16α-hydroxylation of testosterone, androstenedione, and progesterone.

An important question in relation to purified enzyme studies is whether the high selectivity exhibited in a reconstituted system provides an accurate monitor of substrate specificity when the enzyme is bound to the endoplasmic reticulum. Then again, the relative abundance of each isozyme within the liver is a crucial consideration. With these points in mind several other approaches have been used in order to gain insight into the importance of particular isozymes in the liver.

As a first step toward determining the roles of individual P450s *in vivo*, Dannan *et al.* (1986) pretreated rats with various chemicals after which liver microsomes were prepared and assayed for oestradiol 2-hydroxylase activity. Enzyme activity increased in rats pretreated with PB but decreased in rats pretreated with β-naphthoflavone (β-NF) and isosafrole. Similar data have

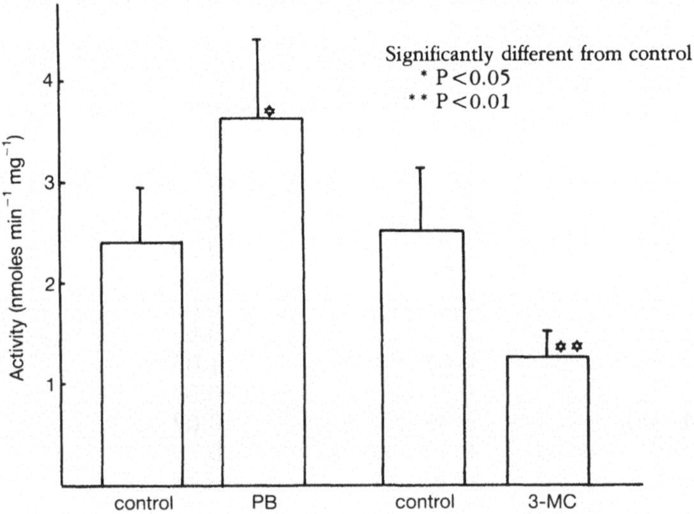

Fig. 23.1. 17β-oestradiol 2-hydroxylase activity of rat liver microsomal preparations. Rats pretreated either with vehicle, phenobarbitone (PB), or 3-methylcholanthrene (3-MC) for 3 days.

been generated in male rats pretreated with PB (increased activity) and 3-MC (decreased activity)—see Fig. 23.1. Induction of 2-hydroxylase activity by PB clearly suggests the involvement of one or more PB-inducible P450 forms (consistent with reconstituted isozyme findings). The lack of enhancement of hydroxylase activity by β-NF or 3-MC indicates that the isozymes MC1a and MC1b do not contribute much to hepatic oestradiol 2-hydroxylase activity. Since it is known that in the rat β-NF suppresses UT-A (PB2a), the implications are that PB2a is a major isozyme involved in oestradiol 2-hydroxylation in the male rat.

So how does smoking affect oestrogen metabolism? Both β-NF and 3-MC are polycyclic aromatic hydrocarbons which despite inducing some substrates (Steinberg *et al.* 1987) suppress hepatic oestrogen 2-hydroxylation in rats. Cigarette smoke is a complex mixture of chemicals including polycyclic aromatic hydrocarbons and thus if the rat data are extrapolated directly to man it could be concluded that induction of oestrogen 2-hydroxylase may not be as important as previously considered. However, caution needs to be observed in extrapolating findings from rat to man.

23.3. Oestrogen 2-hydroxylase activity of human liver

Bolt *et al.* (1975) examined oestradiol hydroxylation in hepatic microsomes obtained from biopsy specimens and found that A-ring hydroxylation greatly exceeded that in the B-ring. Guengerich *et al.* (1986) have reported

Table 23.3. Oestradiol and ethinyloestradiol 2-hydroxylase activity of human liver microsomes

Liver	Cytochrome P-450 (nmol mg^{-1} protein)	Oestradiol 2-hydroxylase	Ethinyloestradiol 2-hydroxylase
		(nmol min^{-1} mg^{-1} protein)	
L2 (M, 28)	0.33	0.37	0.12
L3 (M, 35)	0.37	0.59	0.20
L4 (F, 66)	0.90	1.14	0.35
L5 (M, 60)	0.41	0.62	0.22
L7 (M, 29)	0.71	0.92	0.35
L8 (F, 46)	0.87	1.03	0.45
L9 (M, 27)	0.50	0.67	0.22
L13 (M, 38)	0.36	0.67	0.17
C2 (F, 60)	0.38	0.79	0.21
WI (F, 17)	0.46	0.77	0.34

oestradiol 2-hydroxylase activity of human liver microsomes using the release of tritium method originally described by Fishman *et al.* (1980). Recently, Ball *et al.* (1988a) have reported oestradiol 2-hydroxylase activity of human liver microsomes prepared from livers obtained from kidney transplant donors. Table 23.3 shows these and additional data from a total of 10 subjects. Also given is ethinyloestradiol 2-hydroxylase activity. An approximate threefold variability is evident in oestradiol 2-hydroxylase activity in the 10 livers (4 female, 6 male).

In order to examine the roles of individual isozymes of human liver in oestrogen 2-hydroxylation, studies have been performed with human microsomes and polyclonal rabbit and anti-rat antibodies raised against purified rat enzymes (Back *et al.*, unpublished data). It should be emphasized that any results based on antibody inhibition experiments are only as reliable as the specificities of the anti-P450 antibodies employed. Potential cross reactivities with uncharacterized P450 forms or with closely related isozymes have to be considered (Waxman 1988). Results from such a study are shown in Figs 23.2 and 23.3. Differential immunoinhibition of human liver microsomal oestrogen metabolism is clearly demonstrated with anti-MC1b causing marked inhibition of oestradiol 2-hydroxylation but having only a small effect on ethinyloestradiol 2-hydroxylation. In contrast, anti-PB1a inhibited ethinyloestradiol metabolism to a greater degree than oestradiol. Since rat liver MC1b and PB1a were good catalysts of oestradiol and ethinyloestradiol 2-hydroxylase in the reconstituted system (Table 23.2) it may be that immunochemically similar forms are structurally and catalytically homologous between rat and man. It is suggested therefore, that an MC1b-like enzyme is important in human liver oestradiol 2-hydroxylation. In addition

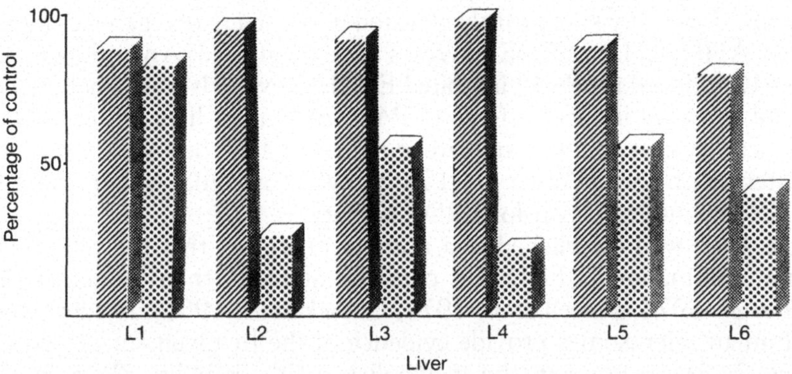

Fig. 23.2. Immunoinhibition of ethinyloestradiol (shaded bars) and oestradiol (stippled bars) 2-hydroxylase activity of human liver microsomes by anti-MC1b.

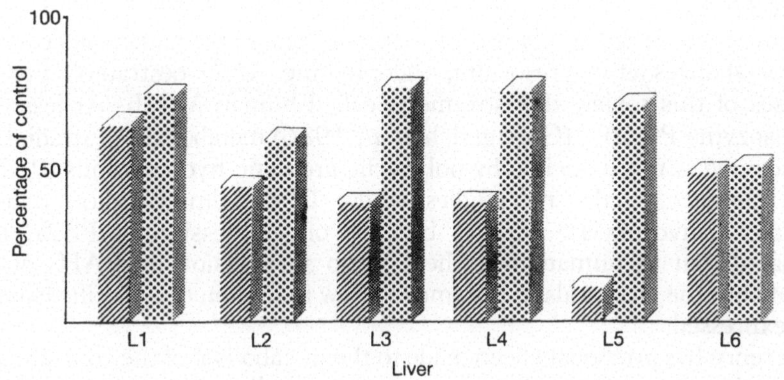

Fig. 23.3. Immunoinhibition of ethinyloestradiol (shaded bars) and oestradiol (stippled bars) 2-hydroxylase activity of human liver microsomes by anti-PB1a.

to these data, the finding of Guengerich *et al.* (1986) that anti-$P450_{NF}$ inhibits oestradiol 2-hydroxylase activity of human liver microsomes also implicates $P450_{NF}$ (rat PCN/PB2a) in metabolism. It is possible that both enzymes have this activity.

23.4. Smoking and induction of P450 enzymes

There are numerous studies on the effects of cigarette smoking on drug metabolism but one of considerable significance is that of Pelkonen *et al.* (1986). Four cytochrome P450 enzyme activities, 7-ethoxyresorufin *o*-deethylase (ERDE), coumarin 7-hydroxylase (CH), 7-ethoxycoumarin *o*-deethylase (ECDE), and aryl hydrocarbon hydroxylase (AHH), were measured in human liver needle biopsy samples from smokers and non-smokers. They found ERDE activity significantly elevated in the livers of cigarette smokers, whereas AHH, CH, or ECDE activities were unaffected. An antibody raised to a 3-MC induced rat P450 inhibited ERDE activity. It was concluded that cigarette smoking induces a form of P450 in human liver, responsible for ERDE activity that contains an epitope recognized by the anti-MC antibody. Consistent with this, Wolf *et al.* (1986) have shown that MC1b is a major catalytic enzyme in the rat for ERDE activity.

It has been well established in a number of studies that the rate of theophylline elimination is higher in cigarette smokers than in non-smokers (Hunt *et al.* 1976; Powell *et al.* 1977; Cusack *et al.* 1985). *In vitro* studies with human microsomes provide evidence of the involvement of two cytochrome P450 isozymes in the metabolism of theophylline (Robson *et al.* 1987). Campbell *et al.* (1987) have implicated a polycyclic aromatic hydrocarbon-inducible P450 in the metabolism of theophylline; for example they showed that theophylline was competitively inhibited by ethoxyresorufin and vice-versa.

So, evidence is accumulating in man that smoking induces an isozyme that metabolizes ethoxyresorufin, theophylline *AND* oestradiol. For the purposes of this review the isozyme is called human MC1b. At least one other isozyme P-450_{NF} (Guengerich *et al.* 1986) metabolizes oestradiol but this isozyme is not inducible by polycyclic aromatic hydrocarbons (PAHs). With reference to the rat studies where β-NF administration reduced oestradiol 2-hydroxylase activity because of suppression of PB2a, it is postulated that in human liver there is no suppression by PAHs of any isozyme but the chemicals in the smoke allow induction of a specific isozyme to be expressed.

Reference has previously been made to the metabolism of the contraceptive steroid ethinyloestradiol. The comparative oestradiol, ethinyloestradiol data in Table 23.2 show that whereas oestradiol 2-hydroxylation is catalysed by both PB and 3-MC inducible forms of cytochrome P450, ethinyloestradiol does not appear to be metabolized by MC inducible (therefore PAH inducible) forms of the enzyme. The major isozymes responsible for ethinyloestradiol 2-hydroxylation are human P-450_{NF} (Guengerich 1988) and the human orthologue of rat PB1a possibly P450 MP (see Fig. 23.3). The evidence for the conclusion of Guengerich included results from studies using enzyme reconstitution, immunoinhibition, correlation of nifedipine oxidase, and oestradiol 2-hydroxylase activities and inhibitors. Given the above findings, marked changes in ethinyloestradiol disposition in smokers would not be expected. This is indeed true. Crawford *et al.* (1981) examined a total of 311 oral contraceptive users (102 smokers, 209 non-smokers) and found no significant difference in ethinyloestradiol plasma concentrations. Recently, Kanarkowski *et al.* (1988) have failed to show any significant difference in ethinyloestradiol plasma concentration profiles in smokers and non-smokers.

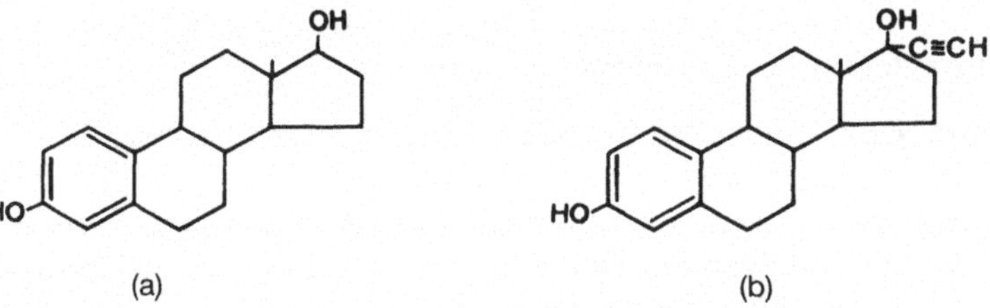

Fig. 23.4. Structures of (a) oestradiol and (b) ethinyloestradiol.

These findings obviously contrast to those of Michnovicz *et al.* (1986) and Jensen *et al.* (1985) where evident differences in oestradiol disposition in smokers and non-smokers are described.

It is clear that the 17α-ethinyl substituent on oestradiol (Fig. 23.4) markedly affects the selectivity of purified reconstituted enzymes towards the otherwise structurally identical steroids. Similar observations have been made by other workers. For example, it has been shown that reconstituted PB2a catalyses the 2α-hydroxylation of progesterone (C-17 substituent of 17β-acetyl) three times as rapidly as testosterone (17β-OH substituent) (Waxman 1988). Androstenedione (17-oxo substituent) is hardly metabolized at all by PB2a. Thus, steroid D-ring modifications have a profound effect on metabolism in the A-ring.

23.5. Conclusions

1. In 1984, Baron in a review on smoking and oestrogen-related disease said that while microsomal enzyme induction is thought to explain the enhanced metabolism of some drugs in smokers, it is not known whether smoking induces the particular enzymes involved in oestrogen disposition. The evidence contained in the present review supports the role of induction of oestradiol 2-hydroxylase by cigarette smoke.

2. The importance of PB-inducible P450s in the metabolism of the contraceptive steroid ethinyloestradiol and the lack of catalytic activity of PAH-induced forms is wholly consistent with clinical data. There is substantial evidence that PB interacts with oral contraceptives leading to an increase in the rate of elimination (Back *et al.* 1981; Back and Orme 1984) whereas smoking does not affect ethinyloestradiol plasma levels.

3. This review has focused alteration on oestrogen 2-hydroxylation. Clearly, additional data are needed on 16α-hydroxylation since this is important in oestrogen metabolism. However if findings can be extrapolated from rat isozymes with androstenedione and testosterone (Waxman 1988)

then it is PB2a and PB3a which are the important isozymes in 16α-hydroxylation, i.e. non-PAH-inducible forms. Smoking is unlikely to induce 16α-hydroxylation of oestrogens.

4. Two recent studies by Vestal *et al.* (1987) and Crowley *et al.* (1988) have indicated that smoking markedly influences theophylline disposition without any effect on the excretion of 6β-hydroxycortisol. This is further evidence for the involvement of different isozymes in the 6β-hydroxylation of cortisol and the 2-hydroxylation of oestradiol.

5. Whilst this chapter has concentrated on hepatic oestradiol 2-hydroxylation other workers have suggested alternative mechanisms. Barbieri *et al.* (1986) provided evidence that nicotine, cotinine, and anabasine all inhibited androstenedione conversion to oestrogen (i.e. aromatase enzyme) in a dose-dependent fashion in choriocarcinoma cell cultures. Similarly in term placental microsomes, there was inhibition of the conversion of testosterone to oestrogen. Recently, Khaw *et al.* (1988) examined the relationship between cigarette smoking and hormone levels in post-menopausal women. They concluded that there was decreased oestrogenic activity in smokers due to an increase in oestrogen protein binding. It is therefore very difficult at this point in the understanding of smoking and oestrogen levels to pin an exclusive tag on any one mechanism.

Acknowledgements

We are extremely grateful to our clinical colleagues Professor M.L'E. Orme and Mr. R. Sells for provision of human liver.

References

Back, D. J. and Orme, M. L'E. (1984). Interindividual variability in oral contraceptive disposition. *Trends in Pharmacological Sciences*, **5**, 480–4.

Back, D. J., Breckenridge, A. M., Crawford, F. E., MacIver, M., Orme, M. L'E., and Rowe, P. H. (1981). Interindividual variation and drug interactions with hormonal steroid contraceptives. *Drugs*, **21**, 46–61.

Ball, S., Back, D. J., and Orme, M. L'E. (1988a). Characterisation and inhibition of estrogen 2-hydroxylase activity in human liver microsomes. *British Journal of Clinical Pharmacology*, **25**, 643–4P.

Ball, S. E., Forrester, L., Wolf, C. R., and Back, D. J. (1988b). Characterisation of the form(s) of cytochrome P-450 involved in oestrogen 2-hydroxylation. *British Journal of Pharmacology*, **94**, 449P.

Barbieri, R. L., Gochberg, J., and Ryan, K. J. (1986). Nicotine, cotinine and anabasine inhibit aromatase in human trophoblast *in vitro*. *Journal of Clinical Investigations*, **77**, 1727–33.

Baron, J. A. (1984). Smoking and estrogen-related disease. *American Journal of Epidemiology*, **119**, 9–22.

Bolt, H. M., Kappus, H., and Bolt, M. (1975). Effect of rifampicin treatment on the metabolism of oestradiol and 17α-ethinyloestradiol by human liver microsomes. *European Journal of Clinical Pharmacology*, **8**, 301–7.

Campbell, M. E., Grant, D. M., Inaba, T., and Kalow, W. (1987). Biotransformation of caffeine, paraxanthine, theophylline and theobromine by polycyclic aromatic hydrocarbon-inducible cytochrome(s) P450 in human liver microsomes. *Drug Metabolism and Disposition*, **15**, 231–49.

Cheng, K-C. and Schenkman, J. B. (1984). Metabolism of progesterone and estradiol by microsomes and purified cytochrome P-450 RLM_3 and RLM_5. *Drug Metabolism and Disposition*, **12**, 222–34.

Crawford, F. E., Back, D. J., Orme, M. L'E., and Breckenridge, A. M. (1981). Oral contraceptive steroid plasma concentrations in smokers and non-smokers. *British Medical Journal*, **282**, 1829–30.

Crowley, J. J., Cusack, B. J., Jue, S. G., Koup, J. R., Park, B. K., and Vestal, R. E. (1988). Ageing and drug interactions II. Effect of phenytoin and smoking on the oxidation of theophylline and cortisol in healthy men. *Journal of Pharmacology and Experimental Therapeutics*, **245**, 513–23.

Cusack, B. J., Dawson, G. W., Mercer, G. D., and Vestal, R. E. (1985). Cigarette smoking and theophylline metabolism: Effects of cimetidine. *Clinical Pharmacology and Therapeutics*, **37**, 330–6.

Dannan, G. A., Porubek, D. J., Nelson, S. D., Waxman, D. J., and Guengerich, F. P. (1986). 17β-estradiol 2- and 4-hydroxylation catalysed by rat hepatic cytochrome P-450: Roles of individual forms, inductive effects, developmental patterns and alterations by gonadectomy and hormone replacement. *Endocrinology*, **118**, 1952–60.

Fishman, J., Bradlow, H. L., Schneider, J., Anderson, K. E., and Kappas, A. (1980). Radiometric analysis of biological oxidations in man: sex differences in estradiol metabolism. *Proceedings of the National Academy of Science*, **77**, 4957–60.

Guengerich, F. P. (1988). Oxidation of 17α-ethynylestradiol by human liver cytochrome P-450. *Molecular Pharmacology*, **33**, 500–8.

Guengerich, F. P., Dannan, G. A., Wright, S. J., Martin, M. V., and Kaminsky, L. S. (1982). Purification and characterization of liver microsomal cytochromes P-450: electrophoretic, spectral, catalytic and immunochemical properties and inducibility of eight isozymes isolated from rats treated with phenobarbital or beta-naphthoflavone. *Biochemistry*, **21**, 6019–30.

Guengerich, F. P., Martin, M. V., Beaune, P. H., Kremers, P., Wolff, T., and Waxman, D. J. (1986). Characterization of rat and human liver microsomal cytochrome P-450 forms involved in nifedipine oxidation, a prototype for genetic polymorphism in oxidative drug metabolism. *Journal of Biological Chemistry*, **261**, 5051–60.

Hunt, S. N., Jusko, W. J., and Yurchak, A. M. (1976). Effect of smoking on theophylline disposition. *Clinical Pharmacology and Therapeutics*, **19**, 546–51.

Jansson, I., Tamburini, P. P., Favreau, L. V., and Schenkman, J. B. (1985). The interaction of cytochrome b5 with four cytochrome P-450 enzymes from the untreated rat. *Drug Metabolism and Disposition*, **13**, 453–8.

Jensen, J., Christiansen, C., and Rodbro, P. (1985). Cigarette smoking, serum estrogens and bone loss during hormone-replacement therapy early after menopause. *New England Journal of Medicine*, **313**, 973–5.

Kanarkowski, R., Tornatore, K. M., D'Ambrosio, R., Gardner, M. J., and Jusko, W. J. (1988). Pharmacokinetics of single and multiple doses of ethinylestradiol and levonorgestrel in relation to smoking. *Clinical Pharmacology and Therapeutics*, **43**, 23–31.

Khaw, K-T., Tazuke, S., and Barrett-Connor, E. (1988). Cigarette smoking and levels of adrenal androgens in postmenopausal women. *New England Journal of Medicine*, **318**, 1705–9.

Michnovicz, J. J., Hershcopf, R. J., Naganuma, H., Bradlow, H. L., and Fishman, J. (1986). Increased 2-hydroxylation of estradiol as a possible mechanism for the anti-estrogenic effect of cigarette smoking. *New England Journal of Medicine*, **315**, 1305–9.

Nebert, D., *et al.* (1987). The P-450 gene superfamily: recommended nomenclature. *DNA*, **6**, 1–11.

Pelkonen, O., *et al.* (1986). The effect of cigarette smoking on 7-ethoxyresorufin o-deethylase and other monooxygenase activities in human liver: analyses with monoclonal antibodies. *British Journal of Clinical Pharmacology*, **22**, 125–34.

Powell, J. R., Thiercelin, J. F., Vozeh, S., Sansom, L., and Riegelman, S. (1977). The influence of cigarette smoking and sex on theophylline disposition. *American Review of Respiratory Disease*, **116**, 17–23.

Robson, R. A., *et al.* (1987). Characterisation of theophylline metabolism in human liver microsomes. *British Journal of Clinical Pharmacology*, **24**, 293–300.

Ryan, D. E., Thomas, P. E., and Levin, W. (1982). Purification and characterisation of a minor form of hepatic microsomal cytochrome P-450 from rats treated with polychlorinated biphenyls. *Archives of Biochemistry and Biophysics*, **216**, 272–88.

Ryan, D. E., Iida, S., Wood, A. W., Thomas, P. E., Lieber, C. S., and Levin, W. (1984). Characterisation of three highly purified cytochromes P-450 from hepatic microsomes of adult male rats. *Journal of Biological Chemistry*, **259**, 1239–50.

Steinberg, P., Latranconi, W. M., Wolf, C. R., Waxman, D. J., Oesch, F., and Friedberg, T. (1987). Xenobiotic metabolising enzymes are not restricted to parenchymal cells in rat liver. *Molecular Pharmacology*, **32**, 463–70.

Vestal, R. E., Cusack, B. J., Mercer, G. D., Dawson, G. W., and Park, B. K. (1987). Aging and drug interactions I. Effect of cimetidine and smoking on the oxidation of theophylline and cortisol in healthy men. *Journal of Pharmacology and Experimental Therapeutics*, **241**, 488–500.

Waxman, D. J. (1986). Rat hepatic cytochrome P-450: comparative studies of multiple isozymic forms. In: *Cytochrome P-450: structure, mechanism and biochemistry* (ed. P. R. Ortiz de Montellano), pp. 525–39. Plenum Press, New York.

Waxman, D. J. (1988). Interactions of hepatic cytochromes P-450 with steroid hormones. Regioselectivity and stereospecificity of steroid metabolism and hormonal regulation of rat P-450 enzyme expression. *Biochemical Pharmacology*, **37**, 71–84.

Waxman, D. J., Lapenson, D. P., Park, S. S., Attisano, C., and Gelboin, H. V. (1987). Monoclonal antibodies inhibitory to rat hepatic cytochromes P-450:

P-450 form specificities and use as probes for cytochrome P-450-dependent steroid hydroxylations. *Molecular Pharmacology*, **32**, 615–24.

Wolf, C. R. (1986). Cytochrome P-450s: polymorphic multigene families involved in carcinogen activation. *Trends in Genetics*, **20**, 209–14.

Wolf, C. R., Seilman, S., Oesch, F., Mayer, R. T., and Burke, M. D. (1986). Multiple forms of cytochrome P-450 related to forms induced marginally by phenobarbital. Difference in structure and in the metabolism of alkoxyresorufins. *Biochemistry Journal*, **240**, 27–33.

IX

Summary and Implications

24. Smoking and hormone related disorders: a summary of the evidence with implications for public health policy and future research

Nicholas Wald, John Baron, and Sir Richard Doll

From the epidemiological perspective it was recognized at the outset that a principal aim of this Symposium was:

(1) to determine whether there was a real association between certain specified conditions and smoking, and, if there was,
(2) to estimate the magnitude of these effects,
(3) to determine the nature of the effects, that is, whether causal or not, and
(4) if possible, to determine the mechanism underlying the association.

The findings presented during the Symposium confirmed that smoking had an effect on the incidence of certain hormone related disorders leading to an increase or a decrease in risk. Table 24.1 lists the various conditions examined (all medical disorders apart from age at menopause) and gives for each a judgement on whether the conditions have a real association with smoking and, if so, whether the association is positive or negative. If a real association was judged to be present, an estimate is given of the relative risk in smokers compared with that of lifelong non-smokers. The nature of each of the associations is also specified (i.e. whether it was thought to be causal) and, if causal, whether there was at least one known plausible mechanism that could account for it.

The findings summarized in Table 24.1 are, in general, more important for their scientific than for their public health implications. Scientifically, the observation that constituents of tobacco smoke both modify hormonal activity and influence the incidence of some diseases of otherwise unknown aetiology may be of great importance to the development of understanding of the mechanisms of human physiology and pathology. However, in terms of absolute risk, only an effect on osteoporotic fractures (particularly of the hip) is large in comparison with the impact smoking has on the incidences of cancer, cardiovascular, and respiratory disease. The few possibly protective

Table 24.1. Summary of smoking and hormone-related disorders or conditions

Disorder	Is there an association with smoking: if so, is the association positive (↑) or negative (↓)	RR estimate (smokers vs. non-smokers)	Nature of association	Is there at least one known plausible mechanism
Age at menopause	Definite*: smokers have earlier menopause	1.8	Probably causal	Yes
Fibroids	Definite: ↓	0.5	Possibly causal	Yes
Hyperemesis gravidarum	Definite: ↓	0.6	Probably causal	Yes
Benign breast disease	Not known	—	—	—
Osteoporotic fracture	Definite: ↑	1.6	Probably causal	Yes
Gallstones	Suggestive: ↑	2.0	Unknown	—
Skin atrophy	Not known	—	—	—
Prostate hypertrophy	Not known	—	—	—
Ulcerative colitis	Definite: ↓	0.5	Possibly causal	No
Crohn's disease	Definite: ↑	2.0	Probably causal	No
Parkinson's disease	Definite: ↓	0.5	Probably causal	Yes
Endometrial cancer	Definite: ↓	0.5	Probably causal	Yes
Breast cancer	No	(1.1)	—	—
Colon cancer	No	—	—	—
Rectum cancer	Suggestive: ↑	1.7	Unknown	No

* A 'definite' association is one that is unlikely to have arisen by chance.

relationships discussed at this Symposium cannot weigh heavily in the determination of public policy. The reduction in the age at menopause may, in different circumstances, be thought to be harmful or beneficial, but is in any case too small to be a serious consideration either way. A beneficial effect on ulcerative colitis and on parkinsonism should be obtainable by pharmacological means, once the responsible chemical is identified instead of exposing patients to whole smoke.

No evidence has been produced to suggest that any of the findings summarized in Table 24.1 are affected by tar and nicotine levels. From a practical point of view, they are probably of minor importance, as the effect of 'compensatory' smoking (considered in detail in the proceedings of the last ISCSH Symposium) (Wald and Froggatt 1989) results in achieving similar intakes of nicotine as would have been achieved with cigarettes delivering larger amounts.

A central question arising from the Symposium was: 'Does cigarette smoking have an anti-oestrogenic effect and, if so, to whom does it apply, and for what conditions or disorders?' The Symposium has gone a long way to providing answers, but there is still need for further clarification and for the detail of the mechanism to be elucidated.

The epidemiological evidence for an anti-oestrogenic effect of smoking is largely based on three sets of observations: the negative association between cigarette smoking and endometrial cancer, the positive association between cigarette smoking and osteoporosis and osteoporotic fractures, and the negative association between smoking and a variety of relatively 'minor' disorders such as uterine fibroids. The well-established association between cigarette smoking and an early menopause has been omitted from this list because, in itself, this seems mainly to be a mechanism by which an anti-oestrogenic effect might be produced.

The results showing that post-menopausal women who smoke have a lower risk of endometrial cancer are remarkably consistent (Weiss, Chapter 14). The evidence that osteoporotic fractures are more common in smokers is less consistent, and further data are needed to estimate the magnitude of the association after account has been taken of such potentially confounding factors as alcohol consumption and drug use (Cooper and Wickham, Chapter 8). Weight can, at least in part, be regarded as an element in a causal chain rather than as a confounding factor, since smoking can reduce weight which, in the elderly, can protect against fracture of the hip. The data regarding the 'minor' disorders (such as fibroids, endometriosis, and benign breast disease) are fairly consistent, but are subject to variation in case ascertainment. These disorders could be underdiagnosed in smokers, who may perhaps be less likely than non-smokers to seek medical attention in response to minor symptoms. The causal implications of the association are, therefore, still uncertain.

The Symposium provided no support for the view that smoking had a protective effect against breast cancer (MacMahon, Chapter 15). Nor did it protect against gallstones or other gall-bladder diseases (Baron and Logan, Chapter 9). Breast cancer, in general, is not as strongly related to oestrogens as endometrial cancer; the lack of a negative association with breast cancer is, therefore, not strong evidence against an anti-oestrogenic effect of cigarette smoking. The fact that smoking may, if anything, be positively associated with gallstones is more difficult to reconcile with the anti-oestrogen hypothesis. Further study of the relationships between cigarette smoking, serum lipids, bile composition, and gallstones would be helpful.

Details of the epidemiology may provide clues as to the underlying mechanism. For example, the risk of hormone-related disorders in ex-smokers will indicate whether the effects of smoking may be reversible. Also the relative strength of the association in pre-menopausal and post-menopausal women will indicate the importance of ovarian vs. other sources of oestrogens. Except for endometrial cancer, these issues have hardly been addressed.

One observation that conflicts with the hypothesis that smoking is anti-oestrogenic is that circulating total oestradiol levels are not decreased in women who smoke (Barrett-Connor, Chapter 17). There is evidence that adrenal androgen levels are increased in smokers, though they have very little agonist activity in themselves and must be converted to either oestradiol or testosterone to have significant hormonal effects. The observation that circulating total oestradiol levels are not decreased in female smokers suggests that an increase in testosterone levels may have important effects. The data, though few, suggest that a small increase may indeed occur. Consequently, further investigation of testosterone levels in women in relation to smoking and hormone-related disorders is important. Because of the binding of both oestradiol and testosterone to sex hormone binding globulin (SHBG), the study of the levels of the free hormone in smokers vs. non-smokers is of interest, though current indications are that smoking does not affect SHBG greatly, if at all. Study of sex hormone-related physiological variables, such as the maturation index of vaginal cytology or skin thickness, would provide an in-built 'bioassay' of the hormonal environment and would be a useful complement to serum levels.

In summary, the anti-oestrogenic theory of smoking holds epidemiologically but requires further biochemical support. The observations made by Barbieri and his colleagues (Canick and Barbieri, Chapter 19) and by Michnovicz *et al*. (Chapter 22) of the effects of tobacco smoke on oestrogen metabolism may provide clues, but their physiological relevance needs to be determined.

Intervention studies offer a means to study the effects of specific smoke constituents. For example, the use of nicotine chewing gum (or the nicotine patch currently under development) would test whether the *in vitro* work by Barbieri and colleagues is an effect of nicotine which may be clinically significant and whether nicotine is responsible for the apparent effect of smoking on ulcerative colitis or Parkinson's disease.

The evidence that smoking exacerbates some diseases of hormonal or unknown aetiology strengthens the arguments in favour of discouraging smoking. The evidence that it relieves or diminishes the risks of some other diseases provides valuable clues to the possibility of their cure or prevention by pharmacological means. The most useful applications of the work summarized in this book may result from the leads that it provides for the study of the aetiology, prevention and treatment of several important and common diseases of adult life. The study of smoking-related diseases promises to yield information of general medical interest that extends far beyond the simple assessment of the toxicity of tobacco smoke.

References

Wald, N. J. and Froggatt, P. (1989). *Nicotine, smoking and the low tar programme* (ed. N. J. Wald and P. Froggatt). Oxford University Press, Oxford.

Index

The manufacturer's authorised representative in the EU for product safety is Oxford University Press España S.A. of El Parque Empresarial San Fernando de Henares, Avenida de Castilla, 2 - 28830 Madrid (www.oup.es/en or product.safety@oup.com). OUP España S.A. also acts as importer into Spain of products made by the manufacturer.
Printed and bound by CPI Group (UK) Ltd, Croydon, CR0 4YY
14/09/2026
02216286-0004